# ADVANCES IN

# Surgery

**Editor-in-Chief**
**John L. Cameron, MD**

ELSEVIER

PHILADELPHIA LONDON TORONTO MONTREAL SYDNEY TOKYO

# ADVANCES IN
## Surgery

VOLUMES 1 THROUGH 51 (OUT OF PRINT)

## VOLUME 54

13. Fascial Closure: New Surgery Paradigms *by Gregory A. Dumanian and Simon Moradian*
14. Enteral Feeding: Percutaneous Endoscopic Gastrostomies, Tubes, and Formulas, *by Colin G. DeLong and Eric M. Pauli*
15. Increasing Importance of Ethics in Surgical Decision Making *by Anghela Z. Paredes, Christopher T. Aquina, Luke V. Selby, Stephanie DiFilippo, and Timothy M. Pawlik*
16. Per Oral Pyloromyotomy for Gastroparesis, *by John H. Rodriguez and Jeffrey Ponsky*
17. What Is the Role of Neoadjuvant Radiation Therapy for Retroperitoneal Sarcoma? *by Sophia K. McKinley, Thomas F. DeLaney, and John T. Mullen*
18. New Models of Surgical Training, *by Christopher C. Stahl and Rebecca M. Minter*

## VOLUME 53

1. Laparoscopic Hernia Repair *by Javier Otero, Andrew T. Huber, and B. Todd Heniford*
2. Ductal Carcinoma In Situ of the Breast: Controversies and Current Management *by Andrea V. Barrio and Kimberly J. Van Zee*
3. What Is the Role for Carotid Stenting Versus Endarterectomy? *by Kyla M. Bennett and John E. Scarborough*
4. Managing Complications of Bariatric Surgery, *by Richard M. Peterson and John D. Scott*
5. Trends in Palliative Surgical Care, *by Allison R. Wilcox and Sandra L. Wong*
6. Management of Difficult Dialysis Access Issues for Dialysis Patients *by Matthew J. Dougherty, Douglas A. Troutman, and Krystal C. Maloni*
7. Has Personalized Medicine for Pancreatic Cancer Arrived? *by Ashley Krepline and Susan Tsai*
8. Is Hyperthyroidism Diagnosed and Treated Appropriately in the United States?, *by Ammar Asban, Sophie Dream, and Brenessa Lindeman*
9. How Do We Prevent Burnout in Surgery? *by Gerard M. Doherty*
10. Elimination of Bile Duct Injury in Cholecystectomy, *by Maria S. Altieri and L. Michael Brunt*

**VOLUME 52**

Editor: John Vassallo
Developmental Editor: Arlene Campos



Editorial Office:
Elsevier
1600 John F. Kennedy Blvd,
Suite 1800
Philadelphia, PA 19103-2899

International Standard Serial Number: 0065-3411
International Standard Book Number: 978-0-323-81365-5

Printed in India

# ADVANCES IN
## Surgery

## CONTRIBUTORS

H. RICHARD ALEXANDER Jr, MD, Division of Surgical Oncology, Rutgers Cancer Institute of New Jersey, Jersey City, New Jersey

JOHN R. BERGQUIST, MD, MS, Department of Surgery, Section of Surgical Oncology, Stanford University, Stanford, California

JAMES H. BLACK III, MD, The David Goldfarb, MD Professor of Surgery, Division of Vascular Surgery and Endovascular Therapy, Johns Hopkins School of Medicine, Baltimore, Maryland

COLE S. BROWN, The University of North Carolina at Chapel Hill, Chapel Hill, North Carolina

RICHARD A. BURKHART, MD, Assistant Professor, Department of Surgery, Division of Hepatobiliary and Pancreatic Surgery, Johns Hopkins University, Baltimore, Maryland

ANDREW M. CAMERON, MD, PhD, Department of Surgery, Johns Hopkins School of Medicine, Baltimore, Maryland

MELISSA CAMP, MD, MPH, Assistant Professor, Department of Surgery, Johns Hopkins, Baltimore, Maryland

JONATHAN CARTER, MD, FASMBS, Department of Surgery, University of California, San Francisco, San Francisco, California

CATHERINE H. DAVIS, MD, MPH, Division of Surgical Oncology, Rutgers Cancer Institute of New Jersey, Jersey City, New Jersey

HANNAH DECKER, MD, Resident, General Surgery, Department of Surgery, University of California, San Francisco, San Francisco, California

NADEGE T. FACKCHE, MD, General Surgery Resident, Howard University Hospital, Washington, DC

JULIO GARCIA-AGUILAR, MD, PhD, Benno C. Schmidt Chair in Surgical Oncology, Chief of Colorectal Service, Department of Surgery, Memorial Sloan Kettering Cancer Center, Professor of Surgery, Weill Cornell Medical College, New York, New York

KATHERINE HE, MD, MS, Resident, Department of General Surgery, Brigham and Women's Hospital, Harvard Medical School, Boston, Massachusetts

CHARLOTTE HORNE, MD, Assistant Professor of Surgery, Penn State Hershey Medical Center, Milton S. Hershey Medical Center, Hershey, Pennsylvania

FABIAN M. JOHNSTON, MD, MHS, Associate Professor of Surgery, Division Chief, Gastrointestinal (GI) Oncology, Program Director, Surgical Oncology Fellowship, Johns Hopkins Hospital, Baltimore, Maryland

ALI KHALIFEH, MD, Division of Vascular and Endovascular Surgery, Mayo Clinic, Rochester, Minnesota

AMY Y. LI, MD, Department of Surgery, Section of Surgical Oncology, Stanford University, Stanford, California

MALCOLM MACCONMARA, MB BCh, FACS, Assistant Professor, Division of Surgical Transplantation, Department of Surgery, The University of Texas Southwestern Medical Center, Dallas, Texas

LAURA MAZER, MD, MHPE, Department of Surgery, Division of Minimally Invasive Surgery, University of Michigan, Ann Arbor, Michigan

AMANDA MUELLER, MD, Department of Surgery, University of California, San Francisco, San Francisco, California

KRISTOFOR A. OLSON, MD, PhD, Department of Surgery and Perioperative Care, The University of Texas at Austin Dell Medical School, Austin, Texas

SARAH PALILLA, PA, Department of Surgery, University of California, San Francisco, San Francisco, California

ERIC PAULI, MD, FACS, FASGE, Professor of Surgery, Penn State Hershey Medical Center, Milton S. Hershey Medical Center, Hershey, Pennsylvania

SUSAN C. PITT, MD, MPHS, FACS, Assistant Professor, Department of Surgery, University of Wisconsin-Madison, Madison, Wisconsin

REESE W. RANDLE, MD, FACS, Assistant Professor, Department of Surgery, Wake Forest Baptist Health, Winston-Salem, North Carolina

SHAWN J. RANGEL, MD, MSCE, Attending Surgeon, Department of Pediatric and Thoracic Surgery, Boston Children's Hospital, Harvard Medical School, Boston, Massachusetts

TODD E. RASMUSSEN, MD, Professor of Surgery, Division of Vascular and Endovascular Surgery, Mayo Clinic, Rochester, Minnesota

THOMAS SCALEA, MD, Honorable Francis X. Kelly Distinguished Professor of Trauma Surgery, Physician-in-Chief, System Chief for Critical Care Services, Director, R Adams Cowley Shock Trauma Center, University of Maryland Medical System, Program in Trauma, University of Maryland School of Medicine, Baltimore, Maryland

TONI T. SEPPÄLÄ, MD, PhD, Adjunct Professor, Department of Surgery, Johns Hopkins University, Baltimore, Maryland; Department of Surgery, Helsinki University Hospital, Helsinki, Finland

MATTHEW SYMER, MD, MS, Department of Surgery, NewYork-Presbyterian Hospital, Weill Cornell Medicine, New York, New York

WILLIAM A. TEETER, MD, Assistant Professor and Director of Education, Multi-trauma Critical Care ICU, Staff Intensivist, Department of Emergency Medicine, University of Maryland School of Medicine, Program in Trauma and Critical Care, R Adams Cowley Shock Trauma Center, Baltimore, Maryland

PEDRO G. TEIXEIRA, MD, Associate Professor, Department of Surgery and Perioperative Care, The University of Texas at Austin Dell Medical School, Austin, Texas

DANA A. TELEM, MD, MPH, FACS, Lazar J Greenfield Professor, Department of Surgery, Division of Minimally Invasive Surgery, University of Michigan, Ann Arbor, Michigan

PARSIA A. VAGEFI, MD, FACS, Ernest Poulos, M.D. Distinguished Chair in Surgery, Chief, Division of Surgical Transplantation, Department of Surgery, The University of Texas Southwestern Medical Center, Dallas, Texas

BRENDAN C. VISSER, MD, Department of Surgery, Section of Surgical Oncology, Stanford University, Stanford, California

ELIZABETH WICK, MD, Professor, Department of Surgery, University of California, San Francisco, San Francisco, California

CHRISTOPHER L. WU, MD, Professor, Department of Anesthesiology, Hospital for Special Surgery, Department of Anesthesiology, Weill Cornell Medicine, New York, New York

HEATHER L. YEO, MD, MBA, MHS, Department of Healthcare Policy and Research, NewYork-Presbyterian, Weill Cornell Medicine, New York, New York

JONATHAN B. YUVAL, MD, Colorectal Service, Department of Surgery, Memorial Sloan Kettering Cancer Center, New York, New York

BARA ZUHAILI, MD, Michigan Vascular Center, Michigan State University, Flint, Michigan

CONTENTS

VOLUME 55 • 2021

## What is the Current Role of Hyperthermic Intraperitoneal Chemotherapy in Colorectal Cancer?

Catherine H. Davis and H. Richard Alexander Jr.



## Machine Perfusion in Liver Transplantation

Malcolm MacConmara and Parsia A. Vagefi

Video content accompanies this article at http://www.advancessurgery.com

**Necrosectomy in the Management of Necrotizing Pancreatitis**

Amy Y. Li, John R. Bergquist, and Brendan C. Visser

Video content accompanies this article at http://www.advancessurgery.com



**Vascular Reconstructions for Traumatic Injuries**

Ali Khalifeh and Todd E. Rasmussen



**Evolution of Point-Of-Care Ultrasound in Surgical Management**

William A. Teeter and Thomas Scalea

Advances in Surgery 55 (2021) 1–8

ADVANCES IN SURGERY

ELSEVIER
MOSBY

# Optimal Surgical Treatment for Type 2 Diabetes

## Sleeve Gastrectomy or Gastric Bypass?

Amanda Mueller, MD, Sarah Palilla, PA, Jonathan Carter, MD*

Department of Surgery, University of California – San Francisco, 513 Parnassus Avenue, HSW1601, San Francisco, CA 94143, USA

**Keywords**

• Gastric bypass • Sleeve gastrectomy • Bariatric surgery • Type 2 diabetes • Diabetes remission • Obesity

**Key points**

- Randomized trials have shown that sleeve gastrectomy and gastric bypass induce similar improvements in type 2 diabetes after 5 years of follow-up.
- Many of the mechanisms of diabetes improvement first described in gastric bypass patients have now been described in sleeve gastrectomy patients.

## INTRODUCTION

Bariatric surgery markedly improves glucose homeostasis and can induce improvement or remission of diabetes mellitus [1]. Although all bariatric procedures improve diabetes to the extent that they induce weight loss, some bariatric operations are known to improve diabetes even before significant weight loss has occurred. For example, gastric bypass can induce complete remission of diabetes within a week of the operation, in contradistinction to other gastrointestinal operations, such as colectomy, which have no effect on diabetes [2,3]. This intriguing observation, made decades ago, inspired intense research into the mechanisms of diabetes resolution after gastric bypass. We now understand that diabetes resolution after bypass is the result of many complementary mechanisms: alterations in gut hormone secretion, changes in the gut microbiome, alterations in bile acid processing, bypass of the duodenum, reductions in inflammation, weight loss in general, and cognitive changes in food intake, to name a few [4,5].

*Corresponding author. *E-mail address:* jonathan.carter@ucsf.edu

https://doi.org/10.1016/j.yasu.2021.05.001
0065-3411/21/Published by Elsevier Inc.

Sleeve gastrectomy is a relatively newer operation, but is now the most popular bariatric operation in the United States because of its simplicity, low complication rate, and effectiveness [6,7]. Although sleeve gastrectomy was originally conceptualized as a purely restrictive operation without much hormonal effect, we now know that many of the neurohormonal changes observed after gastric bypass also occur after sleeve gastrectomy [8]. Here, we review recent evidence from randomized controlled trials specifically designed to elucidate whether clinically important differences exist between gastric bypass and sleeve gastrectomy with respect to diabetes resolution. We also summarize the current understanding of the physiologic basis for diabetes improvement after gastric bypass and sleeve gastrectomy.

## CLINICAL EVIDENCE FROM RANDOMIZED, CONTROLLED TRIALS

Although the literature is filled with retrospective comparisons of diabetes outcomes for patients who underwent sleeve gastrectomy or gastric bypass, several high-quality, well-conducted, prospective, randomized studies have been performed. We summarize these studies here.

In a multicenter, randomized, controlled trial, Wallenius and colleagues [9] randomized 49 patients with severe obesity and type 2 diabetes to sleeve gastrectomy or gastric bypass and followed up them for 2 years. Remission rates, defined as a hemoglobin A1c (A1c) of 6% or less without the use of diabetes medications, were not statistically different between the sleeve gastrectomy or gastric bypass groups at 1 year (44% and 46%, $P = .897$) or 2 years (48% and 54%, $P = .654$). There were no significant differences in the degree of A1c reduction between groups, and the average A1c did not differ significantly between groups at 2 years. The study concluded that gastric bypass and sleeve gastrectomy produced similar diabetes improvement.

In the SLEEVEPASS trial, Salminen and colleagues [10] conducted a multicenter, randomized trial of 240 patients with obesity assigned to either sleeve gastrectomy or gastric bypass; 42% of trial participants had type 2 diabetes. Follow-up checkpoints were at 1, 2, 3, and 5 years. Of the patients with type 2 diabetes, complete or partial remission was seen in 37% after sleeve gastrectomy and 45% after gastric bypass at 5 years ($P>.99$). The mean A1c across the entire follow-up time was also the same: 6.6% in the sleeve group and 6.6% in the gastric bypass group. Although the study was underpowered to detect differences in diabetes resolution rates, there were no significant differences between groups, for any diabetes end point, after 5 years.

The SM-BOSS trial conducted by Peterli and colleagues [11] randomized 217 patients with obesity to sleeve gastrectomy or gastric bypass with a 5-year follow-up period. At baseline, 26 of 101 patients in the sleeve group and 28 of 104 patients in the bypass group had type 2 diabetes. After 5 years, complete diabetes remission was seen in 62% of sleeve gastrectomy patients and 68% of gastric bypass patients ($P>.99$). There was no significant difference in average fasting glucose levels (114 mg/dL in sleeve vs 101 mg/dL in bypass, $P = .21$) or average A1c (6.2% in sleeve vs 5.9% in bypass, $P = .09$).

A trial by Murphy and colleagues [12] specifically set out to examine type 2 diabetes remission rates after sleeve gastrectomy or silastic ring-reinforced gastric bypass. In this trial, 114 patients with type 2 diabetes of at least 6 months duration were randomized to sleeve gastrectomy or gastric bypass. The primary outcome was diabetes remission, defined by several different A1c thresholds at 1 year. In the sleeve gastrectomy group, 52% of patients achieved an A1c of less than 6% without the use of diabetes medications, compared with 49% in the gastric bypass group ($P = .85$). There were no significant differences seen in postoperative A1c or diabetes medication use between groups after 1 year.

The STAMPEDE trial [13] randomized 150 patients with both obesity and type 2 diabetes to medical treatment, sleeve gastrectomy, or gastric bypass, and followed up them for 5 years. The primary end point of the study was diabetes resolution, defined as A1c <6% without the need for medications. At 5 years, 22% of bypass patients and 15% of sleeve patients met the primary end point, a difference that was not statistically significant, $P = .34$. Although a greater percentage of gastric bypass patients were able to discontinue all diabetes medications (45% vs 25%, $P < .05$), average A1c at 5 years was almost identical between sleeve and bypass groups (7.3% vs 7.4%, $P =$ NS).

Finally, Yang and colleagues [14] randomized 64 patients with type 2 diabetes and A1c >7% who were also overweight or obese to sleeve gastrectomy or gastric bypass and followed up them for 3 years. The primary end point was A1c at each follow-up visit. There were no significant differences in diabetes remission rates, medication use, or A1c between groups at 3 years.

Taken in sum, these trials indicate that sleeve gastrectomy and gastric bypass are similarly effective for type 2 diabetes treatment. Although one might argue that all the trials had a small sample size and were underpowered, with a possibility of a type II error, in aggregate, they place an upper boundary on any true difference that could exist between the two procedures. That is, to say, if there is a true difference in diabetes outcomes between sleeve gastrectomy and gastric bypass, it is likely to be small, and not clinically relevant.

## THE PHYSIOLOGY OF OBESITY AS IT RELATES TO DIABETES

To understand how sleeve gastrectomy or gastric bypass can ameliorate diabetes in patients with obesity, one must first understand some of the physiologic changes associated with obesity and glucose homeostasis. In patients with obesity, adipose tissue releases increased amounts of nonesterified fatty acids, glycerol, hormones, proinflammatory cytokines, and other factors that result in insulin resistance [15]. When insulin resistance is accompanied by dysfunction of pancreatic beta cells, insufficient insulin is released, and blood glucose rises [15]. Importantly, inflammation appears to play a central role in the development of obesity-related metabolic diseases. Adipose tissue from obese patients exhibits characteristics of chronic inflammation, which has been shown to cause physiologic dysfunction. For example, adipose cells in obese patients exhibit impaired triglyceride storage and release of circulating fatty acids, resulting in insulin resistance in fat, muscle, and liver [16]. Adipose tissue-derived cytokines and products, including adiponectin, TNFα, PAI-1, and IL-6, appear to play a role in energy homeostasis and glucose metabolism; these systems are altered in the obese state. Adiponectin, in particular, has anti-inflammatory functions and protective effects against multiple obesity-related diseases. Circulating adiponectin has been found to be decreased in patients with obesity [17].

In addition, gut and adipose tissue signal the hypothalamus via hormonal and neural pathways, and these pathways can become altered in the setting of obesity. The hypothalamus integrates satiety signals with adiposity signals and other inputs: time of day, social signals, stressors, available nutrients, taste sensation, and other factors. The hypothalamus then communicates to other areas of the brain to influence multiple pathways of energy homeostasis, including initiation of meals and meal size [18]. For example, adipose tissue secretes leptin, a hormone that has been shown to act in the brain to regulate food intake, energy expenditure, and body weight [19]. Leptin deficiency has been shown to cause severe obesity with hyperphagia, and obese individuals appear to exhibit leptin resistance [20]. Ghrelin, a gut-derived hormone, plays an important role in appetite regulation, and seems to induce hunger and function as a meal initiator. In patients with obesity, ghrelin levels do not fall after meals as they should [21].

Interestingly, even the gut microbiome is altered in obesity. An animal model demonstrated that the obese microbiome has an increased capacity to harvest energy from the diet [22]. Furthermore, this trait appears to be transmissible, and introducing "obese microbiota" to lean mice results in an increase in total body fat [22].

## MECHANISMS OF DIABETES RESOLUTION AFTER SLEEVE GASTRECTOMY OR GASTRIC BYPASS

Fig. 1 shows how both sleeve gastrectomy and gastric bypass affect glucose homeostasis to result in a reduction of fasting blood glucose and A1c. Both sleeve gastrectomy and gastric bypass cause increased release of ghrelin, peptide YY, incretins, and bile acids–all of which contribute to diabetes improvement via more insulin secretion or less insulin resistance. The only pathway unique to gastric bypass is duodenal exclusion. We discuss each pathway below:

### Ghrelin

Ghrelin, a hunger-causing hormone released from the oxyntic glands located in the gastric fundus, has a multitude of functions: it acts as a sensor that alerts the body to the presence of nutrients, it stimulates the secretion of growth hormone, it inhibits insulin secretion, it stimulates gastric emptying, and it potently increases food intake [23]. Ghrelin peaks just before a meal and is suppressed by eating. When body fat is reduced because of caloric limitation, ghrelin stimulates growth hormone secretion, which maintains glucose production even in the setting of food restriction [23]. Ghrelin levels have been shown to markedly decrease after gastric bypass [24]. Similarly, sleeve gastrectomy reduces ghrelin to an even greater extent, possibly explained by the removal of ghrelin-secreting stomach tissue [25]. Ghrelin-mediated appetite suppression ultimately results in weight loss, which in turn lowers insulin resistance and improves diabetes.

### PYY3-36

PYY3-36 (PYY) is a satiety-causing hormone released by the distal gastrointestinal tract by the presence of food. PYY reduces eating via appetite circuits in the hypothalamus. It is often called the "ileal brake" hormone. Endogenous levels have been shown to be low in patients with obesity [26], although their sensitivity to it remains intact [21]. After gastric bypass, levels of PYY after meals increase significantly [27]. Interestingly, increases in meal-stimulated PYY levels also occur after sleeve gastrectomy, despite the fact that sleeve gastrectomy does not alter the anatomy of the intestines in any way [28]. Indeed, postprandial PYY levels after sleeve gastrectomy have been shown to be equivalent to those after gastric bypass [28]. Through receptors in the brain, PYY reduces food intake and results in weight loss, which then improves insulin sensitivity and diabetes.

### Incretins

Incretins are hormones secreted from the gastrointestinal tract that causes the pancreas to secrete more insulin. Some also act on the brain, adipose tissue, muscle, and liver to affect glucose levels. Glucose-dependent insulinotropic peptide (GIP) is an incretin secreted from the K cells, located mainly in the duodenum, and stimulates glucose-dependent insulin secretion from the pancreas. Patients with type 2 diabetes have been shown to have a relative resistance to its effects [29]. GIP levels become elevated after both gastric bypass and sleeve gastrectomy in the first 2 days to 3 weeks after surgery, with no appreciable difference between the two procedures [30].

GLP-1 is another potent incretin hormone produced by the L-cells in the distal ileum and colon and is released in response to nutrient ingestion. GLP-1 has been shown to affect gut motility, inhibit gastric acid secretion, inhibit glucagon secretion, induce expansion of insulin-secreting β-cell mass, and induce satiety [31]. A potent stimulator of insulin secretion, GLP-1 is also released in response to GIP. The effects of GLP-1 are diminished in patients with type 2 diabetes. After gastric bypass, postprandial systemic GLP-1 levels increase substantially and remain elevated over time [29]. Similarly, after sleeve gastrectomy, postprandial GLP-1 increases, although fasting levels remained unchanged [28,32]. Hence, both sleeve gastrectomy and gastric bypass cause increased incretin excretion in response to meals, which then directly ameliorates diabetes.

### Bile acids and gut microbiome

Gut bacteria are known to play a significant role in the synthesis and metabolism of bile acids, and there is strong evidence that bile acids play an

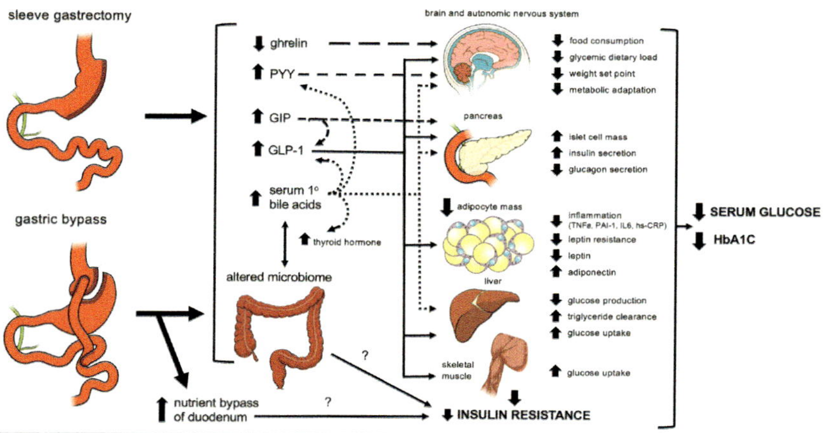


**Fig. 1.** Several of the pathophysiologic mechanisms of diabetes improvement after gastric bypass and sleeve gastrectomy are shown. Both procedures induce changes in ghrelin, GIP, peptide YY (PYY), glucagon-like peptide-1 (GLP-1), and serum primary bile acid levels, as well as induce alterations in the gut microbiome. Downstream effects within the brain, pancreas, adipocyte mass, muscle, and liver then result in amelioration of diabetes, with described pathways shown by arrows. One mechanism specific to gastric bypass is nutrient bypass of the duodenum, which improves diabetes through an incompletely understood mechanism.

important role in glucose homeostasis [33]. Bile acids have been shown to increase the secretion of GLP-1, PYY, and thyroid hormones. Bile acids also have nuclear receptors in the brain, pancreas, and liver. These receptors potentiate insulin action and reduce insulin resistance [33]. Bile acid levels increase after sleeve gastrectomy and gastric bypass [4,34]. Furthermore, alterations in bile acid physiology affect the gut microbiome, and the gut microbiome, in turn, influences obesity, diabetes, and energy extraction from food through unknown pathways that are currently being evaluated [22]. Both gastric bypass and sleeve gastrectomy have been shown to alter gut microbiota and increase bile acid levels [35,36]. Such changes act to improve diabetes.

### Duodenal bypass

There is one mechanism unique to gastric bypass: duodenal exclusion. The exclusion of food from the duodenum has an antidiabetes effect mediated by a mechanism that is yet to be described [37]. As gastric bypass involves bypassing the duodenum, this is another reason for diabetes improvement.

## SUMMARY

Available clinical evidence from prospective, randomized trials has shown that sleeve gastrectomy and gastric bypass produce similar improvements in type 2 diabetes after up to 5 years of follow-up. Mechanistically, many of the pathways for diabetes improvement that were originally described for gastric bypass have now been shown to occur after sleeve gastrectomy. As such, based on current evidence, we recommend clinicians and patients choose between bypass or sleeve based on factors other than long-term diabetes control.

## Disclosure

The authors have nothing to disclose.

## References

[1] Rubino F, Kaplan LM, Schauer PR, et al. The diabetes surgery summit consensus conference: Recommendations for the evaluation and use of gastrointestinal surgery to treat type 2 diabetes mellitus. Ann Surg 2010;251:399–405.
[2] Pories WJ, Swanson MS, MacDonald KG, et al. Who would have thought it? An operation proves to Be the most effective therapy for adult-onset diabetes mellitus, vol. 222. Lippincott-Raven Publishers; 1995.
[3] Pories WJ, Swanson MS, MacDonald KG, et al. Who would have thought it? An operation proves to be the most effective therapy for adult-onset diabetes mellitus. Ann Surg 1995;222(3):339–50, discussion 350-2.
[4] Kohli R, Stefater MA, Inge TH. Molecular insights from bariatric surgery. Rev Endocr Metab Disord 2011;12(3):211–7.
[5] Kamvissi-Lorenz V, Raffaelli M, Bornstein S, et al. Role of the Gut on Glucose Homeostasis: Lesson Learned from Metabolic Surgery. Curr Atheroscler Rep 2017;19(2); https://doi.org/10.1007/s11883-017-0642-5.
[6] English WJ, DeMaria EJ, Hutter MM, et al. American Society for Metabolic and Bariatric Surgery 2018 estimate of metabolic and bariatric procedures performed in the United States. Surg Obes Relat Dis 2020;16(4):457–63.
[7] Kumar SB, Hamilton BC, Wood SG, et al. Is laparoscopic sleeve gastrectomy safer than laparoscopic gastric bypass? a comparison of 30-day complications using the MBSAQIP data registry. Surg Obes Relat Dis 2018;14(3):264–9.
[8] Scott WR, Batterham RL. Roux-en-Y gastric bypass and laparoscopic sleeve gastrectomy: understanding weight loss and improvements in type 2 diabetes after bariatric surgery. Am J Physiol Regul Integr Comp Physiol 2011;301:15–27.
[9] Wallenius V, Alaraj A, Björnfot N, et al. Sleeve gastrectomy and Roux-en-Y gastric bypass in the treatment of type 2 diabetes. Two-year results from a Swedish multicenter randomized controlled trial. Surg Obes Relat Dis 2020;16(8):1035–44.
[10] Salminen P, Helmio M, Ovaska J, et al. Effect of laparoscopic sleeve gastrectomy vs laparoscopic roux-en-y gastric bypass onweight loss at 5 years among patients with morbid obesity the SLEEVEPASS randomized clinical trial. JAMA 2018;319(3):241–54.
[11] Peterli R, Wolnerhanssen BK, Peters T, et al. Effect of laparoscopic sleeve gastrectomy vs laparoscopic roux-en-y gastric bypass onweight loss in patients with morbid obesity the sm-boss randomized clinical trial. JAMA 2018;319(3):255–65.
[12] Murphy R, Clarke MG, Evennett NJ, et al. Laparoscopic Sleeve Gastrectomy Versus Banded Roux-en-Y Gastric Bypass for Diabetes and Obesity: a Prospective Randomised Double-Blind Trial. Obes Surg 2018;28(2):293–302.
[13] Schauer PR, Bhatt DL, Kirwan JP, et al. Bariatric Surgery versus Intensive Medical Therapy for Diabetes — 5-Year Outcomes. N Engl J Med 2017;376(7):641–51.
[14] Yang J, Wang C, Cao G, et al. Long-term effects of laparoscopic sleeve gastrectomy versus roux-en-Y gastric bypass for the treatment of Chinese type 2 diabetes mellitus patients with body mass index 28-35 kg/m2. BMC Surg 2015;15(1); https://doi.org/10.1186/s12893-015-0074-5.
[15] Kahn SE, Hull RL, Utzschneider KM. Mechanisms linking obesity to insulin resistance and type 2 diabetes. Nature 2006;444(7121); https://doi.org/10.1038/nature05482.

[16] Nishimura S, Manabe I, Nagasaki M, et al. CD8+ effector T cells contribute to macrophage recruitment and adipose tissue inflammation in obesity. Nat Med 2009;15(8):914–20.
[17] Ohashi K, Yuasa D, Shibata R, et al. Adiponectin as a Target in Obesity-related Inflammatory State. Endocr Metab Immune Disorders-Drug Targets 2015;15(2):145–50.
[18] Woods SC, D'Alessio DA. Central Control of Body Weight and Appetite. J Clin Endocrinol Metab 2008;93(11_supplement_1):s37–50.
[19] Seeley R, van Dijk G, Campfield L, et al. Intraventricular Leptin Reduces Food Intake and Body Weight of Lean Rats but Not Obese Zucker Rats. Horm Metab Res 1996;28(12): 664–8.
[20] Liu J, Yang X, Yu S, et al. The Leptin Resistance. Adv Exp Med Biol 2018;1090:145–63.
[21] Field BCT, Chaudhri OB, Bloom SR. Bowels control brain: gut hormones and obesity. Nat Rev Endocrinol 2010;6(8):444–53.
[22] Turnbaugh PJ, Ley RE, Mahowald MA, et al. An obesity-associated gut microbiome with increased capacity for energy harvest. Nature 2006;444(7122):1027–31.
[23] Müller TD, Nogueiras R, Andermann ML, et al. Ghrelin. Mol Metab 2015;4(6):437–60.
[24] Cummings DE, Weigle DS, Frayo RS, et al. Plasma Ghrelin Levels after Diet-Induced Weight Loss or Gastric Bypass Surgery. N Engl J Med 2002;346(21):1623–30.
[25] Karamanakos SN, Vagenas K, Kalfarentzos F, et al. Weight Loss, Appetite Suppression, and Changes in Fasting and Postprandial Ghrelin and Peptide-YY Levels After Roux-en-Y Gastric Bypass and Sleeve Gastrectomy. Ann Surg 2008;247(3):401–7.
[26] Batterham RL, Cohen MA, Ellis SM, et al. Inhibition of Food Intake in Obese Subjects by Peptide YY $_{3-36}$. N Engl J Med 2003;349(10):941–8.
[27] Korner J, Bessler M, Cirilo LJ, et al. Effects of Roux-en-Y Gastric Bypass Surgery on Fasting and Postprandial Concentrations of Plasma Ghrelin, Peptide YY, and Insulin. J Clin Endocrinol Metab 2005;90(1):359–65.
[28] McCarty TR, Jirapinyo P, Thompson CC. Effect of Sleeve Gastrectomy on Ghrelin, GLP-1, PYY, and GIP Gut Hormones. Ann Surg 2020;272(1):72–80.
[29] Bose M, Oliván B, Teixeira J, et al. Do Incretins Play a Role in the Remission of Type 2 Diabetes after Gastric Bypass Surgery: What are the Evidence? Obes Surg 2009;19(2): 217–29.
[30] Wallenius V, Dirinck E, Fändriks L, et al. Glycemic Control after Sleeve Gastrectomy and Roux-En-Y Gastric Bypass in Obese Subjects with Type 2 Diabetes Mellitus. Obes Surg 2018;28(6):1461–72.
[31] MacDonald PE, El-kholy W, Riedel MJ, et al. The Multiple Actions of GLP-1 on the Process of Glucose-Stimulated Insulin Secretion. Diabetes 2002;51(Supplement 3):S434–42.
[32] Baggio LL, Drucker DJ. Biology of Incretins: GLP-1 and GIP. Gastroenterology 2007;132(6): 2131–57.
[33] Ahmad TR, Haeusler RA. Bile acids in glucose metabolism and insulin signalling — mechanisms and research needs. Nat Rev Endocrinol 2019;15(12):701–12.
[34] Albaugh VL, Banan B, Ajouz H, et al. Bile acids and bariatric surgery. Mol Aspects Med 2017;56:75–89.
[35] Palleja A, Kashani A, Allin KH, et al. Roux-en-Y gastric bypass surgery of morbidly obese patients induces swift and persistent changes of the individual gut microbiota. Genome Med 2016;8(1):67.
[36] Liu H, Hu C, Zhang X, et al. Role of gut microbiota, bile acids and their cross-talk in the effects of bariatric surgery on obesity and type 2 diabetes. J Diabetes Invest 2018;9(1):13–20.
[37] Cummings DE. Endocrine mechanisms mediating remission of diabetes after gastric bypass surgery. Int J Obes 2009;33:S33–40.

Advances in Surgery 55 (2021) 9–33

ADVANCES IN SURGERY

# Advances in the Diagnosis and Management of Appendicitis in Children

Katherine He, MD, MS[a], Shawn J. Rangel, MD, MSCE[b,*]

[a]Department of General Surgery, Brigham & Women's Hospital, Harvard Medical School, 75 Francis Street CA-034, Boston, MA 02115, USA; [b]Department of Pediatric & Thoracic Surgery, Boston Children's Hospital, Harvard Medical School, 300 Longwood Avenue - Fegan 3, Boston, MA 02115, USA

**Keywords**

• Appendicitis • Appendectomy • Child • Diagnosis • Management

**Key points**

- Appendicitis is the most common surgical emergency in childhood and is associated with the greatest relative burden of hospital cost and surgical site infections within pediatric surgery.
- Use of ionizing radiation during diagnosis can be minimized by optimizing ultrasound quality, leveraging the combined predictive value of laboratory, imaging and clinical data, and implementation of standardized clinical pathways.
- Use of same-day discharge and opioid-sparing pain protocols in children with uncomplicated appendicitis have been associated with shorter length of stay and high caregiver satisfaction.
- Nonoperative management has emerged as a safe treatment option for children with early appendicitis although long-term data are lacking for recurrent appendicitis.
- High-quality comparative effectiveness data are needed to define goal-directed end points for antibiotic treatment in children with complicated appendicitis.

## INTRODUCTION

Appendicitis is the most common surgical emergency in childhood and among all pediatric surgical conditions, it is associated with the greatest relative burden of hospital cost, surgical site infections, hospital revisits, and antibiotic

*Corresponding author. *E-mail address:* shawn.rangel@childrens.harvard.edu

https://doi.org/10.1016/j.yasu.2021.05.002
0065-3411/21/

treatment days [1–3]. Over the past decade, significant advances have been made in the ability to diagnose appendicitis while minimizing the need for ionizing radiation. These have included strategies to improve the diagnostic quality of ultrasound (US), leveraging the combined predictive value of multiple sources of diagnostic data, and use of multidisciplinary clinical pathways. Advances in management have included availability of more robust comparative data to guide antibiotic treatment, same-day discharge protocols to improve health care value, and opioid-sparing pain management strategies, among others. Nonoperative management has also emerged as a viable and safe treatment option for children with early, uncomplicated appendicitis. Finally, expansion of the American College of Surgeon's Pediatric National Surgical Quality Improvement Program (NSQIP-Pediatric) to capture appendectomy measures has led to the development of performance and resource utilization benchmarks to help hospitals prioritize their quality improvement efforts. The purpose of this review is to summarize these recent advances and review ongoing controversies as a framework for future investigation.

## RELEVANCE AND APPROACH TO SEVERITY CLASSIFICATION

Many criteria for differentiating complicated from uncomplicated appendicitis have been proposed and reported in the literature [4–6]. These have included both intraoperative findings representative of implicit perforation (extraluminal fecalith or a visible hole) and indirect evidence of perforation such as the presence of an intra-abdominal or pelvic abscess, generalized peritonitis, and diffuse fibrinopurulent exudate, among others. These considerations were taken into account by the NSQIP-Pediatric Data Definitions Committee in developing its definition for complicated appendicitis as part of its pilot expansion to collect outcome and resource utilization measures for pediatric appendicitis [7]. The committee's definition was based on the presence of one or more of the following 4 intraoperative findings: visible hole, diffuse fibrinopurulent exudate extending outside the right lower quadrant and pelvis, intra-abdominal abscess, and presence of an extraluminal fecalith. In a validation study of 5002 patients from 22 NSQIP-Pediatric hospitals, each of the 4 findings was found to be independently associated with higher rates of any adverse event, organ space infections (OSIs), revisits, increased resource utilization, and longer length of stay (LOS) [8]. Furthermore, different combinations of intraoperative findings were found to potentiate risk for worse outcomes and higher resource utilization, suggesting that more granular risk-assessment could be supported by these criteria for the purpose of risk-adjustment (Fig. 1) [9]. The results of the validation studies supported the current definition used by NSQIP-Pediatric to risk-adjust outcomes based on disease severity.

## DIAGNOSTIC EVALUATION

Establishing the diagnosis of appendicitis in children can be challenging. Many children presenting with appendicitis lack the "classic" signs of fever, anorexia, nausea, and migratory right lower quadrant pain. Furthermore, these findings

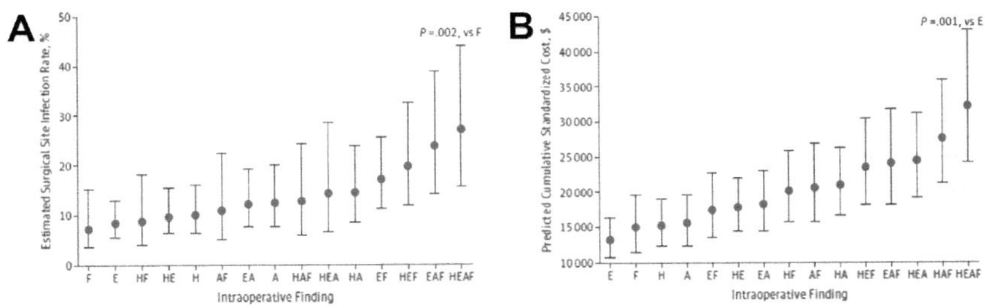


**Fig. 1.** Association of different combinations of intraoperative findings with SSI rates (*A*) and mean hospital cost (*B*) in children with complicated appendicitis. *Abbreviations:* A, abscess; E, diffuse fibropurulent exudate; F, free-floating fecalith; H, visible hole. From Anandalwar SP et al, JAMA Surg. 2018;153(11):1021-1027. Figure used with permission.

have only modest predictive value when present, and the presence or absence of leukocytosis similarly has limited predictive value [10]. Given the limited diagnostic utility of clinical and laboratory data, imaging has become an integral component of diagnostic evaluation. Concern surrounding radiation exposure associated with computed tomography (CT) has led to increasing use of US and MRI. MRI has similar diagnostic accuracy to CT (sensitivity 96%–100% and specificity 96%–99%) [11], although use remains limited because of cost, availability, and technical challenges with imaging younger children [12]. US has become the preferred initial imaging modality as endorsed by the American Academy of Pediatrics and its Section on Surgery [13]; however, the utility of US is operator and hospital dependent, with sensitivities and specificities ranging between 44% to 88% and 90% to 97% among hospitals [11]. Furthermore, rates of nondiagnostic US studies are as high as 51%. Major advances over the past decade have largely focused on improving the quality of US, refinement of clinical prediction rules based on multiple data sources (including US) and use of clinical pathways to standardize the diagnostic process.

### Diagnostic utility of clinical prediction rules and clinical scoring systems

The goal of prediction rules and clinical scoring systems is to estimate the probability of appendicitis based on several sources of data, including vital signs, symptoms, laboratory data, and elements of the clinical history. The two most studied scoring approaches are the Pediatric Appendicitis Score (PAS) and the Alvarado score, although several others have been reported [14]. The major criticism of these tools has been variation in reported predictive value, with sensitivity and specificity ranging between 82% to 93% and 65% to 91% for the PAS and 72% to 93% and 71% to 98% for the Alvarado score, respectively (Table 1) [14]. This variation is likely due to the subjective nature of many clinical scoring criteria and differences in how and in whom hospitals apply them. Based on these considerations, use of these tools should be limited to identifying patients who may benefit from further diagnostic imaging or entry into clinical pathways.

**Table 1**
Test performance characteristics associated with different clinical prediction rules for suspected appendicitis in children

| Authors | Rule name | Sn | Sp | PPV | NPV | LR– | Lower 95% CI on sensitivity | Upper 95% CI for LR– | Outcome frequency | Rule predicted appendicitis frequency | Actual appendicitis frequency |
|---|---|---|---|---|---|---|---|---|---|---|---|
| Validation | | | | | | | | | | | |
| Bond et al, 2011 [28] | Alvarado | 0.90 | 0.71 | 0.83 | 0.81 | 0.15 | 0.82 | 0.25 | 0.62 | 0.67 | 0.62 |
| Escriba et al, 202 [25] | Alvarado | 0.88 | 0.98 | 0.97 | 0.92 | 0.12 | 0.74 | 0.28 | 0.41 | 0.38 | 0.41 |
| Owen et al, 2020 [33] | Alvarado | 0.93 | 0.81 | 0.89 | 0.88 | 0.09 | 0.8 | 0.226 | 0.61 | 0.64 | 0.61 |
| Macklin et al, 2020 [32] | Alvarado | 0.87 | 0.49 | 0.45 | 0.89 | 0.27 | 0.71 | 0.63 | 0.32 | 0.63 | 0.32 |
| Schneider et al, 2018 [26] | Alvarado | 0.72 | 0.81 | 0.66 | 0.85 | 0.34 | 0.66 | 0.37 | 0.34 | 0.37 | 0.34 |
| Bhatt et al, 2020 [23] | PAS | 0.93 | 0.69 | 0.61 | 0.95 | 0.10 | 0.85 | 0.27 | 0.34 | 0.52 | 0.34 |
| Escriba et al, 2020 [25] | PAS | 0.90 | 0.91 | 0.88 | 0.93 | 0.10 | 0.77 | 0.27 | 0.41 | 0.43 | 0.41 |
| Goldman et al, 2017 [24] | PAS | 0.98 | 0.73 | 1.00 | 0.99 | 0.03 | 0.92 | 0.1 | 0.14 | 0.79 | 0.14 |
| Schneider et al, 2018 [26] | PAS | 0.82 | 0.65 | 0.54 | 0.88 | 0.27 | 0.77 | 0.43 | 0.34 | 0.51 | 0.34 |
| Derivation | | | | | | | | | | | |
| Kharbanda et al, 2019 [30] | Kharbanda | 1.00 | 0.34 | 0.47 | 1.00 | 0.00 | 0.98 | [a] | 0.37 | 0.79 | 0.37 |
| Lintula et al, 2012 [31] | Lintula | 0.85 | 0.95 | 0.85 | 0.95 | 0.16 | 0.65 | 0.39 | 0.25 | 0.25 | 0.25 |
| Dado et al, 2014 [29] | Modified Linberg | 0.90 | 0.62 | 0.88 | 0.66 | 0.16 | 0.84 | 0.27 | 0.77 | 0.78 | 0.77 |
| Samuel, 2018 [34] | PAS | 1.00 | 0.96 | 0.97 | 1.00 | 0.00 | 0.99 | [a] | 0.63 | 0.64 | 0.63 |
| Van den broek et al, 2018 [27] | Van den Broek | 1.00 | 0.17 | 0.90 | 0.96 | 0.01 | 0.99 | 0.04 | 0.8 | 0.98 | 0.8 |

*Abbreviations:* CI, confidence interval; LR–, negative likelihood ratio; NPV, negative predictive value; PAS, Pediatric Appendicitis Score; PPV, positive predictive value; Sn, sensitivity; Sp, specificity.

[a] Could not calculate as sensitivity = 1.

(From Kulik DM et al, Journal of Clinical Epidemiology 66 (2013) 95-104. Table used with permission)

### Strategies to optimize the diagnostic quality of US

Several strategies have been reported to increase the diagnostic accuracy of US. In a single-center study of 2347 patients, implementation of an US reporting template to standardize reporting criteria and reduce errors of omission decreased nondiagnostic examinations from 48% to 0.1%, increased sensitivity from 66% to 92%, and decreased CT utilization from 44% to 14% [15]. In another single-center study, use of a standardized US reporting template for appendicitis resulted in a 67% decrease in CT utilization and an annual cost savings of $146,549 [16]. In a single-center study of 294 children, use of a serial US protocol after an initial nondiagnostic examination had a sensitivity of 97% and specificity of 91% [17]. In a study of 230 children, use of standardized sonographic education focusing on proper transducer selection, patient position, graded compression, and optimizing acoustic windows improved appendix visualization from 40.7% to 68.7% [18].

### Strategies to leverage the combined predictive value of US, laboratory and clinical data

Several studies have reported improved predictive value of US by combining imaging results with laboratory and clinical data. In a single-center study of 845 children, incorporation of white blood cell (WBC) count thresholds significantly improved negative predictive value (NPV) in patients with equivocal US findings from 42% to 96% (Table 2) [19]. In another study of 728 children, false-positive US results occurred more frequently with lower PAS scores (PPV 97% in high PAS vs 73% in low PAS) and false-negatives with higher PAS scores (NPV 100% in low PAS vs 81% in high PAS), suggesting that serial examination or further imaging may be warranted in children where US results and clinical assessment are discordant [20]. In a single-center study of 2277 patients, incorporation of symptom duration and WBC profile significantly improved the NPV associated with a nondiagnostic US from 74% to 100% (Fig. 2) [21].

### Role of standardized diagnostic clinical pathways

Diagnostic clinical pathways (DCP) have been used to standardize and streamline the evaluation of children with suspected appendicitis to reduce practice variation and CT utilization. In a prospective study of 227 patients, incorporation of a DCP using a standardized US reporting template and risk stratification using PAS to direct imaging recommendations and surgical consultation resulted in a reduction of CT utilization from 66% to 22% without adversely affecting LOS, rates of complicated appendicitis, or negative appendectomy rates [22]. Incorporating the combined predictive value of US and laboratory data into a decision-support framework can further improve the clinical utility of DCPs. In a single-center study of 416 patients, this approach led to an 86% reduction in CT utilization (21% vs 3%) and a 15% reduction in mean time to appendectomy (8.5–7.2 hours) without an increase in negative appendectomy rate (Fig. 3) [23].

**Table 2**
Influence of white blood cell count and polymorphonucleocyte differential on the predictive value of different ultrasound findings in children with suspected appendicitis

| | Patients n (%) | US findings only | | US findings + WBC/PMN% thresholds | |
|---|---|---|---|---|---|
| | | PPV, % (95% CI) | NPV, % (95% CI) | PPV, % (95% CI) | NPV, % (95% CI) |
| Appendix not visualized, no primary[a] or secondary[b] signs | 240 (28.4) | 15.8 (11.2–20.5) | 41.3 (35.1–47.5) | 23.7(15.9–31.5) | 95.0 (89.5–100.0) |
| Appendix not visualized, fluid present in RLQ or pelvis, no primary or secondary signs | 193 (22.8) | 21.2 (15.4–27.0) | 46.0 (39.0–53.0) | 38.0 (28.1–47.9) | 98.2 (94.8–101.7) |
| Normal appendix visualized, no primary or secondary signs | 57 (6.7) | 22.8 (11.9–33.7) | 51.8 (38.8–64.8) | 55.6 (32.6–78.6) | 100.0 (100.0–100.0) |
| Appendix visualized with primary signs only | 153 (18.1) | 79.1 (717–85.4) | 60.7 (53.0–68.4) | 913 (85.9–96.7) | 68.2 (48.7–87.7) |
| Secondary signs present ± visualized appendix ± primary signs | 202 (23.9) | 89.1 (84.8–93.4) | 66.9 (60.4–73.4) | 96.8 (94.0–99.6) | 50.0 (30.8–69.2) |

*Abbreviations:* NPV, negative predictive value of not having appendicitis when WBC ≤9000/μL and PMNs ≤65%; PMN%, polymorphonuclear leukocyte differential; PPV, positive predictive value of having appendicitis when WBC greater than 9000 μL and PMNs greater than 65%; RLQ, right lower quadrant; US, ultrasound.

[a]Primary signs of appendicitis are hyperemia of appendiceal wall or wall thickness ≥7 mm.

[b]Secondary signs of appendicitis are fecalith or echogenic fat.

(From Anandalwar SP et al, J Am Coll Surg. 2015 Jun;220(6):1010–7. Used with permission.)

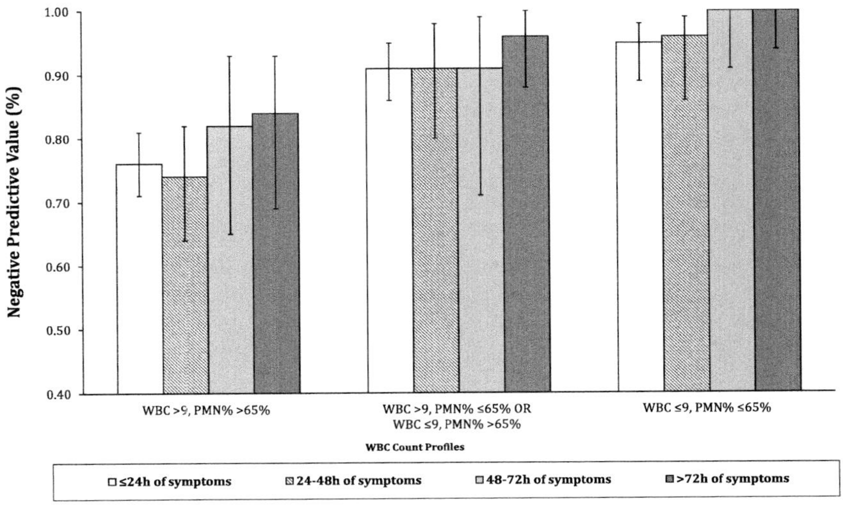


**Fig. 2.** Influence of symptom duration, WBC count, and polymorphonucleocyte shift (PMN%) on the negative predictive value of a nondiagnostic ultrasound in children with suspected appendicitis. From Kashtan MA et al, J Pediatr Surg. 2020 Jun;55(6):1032-1036. Used with permission.

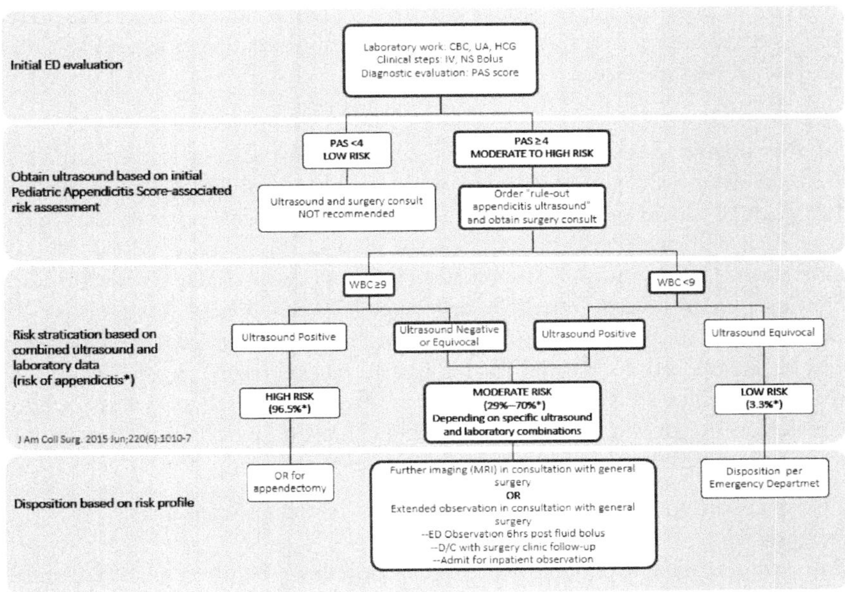


**Fig. 3.** Evidence-based clinical pathway for suspected appendicitis based on the combined predictive value of laboratory, ultrasound, and clinical data. From Anandalwar SP et al, J Surg Res. 2020 Sep 9;257:529-536. Used with permission.

## SURGICAL MANAGEMENT

### Influence of operative timing on outcomes and resource utilization

Many studies have attempted to characterize the influence of treatment delay on perforation risk, although the majority are limited by retrospective, single-center study designs and lack of standardized outcome definitions. The most rigorous evidence to date has come from NSQIP-Pediatrics' procedure-targeted appendectomy data using standardized definitions and chart review methodology. In a study of 2429 children from 29 NSQIP-Pediatric hospitals, no association was found between time from presentation to appendectomy and risk of complicated appendicitis or postoperative complications for patients undergoing appendectomy within 24 hours of presentation (Fig. 4) [24]. In a follow-up study of 18,927 patients from 140 NSQIP-Pediatric hospitals, a modest increase in the rate of complicated appendicitis (based on intraoperative criteria) was found in patients undergoing appendectomy between 16 and 24 hours after presentation compared to those undergoing earlier appendectomy [25]; however, no differences were found in SSIs (3.3% vs 2.8%), ED re-visits (8.5% vs 8.4%), or readmissions (6.0% vs 5.9%). Longer periods of delay have been associated with increased cost and LOS. In a study of 2116 patients from 16 NSQIP-Pediatric hospitals, hospitals associated with the longest quartile of time to appendectomy had longer LOS and 23% higher mean total cost compared with those associated with the shortest quartile (Fig. 5) [26]. Based on these considerations, hospitals should strive to perform appendectomy within 16 hours of presentation to reduce the risk of complicated disease, and preferably as early as resources allow to minimize resource utilization and lost days from work for caregivers.

### Operative approach

Laparoscopy has become the preferred surgical approach, with less than 5% of all children undergoing open appendectomy based on NSQIP-Pediatric data [12]. A 2018 Cochrane review found that compared with open surgery, laparoscopy is associated with lower rates of wound infection (2% vs 7.6%), 19-hour shorter LOS and 0.5-day shorter return to normal activity without any difference in intra-abdominal abscess rate [27]. Single-port laparoscopy has become popular at some institutions although the practice has been associated with longer operative time and the long-term cosmetic benefits are unclear [28]. In a single-center study of 198 patients, single port laparoscopy was found to have superior cosmetic outcomes by both patients and parents at 6 weeks; however, no difference remained after 25 months of follow-up [29].

### Initial medical versus operative management for complicated appendicitis

Many studies have attempted to compare outcomes between early appendectomy and initial nonoperative management for appendicitis associated with abscess or phlegmonous changes. In a meta-analysis of 15 trials including 1243 patients, nonoperative treatment of complicated appendicitis was associated with lower rates of complications and wound infections, whereas immediate

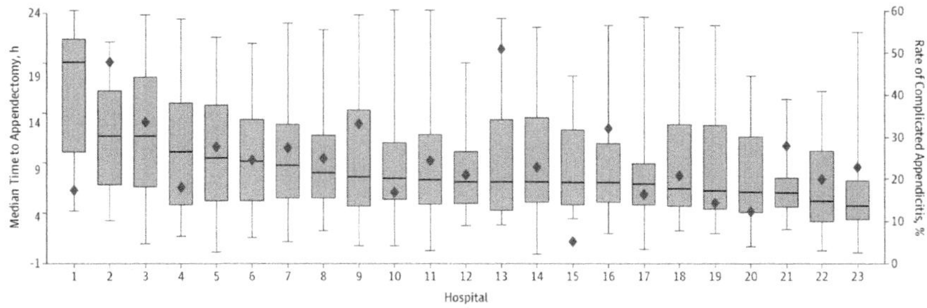


**Fig. 4.** Variation in median time from presentation to appendectomy and rates of complicated appendicitis at 23 hospitals participating in NSQIP-Pediatric. From Serres SK et al, JAMA Pediatr. 2017 Aug 1;171(8):740-746. Used with permission.

appendectomy was associated with shorter LOS (Fig. 6) [30]. It is important to emphasize that the investigators reported significant heterogeneity across studies, which likely reflects variation in disease severity based on differences in patient populations, access to care, and other sociodemographic factors leading to differential outcomes between hospitals.

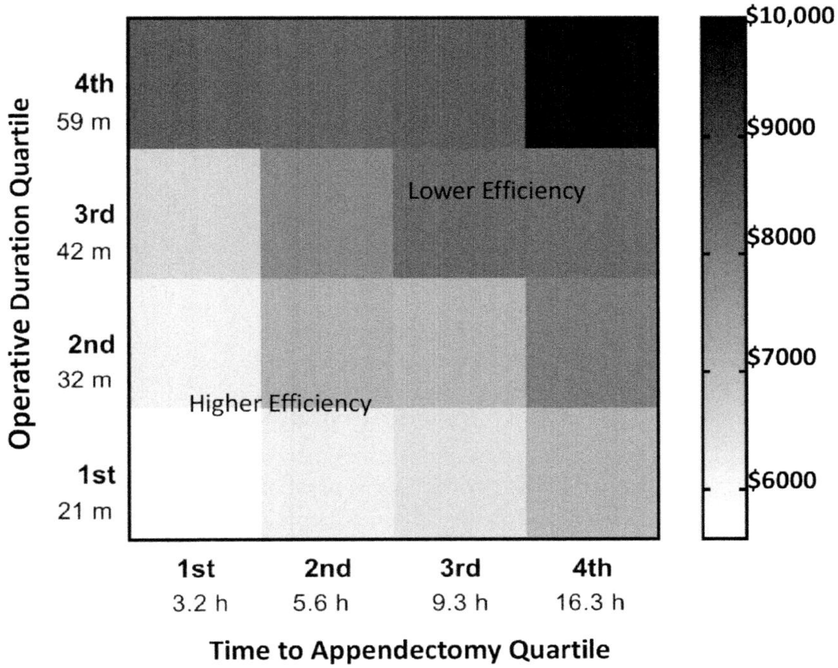


**Fig. 5.** Association of time from ED presentation to appendectomy and case duration on median total hospital cost in children with uncomplicated appendicitis. From Serres SK et al, J Am Coll Surg. 2018 Jun;226(6):1014-1021. Figure used with permission.

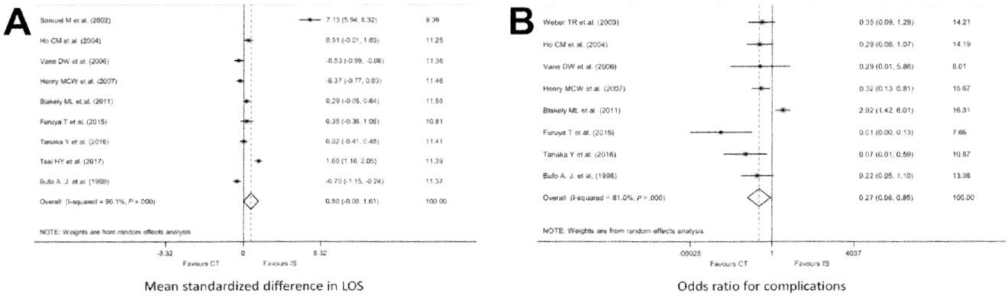


**Fig. 6.** Meta-analyses of studies examining the influence of conservative treatment (CT) and immediate surgery (IS) on (A) standardized mean difference for length of stay and (B) odds ratio for complication rate in children with complicated appendicitis. From Vaos G et al, J Pediatr Surg. 2019 54(7):1365–1371. Used with permission.

## Role of irrigation and drains

In a single-center randomized control trial (RCT) of 220 patients with perforated appendicitis, irrigation with at least 500 mL of normal saline was not associated with lower rates of postoperative abscesses, return to oral intake, or decreased time to discharge as compared with using suction alone [31]. Another RCT of 100 patients comparing betadine to normal saline irrigation demonstrated a small but nonsignificant benefit for preventing postoperative abscesses, ED revisits and reducing LOS, although the study was likely underpowered, limiting the interpretation of results [32]. The largest reported experience evaluating the efficacy of drain placement in pediatric appendicitis has come from the Japanese National Clinical Database. In a propensity-matched, multicenter study of 1762 children with perforated appendicitis, drain placement was not associated with a reduction in complications, OSI, readmission, or reoperation, but did increase LOS (9 vs 7 days) and rate of wound dehiscence (2.4 vs 0.3%) [33].

## Antibiotic management of uncomplicated appendicitis

Recent studies using NSQIP-Pediatric data have provided increasing clarity around optimal antibiotic management for uncomplicated appendicitis. In a study of 1389 patients from 17 NSQIP-Pediatric hospitals, extended-spectrum antipseudomonal agents (piperacillin/tazobactam) were found to be equivalent to nonextended spectrum agents in preventing organ space and incisional SSIs [34]. In a follow-up study of 846 patients from 14 NSQIP-Pediatric hospitals comparing the effectiveness of non-extended spectrum agents, use of ceftriaxone and metronidazole was associated with a 90% lower odds of postoperative SSI compared with cefoxitin [35]. Based on these data, ceftriaxone and metronidazole should be considered the first-line regimen for uncomplicated appendicitis based on treatment efficacy and antimicrobial stewardship.

The decision to re-dose antibiotics in the operating room after antibiotic administration in the ED remains controversial. In a single-center study of 478 patients, re-dosing did not influence rates of superficial SSI and OSI after

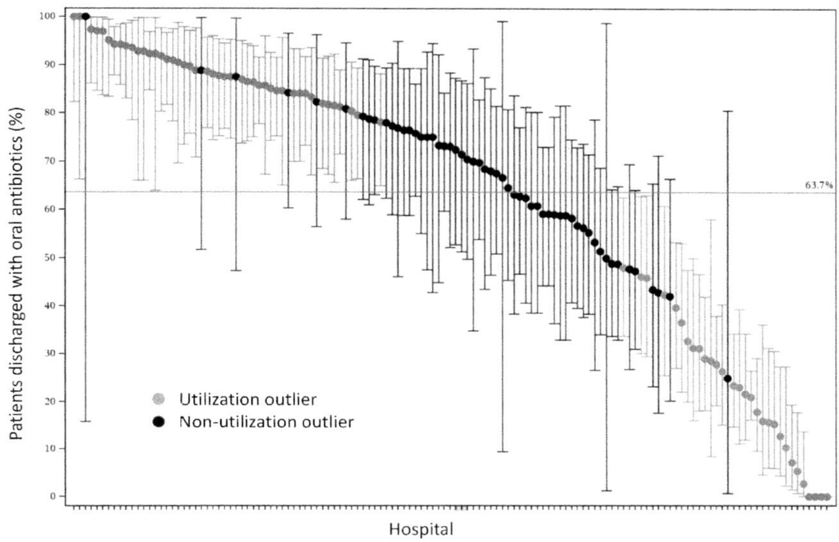


**Fig. 7.** Variation in use of oral antibiotics after discharge in children with complicated appendicitis at 131 hospitals participating in NSQIP-Pediatric.

adjusting for intraoperative severity [36]. The need for postoperative antibiotics in cases of gangrenous appendicitis without frank perforation is also controversial. A 2005 Cochrane review concluded that a single preoperative dose of antibiotics was sufficient for uncomplicated appendicitis but did not stratify results based on disease severity [37]. This remains an important question to address on behalf of antimicrobial stewardship considering that 27% of children with uncomplicated appendicitis receive postoperative antibiotics [34].

## Antibiotic management for complicated appendicitis

Use of antibiotics in the postoperative period is necessary to prevent OSI although excessive use can be associated with increased antimicrobial resistance and patient harm. Lack of robust evidence-based guidelines have led to great practice variation among NSQIP hospitals in the use of antibiotics after discharge, and in the approach used to determine duration of antibiotic treatment (Fig. 7) [12]. With respect to the latter, a recent survey of 78 NSQIP hospitals identified 42 unique approaches to postoperative antimicrobial management for children with complicated appendicitis (Fig. 8) [38]. Selective utilization of outpatient antibiotics based on WBC and other goal-directed end points have become popular, although comparative effectiveness data to support these approaches remain limited. The potential benefits of goal-directed approaches are shorter courses of antibiotic therapy and improved antimicrobial stewardship, whereas risks include inadequate treatment and higher OSI rates. The latter is a particularly important consideration given that use of

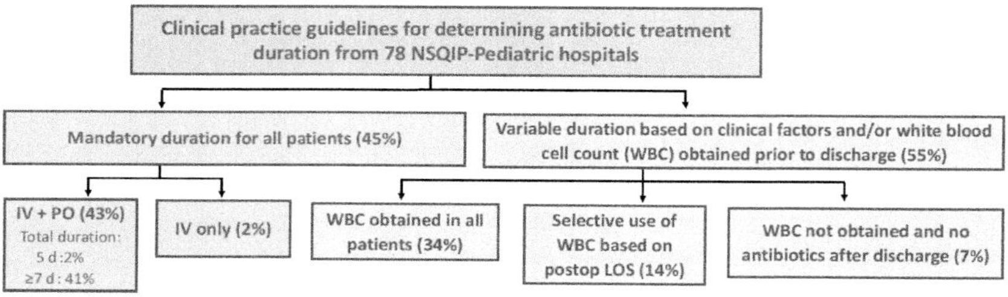


**Fig. 8.** Variation in approach for determining need and duration of oral antibiotics after discharge in children with complicated appendicitis as reported by 78 hospitals participating in NSQIP-Pediatric.

oral antibiotics after discharge has been shown to reduce the odds of OSI by 61% in patients with high severity disease (Fig. 9) [39]. Use of antibiotic treatment after discharge in patients with less severe disease remains uncertain and in need of future investigation.

## Screening and management of OSIs

Consensus guidelines are lacking for use of postoperative imaging and imaging practices vary widely across hospitals. In a study of 1316 patients from 20 NSQIP-Pediatric hospitals, postoperative US and CT utilization ranged from 1.2% to 20.3% and 2.1% to 31.7%, respectively. Furthermore, a nearly three-fold variation in diagnostic efficiency (ratio of imaging studies obtained per OSI diagnosed) was observed, likely reflecting significant differences in the use of selection criteria among centers [40]. Several strategies have been reported to increase the diagnostic yield of postoperative imaging. In a study of 1174 patients from the Pediatric Health Information System (PHIS) database, delay in imaging until POD 7 reduced postoperative imaging utilization by 44% and reduced readmission rates (28% vs 36%) [41]. Choice of imaging is also an important consideration. Efficacy of US in guiding percutaneous

| Outcome | Analysis Cohort | OR [95%CI] | *P*-value |
|---|---|---|---|
| **Organ Space Infection** | All Patients | 0.62 [0.29, 1.31] | .21 |
| | High-Severity Disease | 0.39 [0.15, 0.96] | .04 |
| **Hospital Revisits** | | | |
| All Revisits | All Patients | 1.03 [0.61, 1.74] | .9 |
| | High-Severity Disease | 0.74 [0.4, 1.38] | .35 |
| ED Revisits without readmission | All Patients | 1.34 [0.56, 3.22] | .51 |
| | High-Severity Disease | 0.71 [0.25, 2.01] | .51 |
| Inpatient Readmissions | All Patients | 0.86 [0.4, 1.86] | .71 |
| | High-Severity Disease | 0.83 [0.35, 1.92] | .66 |

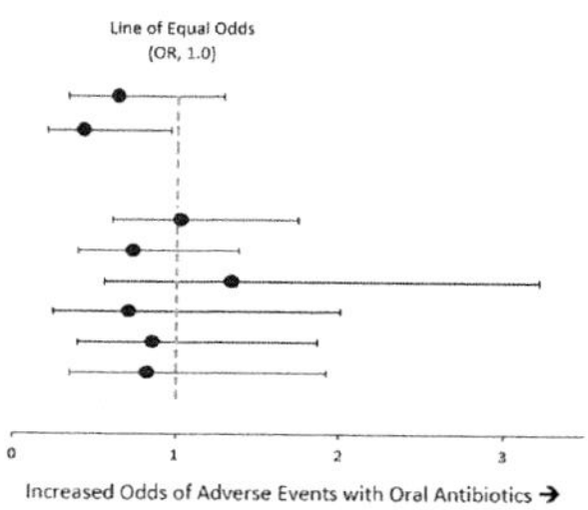


**Fig. 9.** Association between use of oral antibiotics after discharge, organ space infection, and hospital revisits in children with complicated appendicitis. From Anandalwar SP et al, Ann Surg. 2019 Jul 3. Used with permission.

drainage of intra-abdominal abscesses has been reported to be between 85% and 90% and comparable to CT. The Society of Interventional Radiology therefore recommends US as the first-line imaging study in suspected OSI to spare potential radiation exposure [40,42].

## Role of parenteral nutrition

Consensus guidelines for use of parenteral nutrition (PN) in patients with complicated appendicitis are lacking and utilization ranges from 0% to 40% across hospitals [12,43]. Proponents of PN suggest optimizing nutrition may improve immune function and improve healing while opponents cite high cost and associated complications. In a study of 1073 patients from 29 NSQIP-Pediatric hospitals, rates of overall complications, revisits, and SSIs were similar between high and low PN-utilizing hospitals although use of PN was associated with 22% higher hospital cost after adjusting for LOS (Fig. 10) [43]. These data suggest that routine use of PN in patients with complicated appendicitis is not warranted.

## Indications and timing of interval appendectomy for complicated appendicitis

Historically, children with complicated appendicitis initially managed nonoperatively underwent interval appendectomy to prevent recurrence. This practice has come into question with recurrence rates reported to be between 8% and 34%, although follow-up periods are notably variable [44,45]. Furthermore, carcinoid tumors are relatively rare, reported to be less than 1% in a systematic review of 15 studies including 955 patients [46]. The presence of a fecalith has been associated with a 50% recurrence within 4 years based on a recent meta-analysis [47]. These data and their associated uncertainty should be discussed with patients and their caregivers in order for them to make informed decisions on operative versus nonoperative management. For operative management, data are lacking to identify the optimal timeline to balance resolution of the initial inflammatory process with the risk of recurrent appendicitis.

| Outcome | High PN Rate | Low PN Rate | OR [95% CI] | *p* |
|---|---|---|---|---|
| All Complications | 10.5% | 12.3% | 0.80 [0.46, 1.37] | .41 |
| Composite SSI | 8.8% | 11.3% | 0.72 [0.40, 1.32] | .29 |
| Incisional SSI | 1.2% | 1.2% | 0.87 [0.20, 3.83] | .86 |
| OSI | 7.6% | 10.0% | 0.71 [0.38, 1.33] | .29 |
| All Revisits | 15.9% | 14.7% | 1.10 [0.75, 1.61] | .63 |

| Outcome | PN | No PN | RR [95% CI] | *p* |
|---|---|---|---|---|
| Hospital Cost | $25,164 | $20,478 | 1.23 [1.15, 1.32] | <.01 |

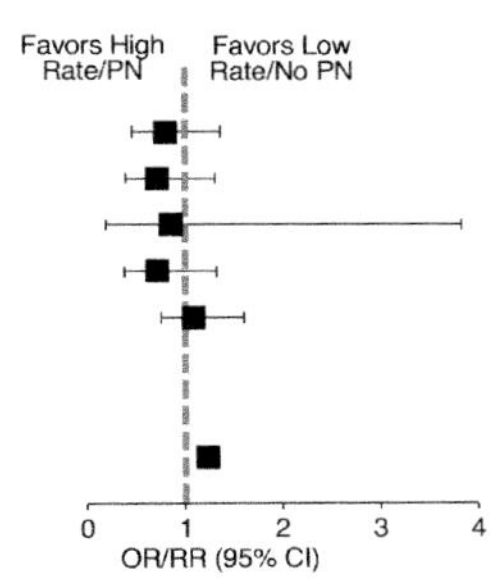


**Fig. 10.** Comparison of complication rates, hospital revisits, and resource utilization in children with complicated appendicitis treated at high and low parenteral nutrition using hospitals before and after matching on clinical characteristics and length of stay.

### Same-day discharge for patients with uncomplicated appendicitis

Same-day discharge protocols can reduce resource utilization and have been proven safe in patients with uncomplicated appendicitis (Table 3) [48–51]. Same-day discharge has been associated with decreased LOS; however, data regarding risk of readmission have been conflicting. An increase in readmission rates from 1.2% to 4.2% was observed in one prospective study of 794 patients [49], whereas others showed no difference [48,51]. In a subgroup analysis, patients with gangrenous or perforated appendicitis had a greater than three times higher odds of readmission, suggesting that patient selection is critical for success [49]. High caregiver satisfaction has been associated with same-day discharge protocols. In one prospective study of 158 patients, when asked at their 2-week follow-up visit, 92% of parents would choose same-day discharge again [51].

### Approach to perioperative pain management

Duration and amount of prescribed opioids have been shown to be highly variable in children with appendicitis, and narcotic prescription has been associated with increased odds of emergency department revisit (13% vs 4.3%) and constipation requiring medical attention (2.1% vs 0%) in a retrospective study of 590 patients [52]. A systematic review of 6 RCTs found that the use of opioids in undifferentiated acute abdominal pain in children did not result in improved pain scores and had a six times increased risk of narcotic-related side-effects [53]. A systemic review of nonopioid agents for postoperative analgesia in pediatric surgical populations found perioperative acetaminophen, nonsteroidal anti-inflammatory drugs, dexamethasone, ketamine, clonidine, and dexmedetomidine may decrease postoperative pain and opioid consumption [54]. Nonpharmacologic interventions to reduce procedural pain and distress in children include passive and active distraction, positive reinforcement, and coaching by caregivers [55]. In a single-center RCT of 184 patients, use of an intraperitoneal local anesthetic was not be found to improve pain scores in children after appendectomy [56].

## MEDICAL MANAGEMENT AS DEFINITIVE TREATMENT FOR EARLY APPENDICITIS

Appendicitis has traditionally been considered a "surgical diagnosis," although nonoperative management has increased in popularity over the past several years. Available data from recent meta-analyses suggest up to a 97% success rate of nonoperative management during initial hospitalization, with longer-term success varying between 68% and 84% depending on the duration of follow-up and whether treatment failure is defined as recurrent appendicitis or appendectomy for any reason after initial hospitalization (Table 4) [47,57–65].

Development of complicated appendicitis as defined by perforation, gangrene, or peritonitis after medical management has been reported to be less than 4% [61,63–65]. In a systematic review of 20 studies including 3618 patients, complication rates after medical management and appendectomy were similar, and was estimated to be 9.6% and 12.5%, respectively [57].

**Table 3**
Published studies reporting outcomes and resource utilization associated with same-day discharge in children undergoing appendectomy for uncomplicated appendicitis

| Study | Criteria for SDD eligibility | SDD (n) | Non-SDD (n) | Study design | Median follow-up | Revisits and readmission | Resource utilization |
|---|---|---|---|---|---|---|---|
| Alkhoury, 2012 [51] | Inclusion: 2–19 y<br>Exclusion: gangrene or perforated appendicitis | 158 | 0 | Prospective protocol implementation | 2 wk | ED visit:<br>SDD: 2%, non-SDD: 3%<br>Readmission:<br>SDD: 0%, non-SDD 0% | Time to discharge:<br>SDD: 4.8 h,<br>non-SDD: 15.8 h |
| Devin, 2020 [48] | Inclusion: <18 y<br>Exclusion: interval appendectomy, complicated appendicitis—perforation, fecalith outside appendix, abscess, or diffuse fibrinopurulent exudate | 268 | 307 | Prospective protocol implementation | 30 d | ED visit:<br>SDD: 5.2%, non-SDD: 5.5%<br>Readmission:<br>SDD: 1.5%, non-SDD 3.3% | Length of stay:<br>SDD: 2.6 h,<br>non-SDD: 10.6 h |
| Putnam, 2014 [49] | Inclusion: <18 y<br>Exclusion: interval appendectomy, gangrenous or perforated appendicitis | 478 | 316 | Prospective vs historic cohort | 30 d | ED visit:<br>SDD: 2.1%, non-SDD: 1.9%<br>Readmission:<br>SDD: 4.2%, non-SDD 1.2% | Length of stay:<br>SDD: 22 h,<br>non-SDD: 35 h |

(continued on next page)

**Table 3**
**(*continued*)**

| Study | Criteria for SDD eligibility | SDD (n) | Non-SDD (n) | Study design | Median follow-up | Revisits and readmission | Resource utilization |
|---|---|---|---|---|---|---|---|
| Farach, 2014 [50] | Inclusion: <21 y<br>Exclusion: suppurative, gangrenous, or perforated appendicitis, fever >38C, hemodynamic changes, inability to void poor oral intake, inadequate pain control, complex comorbidities, social indications, late operation | 206 | 164 | Prospective protocol implementation | 2 wk | Complication rate (including wound infection, intra-abdominal abscess, and ileus/bowel obstruction):<br>SDD: 2.7%<br>non-SDD: 11% | SDD with $4111 lower hospital charges per patient |

*Abbreviation:* SDD, same-day discharge.

**Table 4**
Prospective studies reporting outcomes and resource utilization associated with nonoperative management of uncomplicated appendicitis in children

| Study | Study design | Nonoperative management (n) | Operative management (n) | Follow-up duration | Incidence of complicated appendicitis in nonoperative group | Resource utilization | Success of nonoperative management during index admission/ antibiotic treatment[a] | Success of nonoperative management after discharge from index admission[b] |
|---|---|---|---|---|---|---|---|---|
| Svensson, 2015; Patkova, 2020 [61,62] | Randomized control trial | 24 | 26 | 1 y | 4.2% | Length of stay ($P = .0004$):<br>Nonoperative: 51.5 h<br>Operative: 34.5 h<br>Cost for initial inpatient stay ($P < .0001$):<br>Nonoperative: $30,732<br>Operative: $45,805<br>Total cost of treatment ($P = .11$):<br>Nonoperative: $34,587<br>Operative: $45,805 | 92% | 1 y: 62%<br>5 y: 46% |
| Tanaka, 2015 [63] | Prospective patient choice trial | 78 | 86 | 4.3 y | 1.3% | Length of stay ($P = .81$):<br>Nonoperative: 6.6 d<br>Operative: 6.5 d | 98.7% | 1 y: 79.2%<br>4.3 y: 71.4% |
| Hartwich, 2016 [64] | Prospective patient choice trial | 24 | 50 | 14 mo | 0% | Estimated total cost ($P < .01$):<br>Nonoperative: $2771<br>Operative: $4130 | 87.5% | 1 y: 70.8% |

(continued on next page)

**Table 4**
***(continued)***

| Study | Study design | Nonoperative management (n) | Operative management (n) | Follow-up duration | Incidence of complicated appendicitis in nonoperative group | Resource utilization | Success of nonoperative management during index admission/ antibiotic treatment[a] | Success of nonoperative management after discharge from index admission[b] |
|---|---|---|---|---|---|---|---|---|
| Minneci, 2016 [65] | Prospective patient choice trial | 37 | 65 | 1 y | 2.7% | Length of stay ($P<.001$):<br>Nonoperative: 37 h<br>Operative: 20 h<br>Estimated total cost ($P = .01$):<br>Nonoperative: $4219<br>Operative: $5029 | 94.6% | 30 d: 89.2%<br>1 y: 75.7% |

[a]Patients initially managed nonoperatively that were successfully discharged without undergoing appendectomy.
[b]Patients managed nonoperatively that subsequently underwent appendectomy after discharge from the index hospitalization, with the exception of Tanaka 2015, which defined success as absence of recurrent appendicitis.

Overall outcomes comparing nonoperative and operative treatment vary, with some systematic reviews reporting similar duration of pain and time off work [57] and others reporting nonoperative management to be associated with fewer disability days and appendectomy was associated with higher patient satisfaction [59]. Studies found nonoperative and operative management comparable in regard to LOS, with one meta-analysis concluding initial LOS was 0.5 days shorter after appendectomy [47,58,60]. In a meta-analysis of 5 studies including 404 patients, nonoperative management was associated with lower cost during the initial hospitalization and during the follow-up period [47].

In summary, nonoperative management offers the benefit of an additional treatment option for early appendicitis; however, controversy remains surrounding long-term efficacy, diagnostic accuracy for patients treated medically without a pathologic diagnosis, and the public health implications of prolonged antibiotic treatment required for nonoperative management [66].

## OUTCOME, PROCESS, AND RESOURCE UTILIZATION BENCHMARKS

Outcomes and resource utilization after management of appendicitis in children are highly variable and may be influenced by both disease severity and hospital-level differences in management. The expansion of NSQIP-Pediatric to capture appendectomy-targeted measures has facilitated development of outcome, process, and resource utilization benchmarks derived from its 131 participating hospitals (Table 5) [12]. The benchmarks have provided an ongoing framework for hospitals to identify and prioritize efforts for quality and process improvement as they pertain to both diagnosis and management [22,23,67,68]. Furthermore, the benchmarks have supported ongoing quality improvement collaboratives among NSQIP-Pediatric hospitals to identify and share best practices from high-performing hospitals [69].

## FUTURE DIRECTIONS AND PRIORITIES

Efforts to disseminate diagnostic strategies minimizing the use of ionizing radiation should be a high national priority. Approximately, 1 in 4 children evaluated at NSQIP-Pediatric hospitals still undergo imaging with CT, and rates may be up to 3 times higher at their referring community hospitals [70]. Collaborative efforts to share best practices and imaging protocols between academic hospitals and their referral centers have been reported and should be scaled up and supported on a national scale [71]. With respect to management, longer-term data are needed to characterize the risk of treatment failure for children undergoing nonoperative management for early appendicitis. Although the option of nonoperative treatment should be embraced in the context of expanding treatment options, available trends would suggest treatment failure significantly increases with longer follow-up. This knowledge may influence decision-making on behalf of caregivers, and we must be transparent about the limitations of existing data. Finally, high-quality comparative effectiveness data are needed to define end points for antibiotic treatment duration to optimize the

**Table 5**
Outcome, process, and resource utilization benchmarks for the diagnosis and management of children undergoing appendectomy for suspected appendicitis at 131 hospitals participating in NSQIP-Pediatric

| | NSQIP-Pediatric benchmark | Interquartile range |
|---|---|---|
| Diagnostic evaluation measures | | |
| Computed tomography utilization | 23.6% | 11.1%–35.9% |
| MRI utilization | 3.0% | 0%–1.0% |
| Compliance with ACR guidelines[b] | 64.8% | 51.1%–90.0% |
| Mean time from ED presentation to appendectomy[c] | 7.4 h | 4.9–12.9 h |
| Normal appendix found on pathology examination | 2.4% | 0%–4.5% |
| Uncomplicated appendicitis measures | | |
| Mean case duration | 38 min | 37–46 min |
| Surgical site infection rate | 1.7% | N/A[a] |
| Organ space infection rate | 0.6% | N/A[a] |
| Revisit to the ED or inpatient setting | 4.9% | N/A[a] |
| Complicated appendicitis measures | | |
| Postoperative ultrasound utilization | 12.5% | 1%–22.0% |
| Postoperative computed tomography utilization | 12.6% | 5.2%–18.5% |
| Parenteral nutrition utilization | 6.3% | 0%–12.2% |
| Peripherally inserted central catheter utilization | 8.0% | 0%–16.1% |
| post-discharge oral antibiotic utilization | 63.8% | 49.2%–86.4% |
| post-discharge IV antibiotic utilization | 1.8% | 0%–1.0% |
| Surgical site infection rate | 8.4% | N/A[a] |
| Organ space infection rate | 10.7% | N/A[a] |
| Revisit to the ED or inpatient setting | 12.5% | N/A[a] |

[a]Not reported.
[b]ACR, American College of Radiology guidelines for imaging suspected appendicitis in children.
[c]2016 pilot data from 29 NSQIP-Pediatric hospitals.

balance between SSI prevention and antimicrobial stewardship. This avenue of investigation should also be considered a high-priority goal considering that appendicitis contributes more to the burden of SSIs and antibiotic treatment days than any other surgical disease in childhood.

## CLINICS CARE POINTS

- Ultrasound is the preferred initial imaging modality for suspected appendicitis. Avoid Computed Tomography (CT) as first-line imaging.
- Creation of a multidisciplinary, institution-specific standardized diagnostic clinical pathway has the potential to streamline diagnostic evaluation of children with suspected appendicitis while reducing practice variation and CT utilization.
- Surgeons should strive to perform an appendectomy within 16 hours of presentation to reduce the risk of complicated disease, and preferable as early as resources allow to minimize resource utilization.
- Given the paucity of long-term effectiveness data, decision-making regarding medical management of uncomplicated appendicitis should be tailored to each patient/family's preferences and risk tolerance for recurrent appendicitis.

## DISCLOSURE

The authors have nothing to disclose.

## References

[1] Cameron DB, Graham DA, Milliren CE, et al. Quantifying the burden of interhospital cost variation in pediatric surgery: implications for the prioritization of comparative effectiveness research. JAMA Pediatr 2017;171(2):e163926.
[2] Cameron DB, Serres SK, Glass CC, et al. Leveraging the incidence, burden, and fiscal implications of unplanned hospital revisits for the prioritization of prevention efforts in pediatric surgery. Ann Surg 2020;271(1):191–9.
[3] Kronman MP, Hersh AL, Gerber JS, et al. Identifying antimicrobial stewardship targets for pediatric surgical patients. J Pediatr Infect Dis Soc 2015;4(4):e100–8.
[4] Feng C, Anandalwar S, Sidhwa F, et al. Beyond perforation: Influence of peritoneal contamination on clinical severity and resource utilization in children with perforated appendicitis. J Pediatr Surg 2016;51(11):1896–9.
[5] Yousef Y, Youssef F, Dinh T, et al. Risk stratification in pediatric perforated appendicitis: Prospective correlation with outcomes and resource utilization. J Pediatr Surg 2018;53(2):250–5.
[6] St Peter SD, Sharp SW, Holcomb GW, et al. An evidence-based definition for perforated appendicitis derived from a prospective randomized trial. J Pediatr Surg 2008;43(12):2242–5.
[7] American College of Surgeons National Surgical Quality Improvement Program – Pediatric Operations Manual: Appendectomy Procedure Targeted Variables. American College of Surgeons; Chicago (IL): Published online January 2020.
[8] Cameron DB, Anandalwar SP, Graham DA, et al. Development and implications of an evidence-based and public health-relevant definition of complicated appendicitis in children. Ann Surg 2020;271(5):962–8.
[9] Anandalwar SP, Cameron DB, Graham DA, et al. Association of intraoperative findings with outcomes and resource use in children with complicated appendicitis. JAMA Surg 2018;153(11):1021–7.

[10] Benabbas R, Hanna M, Shah J, et al. Diagnostic accuracy of history, physical examination, laboratory tests, and point-of-care ultrasound for pediatric acute appendicitis in the emergency department: a systematic review and meta-analysis. Acad Emerg Med 2017;24(5):523–51.
[11] Glass CC, Rangel SJ. Overview and diagnosis of acute appendicitis in children. Semin Pediatr Surg 2016;25(4):198–203.
[12] American College of Surgeons National Surgical Quality Improvement Program - Pediatrics. Semiannual Report (NSQIP-P SAR). Dates of surgery Jan 1, 2019 - Dec 31, 2019. American College of Surgeons; 2020.
[13] AAP SOSu – Avoid CT scan as first-line imaging in suspected appendicitis | Choosing Wisely. 2019. https://www.choosingwisely.org/clinician-lists/aap-sosu-avoid-ct-scan-as-first-line-imaging-in-suspected-appendicitis/. Accessed January 3, 2021.
[14] Kulik DM, Uleryk EM, Maguire JL. Does this child have appendicitis? A systematic review of clinical prediction rules for children with acute abdominal pain. J Clin Epidemiol 2013;66(1):95–104.
[15] Nielsen JW, Boomer L, Kurtovic K, et al. Reducing computed tomography scans for appendicitis by introduction of a standardized and validated ultrasonography report template. J Pediatr Surg 2015;50(1):144–8.
[16] Nordin AB, Sales S, Nielsen JW, et al. Standardized ultrasound templates for diagnosing appendicitis reduce annual imaging costs. J Surg Res 2018;221:77–83.
[17] Schuh S, Chan K, Langer JC, et al. Properties of serial ultrasound clinical diagnostic pathway in suspected appendicitis and related computed tomography use. Acad Emerg Med 2015;22(4):406–14.
[18] Reddan T, Corness J, Harden F, et al. Improving the value of ultrasound in children with suspected appendicitis: a prospective study integrating secondary sonographic signs. Ultrasonography 2019;38(1):67–75.
[19] Anandalwar SP, Callahan MJ, Bachur RG, et al. Use of white blood cell count and polymorphonuclear leukocyte differential to improve the predictive value of ultrasound for suspected appendicitis in children. J Am Coll Surgeons 2015;220(6):1010–7.
[20] Bachur RG, Callahan MJ, Monuteaux MC, et al. Integration of ultrasound findings and a clinical score in the diagnostic evaluation of pediatric appendicitis. J Pediatr 2015;166(5):1134–9.
[21] Kashtan M, Graham D, Anandalwar S, et al. Influence of symptom duration and WBC profile on the negative predictive value of a nondiagnostic ultrasound in children with suspected appendicitis. J Pediatr Surg 2020;55(6):1032–6.
[22] Schoel L, Maizlin II, Koppelmann T, et al. Improving imaging strategies in pediatric appendicitis: a quality improvement initiative. J Surg Res 2018;230:131–6.
[23] Anandalwar SP, Graham DA, Kashtan MA, et al. Leveraging the combined predictive value of ultrasound and laboratory data to reduce radiation exposure and resource utilization in children with suspected appendicitis. J Surg Res 2020;257:529–36.
[24] Serres SK, Cameron DB, Glass CC, et al. Time to appendectomy and risk of complicated appendicitis and adverse outcomes in children. JAMA Pediatr 2017;171(8):740–6.
[25] Kovler ML, Pedroso FE, Etchill EW, et al. Prolonged in-hospital time to appendectomy is associated with increased complicated appendicitis in children. Ann Surg 2020; https://doi.org/10.1097/SLA.0000000000004316 Publish Ahead of Print.
[26] Serres SK, Graham DA, Glass CC, et al. Influence of time to appendectomy and operative duration on hospital cost in children with uncomplicated appendicitis. J Am Coll Surg 2018;226(6):1014–21.
[27] Jaschinski T, Mosch CG, Eikermann M, et al. Laparoscopic versus open surgery for suspected appendicitis. Cochrane Database Syst Rev 2018;11; https://doi.org/10.1002/14651858.CD001546.pub4.

[28] St Peter SD, Adibe OO, Juang D, et al. Single incision versus standard 3-port laparoscopic appendectomy: a prospective randomized trial. Ann Surg 2011;254(4):586–90.
[29] Gasior AC, Knott EM, Holcomb GW, et al. Patient and parental scar assessment after single incision versus standard 3-port laparoscopic appendectomy: long-term follow-up from a prospective randomized trial. J Pediatr Surg 2014;49(1):120–2, discussion 122.
[30] Vaos G, Dimopoulou A, Gkioka E, et al. Immediate surgery or conservative treatment for complicated acute appendicitis in children? A meta-analysis. J Pediatr Surg 2019;54(7):1365–71.
[31] St Peter SD, Adibe OO, Iqbal CW, et al. Irrigation versus suction alone during laparoscopic appendectomy for perforated appendicitis: a prospective randomized trial. Ann Surg 2012;256(4):581–5.
[32] Anderson KT, Putnam LR, Bartz-Kurycki MA, et al. Povidone-iodine irrigation for pediatric perforated appendicitis may be protective: a bayesian pilot randomized controlled trial. Ann Surg 2020;271(5):827–33.
[33] Fujishiro J, Fujiogi M, Hirahara N, et al. Abdominal drainage at appendectomy for complicated appendicitis in children: a propensity-matched comparative study. Ann Surg 2020; https://doi.org/10.1097/SLA.0000000000003804 Publish Ahead of Print.
[34] Cameron DB, Melvin P, Graham DA, et al. Extended versus narrow-spectrum antibiotics in the management of uncomplicated appendicitis in children: a propensity-matched comparative effectiveness study. Ann Surg 2018;268(1):186–92.
[35] Kashtan MA, Graham DA, Melvin P, et al. Ceftriaxone combined with metronidazole is superior to cefoxitin alone in the management of uncomplicated appendicitis in children: results from a multicenter collaborative comparative effectiveness study. Ann Surg 2020; https://doi.org/10.1097/SLA.0000000000003704.
[36] Litz CN, Asuncion JB, Danielson PD, et al. Timing of antimicrobial prophylaxis and infectious complications in pediatric patients undergoing appendectomy. J Pediatr Surg 2018;53(3):449–51.
[37] Andersen BR, Kallehave FL, Andersen HK. Antibiotics versus placebo for prevention of postoperative infection after appendicectomy. Cochrane Database Syst Rev 2005;3:CD001439.
[38] Anandalwar SP, Rangel SJ. What's in your CPG: analysis of practice variation to prioritize comparative effectiveness Research in the postoperative management of complicated appendicitis [oral abstract]. In: Presented at the: Annual American College of Surgeons Quality & Safety Conference. 2019 Washington, DC.
[39] Anandalwar S, Graham D, Kashtan M, et al. Influence of oral antibiotics following discharge on organ space infections in children with complicated appendicitis. Ann Surg 2019; https://doi.org/10.1097/SLA.0000000000003441 Publish Ahead of Print.
[40] Kashtan MA, Graham DA, Rangel SJ. Utilization and performance benchmarking for postoperative imaging in children with complicated appendicitis: results from a multicenter collaborative cohort study. Ann Surg 2020; https://doi.org/10.1097/SLA.0000000000004250.
[41] Baumann LM, Williams K, Oyetunji TA, et al. Optimal timing of postoperative imaging for complicated appendicitis. J Laparoendosc Adv Surg Tech A 2018;28(10):1248–52.
[42] Hogan MJ, Marshalleck FE, Sidhu MK, et al. Quality improvement guidelines for pediatric abscess and fluid drainage. J Vasc Interv Radiol 2012;23(11):1397–402.
[43] Kashtan MA, Rangel SJ. Variability, cost, and outcomes associated with the use of parenteral nutrition in children with complicated appendicitis [oral abstract]. In: Presented at the: 50th Annual American Pediatric Surgical Association Meeting. 2014 Boston, MA.
[44] van Amstel P, Sluckin TC, van Amstel T, et al. Management of appendiceal mass and abscess in children; early appendectomy or initial non-operative treatment? A systematic review and meta-analysis. Surg Endosc 2020;34(12):5234–49.
[45] Puapong D, Lee SL, Haigh PI, et al. Routine interval appendectomy in children is not indicated. J Pediatr Surg 2007;42(9):1500–3.

[46] Hall NJ, Jones CE, Eaton S, et al. Is interval appendicectomy justified after successful nonoperative treatment of an appendix mass in children? A systematic review. J Pediatr Surg 2011;46(4):767–71.
[47] Huang L, Yin Y, Yang L, et al. Comparison of antibiotic therapy and appendectomy for acute uncomplicated appendicitis in children: a meta-analysis. JAMA Pediatr 2017;171(5):426–34.
[48] Devin CL, D'Cruz R, Linden AF, et al. Reducing resource utilization for patients with uncomplicated appendicitis through use of same-day discharge and elimination of postoperative antibiotics. J Pediatr Surg 2020;55(12):2591–5.
[49] Putnam LR, Levy SM, Johnson E, et al. Impact of a 24-hour discharge pathway on outcomes of pediatric appendectomy. Surgery 2014;156(2):455–61.
[50] Farach SM, Danielson PD, Walford NE, et al. Same-day discharge after appendectomy results in cost savings and improved efficiency. Am Surg 2014;80(8):787–91.
[51] Alkhoury F, Burnweit C, Malvezzi L, et al. A prospective study of safety and satisfaction with same-day discharge after laparoscopic appendectomy for acute appendicitis. J Pediatr Surg 2012;47(2):313–6.
[52] Anderson KT, Bartz-Kurycki MA, Ferguson DM, et al. Too much of a bad thing: Discharge opioid prescriptions in pediatric appendectomy patients. J Pediatr Surg 2018;53(12):2374–7.
[53] Poonai N, Paskar D, Konrad S-L, et al. Opioid analgesia for acute abdominal pain in children: A systematic review and meta-analysis. Acad Emerg Med 2014;21(11):1183–92.
[54] Zhu A, Benzon HA, Anderson TA. Evidence for the efficacy of systemic opioid-sparing analgesics in pediatric surgical populations: a systematic review. Anesth Analg 2017;125(5):1569–87.
[55] Srouji R, Ratnapalan S, Schneeweiss S. Pain in children: assessment and nonpharmacological management. Int J Pediatr 2010;2010; https://doi.org/10.1155/2010/474838.
[56] Hamill JK, Liley A, Hill AG. Intraperitoneal local anesthetic for laparoscopic appendectomy in children: a randomized controlled trial. Ann Surg 2017;266(1):189–94.
[57] Podda M, Gerardi C, Cillara N, et al. Antibiotic treatment and appendectomy for uncomplicated acute appendicitis in adults and children: a systematic review and meta-analysis. Ann Surg 2019;270(6):1028–40.
[58] Georgiou R, Eaton S, Stanton MP, et al. Efficacy and safety of nonoperative treatment for acute appendicitis: a meta-analysis. Pediatrics 2017; https://doi.org/10.1542/peds.2016-3003.
[59] Kessler U, Mosbahi S, Walker B, et al. Conservative treatment versus surgery for uncomplicated appendicitis in children: a systematic review and meta-analysis. Arch Dis Child 2017;102(12):1118–24.
[60] Maita S, Andersson B, Svensson JF, et al. Nonoperative treatment for nonperforated appendicitis in children: a systematic review and meta-analysis. Pediatr Surg Int 2020;36(3):261–9.
[61] Svensson JF, Patkova B, Almström M, et al. Nonoperative treatment with antibiotics versus surgery for acute nonperforated appendicitis in children: a pilot randomized controlled trial. Ann Surg 2015;261(1):67–71.
[62] Patkova B, Svenningsson A, Almström M, et al. Nonoperative treatment versus appendectomy for acute nonperforated appendicitis in children: five-year follow up of a randomized controlled pilot trial. Ann Surg 2020;271(6):1030–5.
[63] Tanaka Y, Uchida H, Kawashima H, et al. Long-term outcomes of operative versus nonoperative treatment for uncomplicated appendicitis. J Pediatr Surg 2015;50(11):1893–7.
[64] Hartwich J, Luks FI, Watson-Smith D, et al. Nonoperative treatment of acute appendicitis in children: A feasibility study. J Pediatr Surg 2016;51(1):111–6.
[65] Minneci PC, Mahida JB, Lodwick DL, et al. Effectiveness of patient choice in nonoperative vs surgical management of pediatric uncomplicated acute appendicitis. JAMA Surg 2016;151(5):408–15.

[66] Bachur RG, Rangel SJ. The threat of diagnostic uncertainty in the medical management of uncomplicated appendicitis. JAMA Pediatr 2017;171(6):505–6.
[67] Litz CN, Stone L, Alessi R, et al. Impact of outpatient management following appendectomy for acute appendicitis: An ACS NSQIP-P analysis. J Pediatr Surg 2018;53(4):625–8.
[68] AlFraih Y, Robinson T, Stein N, et al. Quality assurance and performance improvement project for suspected appendicitis. Pediatr Qual Saf 2020;5(3):e290.
[69] American College of Surgeons' Pediatric Surgical Quality Collaborative. Reducing use of CT imaging in the diagnostic evaluation of suspected appendicitis in children. https://med.uth.edu/pediatricsurgery/research/research-centers-and-programs/psqc/. Accessed December 28, 2020.
[70] Glass CC, Saito JM, Sidhwa F, et al. Diagnostic imaging practices for children with suspected appendicitis evaluated at definitive care hospitals and their associated referral centers. J Pediatr Surg 2016;51(6):912–6.
[71] Kotagal M, Richards MK, Chapman T, et al. Improving ultrasound quality to reduce computed tomography use in pediatric appendicitis: the Safe and Sound campaign. Am J Surg 2015;209(5):896–900, discussion 900.

Advances in Surgery 55 (2021) 35–48
ADVANCES IN SURGERY

# Malignant Bowel Obstruction

Nadege T. Fackche, MD[a],
Fabian M. Johnston, MD, MHS[b,*]

[a]Howard University Hospital, 2041 Georgia Avenue, NW Suite 4000, Washington, DC 20060, USA; [b]Division of Gastrointestinal (GI) Oncology, Surgical Oncology Fellowship, Johns Hopkins Hospital, 600 N Wolfe Street, Suite Halsted 612, Baltimore, MD 21287, USA

**Keywords**

- Malignant bowel obstruction • Palliative care
- Advanced care planning discussions

**Key points**

- Malignant bowel obstruction (MBO) is a frequent and often lethal condition affecting patients with advanced gastrointestinal cancers.
- Therapeutic strategies should include the early involvement of palliative care specialists and a multidisciplinary approach to achieving goals of care as identified by the patient and their surrogates.
- Multimodal medical therapy using a combination of antiemetics, analgesics, and antisecretory agents is the mainstay treatment of MBO, as it offers adequate symptom control for the lowest morbidity.
- Interventional and surgical palliation are indicated in carefully selected patients in whom the benefits of symptom control outweigh the risks of intervention.

## INTRODUCTION

Malignant bowel obstruction (MBO) is a frequent, and unfortunately, preterminal complication most often seen in advanced gastrointestinal and gynecologic cancers. MBO is defined as the clinical or radiographic evidence of bowel obstruction beyond the ligament of Treitz; this occurs in the setting of primary intraabdominal malignancy or primary extraabdominal malignancy with confirmed peritoneal dissemination [1]. This operative definition was adopted by consensus at the International Conference on MBO in 2007, with the aim of distinguishing MBO from adhesive postoperative and radiation-induced

Funding Sources for Authors: F.M Johnston: AHRQ 1K08HS024736.

*Corresponding author. *E-mail address:* fjohnst4@jhmi.edu

https://doi.org/10.1016/j.yasu.2021.05.003

obstructions, as those carry a more favorable prognosis and thus warrant different management [1,2]. The affected patients may pose a clinical conundrum for clinicians, often presenting with multiple comorbidities and altered physiologic states, thus requiring an individualized and multidisciplinary approach to care. Prompt initiation of advance care planning (ACP) discussions and the palliative care team's early involvement is essential to designing patient-centered care strategies that optimize outcomes.

## EPIDEMIOLOGY AND PATHOPHYSIOLOGY

MBO affects 10% to 30% of patients with gastrointestinal malignancies and up to 60% of patients with gynecologic malignancies and heralds a poor prognosis [3,4]. The average survival ranges from 4 to 5 weeks in patients with inoperable disease to 8 to 10 months when MBO occurs early and in surgically fit patients. Although ovarian and colorectal cancer are the most common causes, intrabdominal entities prone to peritoneal dissemination (gastric and biliopancreatic cancers, abdominal mesothelioma, and pseudomyxoma peritonei), and extra-abdominal cancers (breast, melanoma) are often reported [3–7]. MBO is often associated with peritoneal carcinomatosis, can involve either one or multiple segments, and disproportionally affects the small bowel. The obstruction can be mechanical or functional. Mechanical obstruction is often the consequence of a mass effect from either intraluminal tumor growth or extraluminal compression due to peritoneal or mesenteric tumor deposits. Functional obstruction leading to impaired dysmotility may be the result of tumor infiltration of the enteric nerve plexus [3]. Regardless of the initial mechanism, MBO frequently induces a self-perpetuating cycle. Persistent intestinal distention leads to the intraluminal accumulation of fluid and gases, increasing endoluminal pressure and peristaltic contractions, and more importantly, triggering the release of inflammatory, vasoactive, and nociceptive mediators. The resulting hyperemia and edema of the intestinal wall then further contributes to hypersecretion and accumulation of fluid, subsequently exacerbating intestinal distention [3,4,8].

## EVALUATION OF THE PATIENT WITH MALIGNANT BOWEL OBSTRUCTION

The progression to MBO is often insidious, with many patients reporting weeks of increasingly frequent and prolonged self-remitting subocclusive episodes marked by nausea, emesis, brief obstipation, colicky abdominal pain, and distention. Obstipation lasting more than 72 hours usually signals the progression to more definitive obstruction. Careful history taking and physical examination are paramount, as they may hint at the obstruction level and inform decision-making. For example, although large-volume bilious emesis, anorexia, periumbilical pain, and mild-to-moderate abdominal distention point to a small bowel obstruction, markedly distended abdomen, squalid small volume emesis, and localized pain are more consistent with a large bowel obstruction. In many of these patients, the colicky, crampy abdominal pain induced by intestinal obstruction is superimposed to the background, chronic pain caused by the neoplastic process.

The foremost step in evaluating patients with MBO is the determination of individual goals of care. It is essential to determine the patient's and health care proxy's understanding of their prognosis, their wish or reluctance to pursue aggressive treatment, and their understanding of how the risks and benefits of potential interventions may stack against individual quality-of-life (QOL) measures. To this end, the early involvement of palliative care specialists is essential. The American society of clinical oncology's latest guidelines urges the integration of inpatient and outpatient multidisciplinary palliative care early in the course of the disease (level 1 evidence) [9]. These recommendations are based on reports from multiple randomized controlled trials (RCTs) showing increased QOL, decreased mean depression score at 3 months, and increased satisfaction with care using palliative care services [9–12]. ACP encompasses decisions about medical care preferences, particularly end-of-life care, as discussed and recorded by patients, health care proxy, and their health providers [13,14]. These discussions are paramount in designing care strategies aligned with the patient's individual goals of care. Initiation of ACP has been associated with decreased depression indices, reduced hospitalizations, increased QOL, satisfaction with care, and use of palliative care services [13–16]. In a recent survey of 200 patients with advanced cancer at Johns Hopkins, only 24% of the cohort reported having had ACP discussions [14]. Furthermore, Kubi and colleagues demonstrated that the majority (94%) wished they had these discussions with their care team early in the disease process [14].

Once goals of care have been clearly defined, investigative workup must establish the patient's overall physiologic state and ability to tolerate available interventions. Nutritional status, overall functional capacity, frailty score, and peritoneal disease's extent are essential for optimal risk stratification of the patient with MBO. Functional performance assessment tools such as the Karnofsky Performance Scale (KPS) and the Eastern Cooperative Oncology Group (ECOG) performance status are proven predictive tools that will help determine patients whose predicted remaining life expectancy is long enough to derive substantial benefit from invasive interventions [17–21]. KPS scores greater than 50 have reported median survival times of 172 days versus 29 days when KPS scores are less than 50 [20,21]. Hwang and colleagues demonstrated that combining KPS with QOL and symptom assessment indices led to more accurate prediction of survival in patients with KPS score greater than 50 [21].

Multidetector computed tomography scan (MDCT) with intravenous contrast is the diagnostic tool of choice for MBO [3,4,8,22,23]. Relatively inexpensive and readily available in most clinical settings, MDCT features reported sensitivities and specificity greater than 93% [22–25]. MCDT is essential for identifying the location and number of obstructed segments and the presence of ominous features such as strangulation, perforation, or extensive peritoneal disease [24–27]. In addition to establishing a baseline from which response to therapy can be assessed, the initial scan should be used to rule out nonmalignant causes of obstruction such as postoperative adhesions, hernias, or radiation-induced fibrosis. A few studies have investigated adverse radiographic prognostic factors for MBO. Frequently identified findings correlating with poor outcomes include diffuse mesenteric infiltration, bowel wall thinning, and the presence of ascites [24]. The use of oral water-soluble contrast, which has proved utility as a diagnostic tool and a predictor of nonresolution in patients with adhesive small bowel obstruction, has been advocated by some investigators. However, a recent Cochran review by Syrmis and colleagues was inconclusive due to the scarcity of available data [28–30]. MRI offers a comparable sensitivity and specificity to MCDT and may be superior in evaluating the extent of peritoneal dissemination but is however expensive and of limited availability [8,26,27]. Plain abdominal radiographs, often the initial radiographic test obtained in the clinical setting for patients with bowel obstruction, are less accurate and of limited utility in MBO. They provide little information about the etiologic nature of the obstruction.

## MANAGEMENT

Clinical decision-making in MBO should aim to achieve goals of care as determined by the duly informed patient and their surrogates with the assistance of a multidisciplinary team including primary care physicians, surgeons, oncologists, and palliative care specialists [5,31,32]. The optimal management of this condition requires a thorough understanding of the complex interplay of pathologic processes affecting individual patients. More often than not, MBO occurs in the context of shortened life expectancy due to advanced malignancy and multiple comorbidities. In this setting, the primary aim should be to achieve adequate symptom palliation and optimize the patient's QOL over their remaining lifespan while minimizing the proposed interventions' morbidity. Available therapeutic options for patients with MBO can be broadly grouped into medical therapy, endoluminal and decompressive interventions, and surgical palliation (Fig. 1).

### Medical therapy

Using a combination of gastroenteric drainage, analgesic, antiemetic, antisecretory, and steroid drugs, medical therapy is the cornerstone of managing patients with MBO. This therapeutic strategy features minimal morbidity and aims to control debilitating nausea, emesis, and pain resulting from persistent intestinal distention. Once emergent intervention for either perforation or impeding strangulation is ruled out, a trial of expectant management using a combination of judicious intravenous fluid resuscitation, antiemetics, gastrointestinal decompression via nasoenteric tube, and electrolyte repletion should be the initial strategy. With rates of spontaneous resolution of MBO nearing 30%, and despite a recurrence rate higher than 70%, this approach may allow some much-needed respite in the moribund patient or time for careful individualization of therapy in a patient with longer life

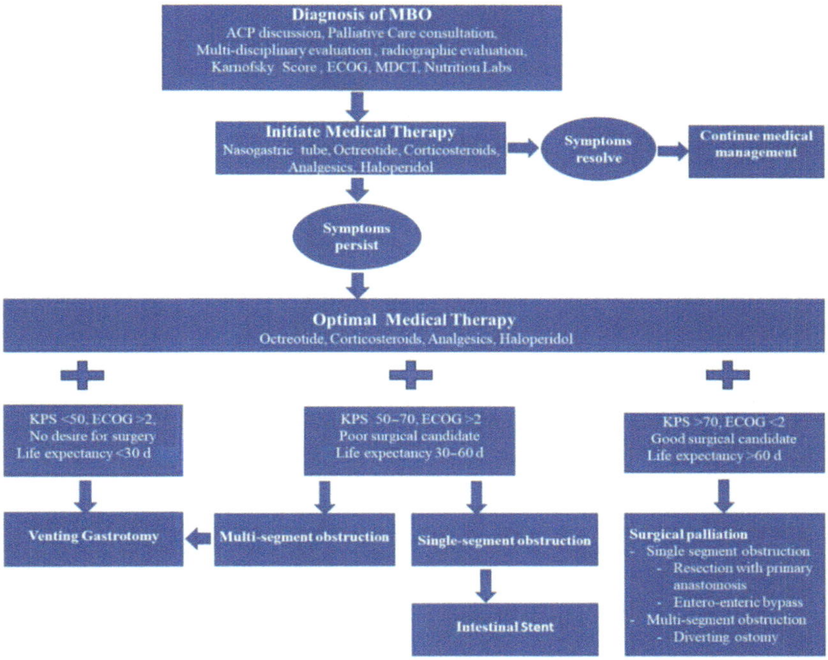


**Fig. 1.** ACP: advanced care planning; ECOG: Eastern Cooperative Oncology Group Performance Scale, a 6-item (0–5) prognosis tool, measures a patient's functional status from fully active (0) to dead (5); MDCT, multidetector computed tomography; Karnofsky Performance Scale classifies patients based on the percentage of functional impairment, where 0% is dead, 10% moribund, and 100% denotes no impairment.

expectancy [3,33,34]. By consensus, the cornerstone of pharmacologic treatment of MBO consists of combining steroids, antiemetics, and antisecretory drugs. Although this strategy has shown some efficacy in various reports, evidence-based data are lacking, as most of these studies were small and inadequately powered.

*Antiemetics*

Intractable and debilitating nausea and emesis affects 30% to 70% of patients with MBO [35]. The cause is often multifactorial, but the most commonly postulated mechanisms include activation of the chemoreceptor trigger zone (CTZ) and of gastrointestinal vagal afferent fibers [3,4,8]. In MBO, CTZ is often stimulated by ongoing oncologic drug regimen, resulting in the vomiting reflex's induction. Similarly, gastrointestinal afferent vagal fibers are activated by bowel edema and distention and induce nausea and emesis via activation of proemetic receptors [36,37]. Currently, dopamine D2 antagonists and serotonin antagonists are the most common drugs used in MBO. By expert consensus, the dopamine receptor antagonist, haloperidol, which has proved effective in postoperative nausea, is the drug of choice for patients with MBO [35,38,39]. Haloperidol is highly selective for the D2 receptors and provides an antiemetic effect with less sedation and side effects. Second-line agents include metoclopramide, olanzapine, ondansetron, and chlorpromazine [35].

*Antisecretory agents*

Antisecretory therapy is the mainstay of medical treatment in MBO and aims at decreasing bowel edema and intraluminal hypersecretion [4,40–42]. Available agents include somatostatin inhibitors (SSI), proton pump inhibitors (PPIs), anticholinergics, and histamine receptor (H2) antagonists. Of these agents, the somatostatin antagonist octreotide is the most studied and currently the preferred therapy for the management of hypersecretion in MBO. Octreotide and SSIs induce potent splanchnic vasoconstriction and inhibition of the vasoactive intestinal peptide, ultimately leading to a significant decrease in gastrointestinal secretions and thus to improved bowel distention and bowel edema [41]. In the last 2 decades, RCTs comparing octreotide with placebo in patients with advances cancers have suggested successful symptom control in the treatment branches [35,41,43,44]. Unfortunately, these studies' small power and variable definitions of what constitutes treatment success across studies have hindered a definitive conclusion about octreotide's efficacy in this setting. In a double-blind RCT comparing octreotide to placebo in 87 patients with MBO, Laval and colleagues demonstrated a higher success rate for octreotide (38% vs 28%). This study's treatment success was defined as decreased episodes of emesis ($<2$) and no need for nasogastric tube (NGT) to anticholinergic at 14 days [44]. Although the more recent study by Currow and colleagues showed no statistical difference in the number of days free of vomiting, there was a significant reduction in the number of vomiting episodes in the octreotide group compared with the placebo group (IRR 0.40, $P = .02$) [45]. Recent reports have also demonstrated that octreotide was superior to anticholinergics in reducing secretions, nausea, and vomiting in patients with MBO from peritoneal carcinomatosis [35,41,46]. Anticholinergic drugs such as scopolamine are used as second-line therapy due in part to their side-effect profile.

An affordable alternative to octreotide is a combination therapy including PPIs, H2 blockers, and steroids. With this approach, PPIs and H2 blockers decrease gastric secretions and distension, whereas glucocorticoids modulate the inflammatory response associated with bowel obstruction [3,5,35]. Although the evidence to support the isolated use of PPIs and H2 blockers is scarce, they are increasingly used as part of a multidrug regimen in MBO. A 2009 metanalysis by Clark and colleagues demonstrated that although both PPIs and H2 blockers effectively reduced secretions, ranitidine, an H2 blocker, was superior, reducing gastric secretions by 0.22 cc/kg ($P<.05$) in patients with MBO [47]. Multisociety French guidelines for the management of bowel obstruction in patients with peritoneal carcinomatosis based on available evidence recommended the routine use of PPIs in this population [48]. A recent

Japanese review of practice patterns in patients with MBO, on the other hand, showed a slightly longer length of NGT use with PPIs (14 days vs 12 days, $P = .01$); their combination with corticosteroid led to a shorter NGT use (9 days vs 13 days $P < .01$) [49]. Various small studies have suggested a benefit to the short-term use of corticosteroids when combined with antisecretory drugs [35,39,44,49–51]. In addition, Cochrane systematic reviews showed a trend toward MBO resolution with the use of corticosteroids. Still, they were ultimately inconclusive due to various issues with the methodologies of available studies [50,52]. Although supporting level 1 evidence is lacking, short courses of intravenous methylprednisolone used in conjunction with antiemetic and antisecretory agents maybe beneficial. Purported benefits include decreasing peritumoral edema and inflammation as well as indirect antiemetic and analgesic effects [4].

*Analgesics*

Pain in patients with MBO is often multifactorial and complex, with colicky abdominal pain from acute obstruction, superimposed to background pain deriving from mucositis, enteric plexus invasion by tumor's side effects of various chemotherapeutic drugs [4,8,39,53]. It has been reported that pain is undertreated in up to 31% of patients with cancer pain [54]. Identified barriers to effective pain management include patient factors such as cultural and religious beliefs and knowledge deficits and clinicians' lack of comfort with the evaluation and management of chronic pain [55–57]. Adequate analgesia in these patients requires a delicate balance of opioids and nonopioids drugs that effectively target each pain syndrome and the treatment team's understanding of the intricacies at play [54,58,59]. For example, short-acting intravenous opioids are the therapy for choice to address intestinal obstruction pain and reduce painful bowel contractions against the obstruction [4,8]. Neuropathic pain, on the other hand, is best managed with a combination of opiates and anticonvulsants such as tramadol or Neurontin [60]. Regardless of the initial regiment, pain and QOL should be reassessed and addressed frequently, as pain in these patients is often evolving with the disease's progression [58].

To conclude, multimodal medical palliation is the mainstay of the management for MBO. It should be considered for patients with inoperable disease who have a reduced predicted lifespan and those who otherwise do not wish to undergo a procedure. Definitive interventions for a given patient are informed by the level and pattern of obstruction–single versus multiple segments–clinical cancer stage, plans for further oncologic therapy, current health and performance status, and overall prognosis.

## Interventional palliation

Patients with MBO who are poor surgical candidates or do not wish to undergo surgery may benefit from endoluminal stenting or definitive gastrointestinal decompression. In these patients, concurrent medical therapy may maximize symptom control [3,8,61,62].

*Endoluminal stenting*

An alternative to surgical intervention, endoscopic stenting for malignant bowel obstruction, offers high rates of technical and clinical success without the prohibitive morbidity of surgical intervention. The rates of effective resolution of obstructive symptoms seen with stenting (75%–90%) are comparable to palliative surgery [61,62]. However, due to shorter luminal patency intervals and high reobstruction rates–up to 40%–, endoscopic stenting is often used as a temporizing measure or as a bridge to surgery [3,8,28]. A recent study comparing endoscopic stenting with surgical palliation reported shorter survival (148 days vs 336 days) and luminal patency duration (27 days vs 145 days). Long-segment obstruction requiring the insertion of multiple stents was associated with a higher likelihood of stent failure (odds ratio 0.2 confidence interval 0.05–0.79 $P = .02$) [61]. Current indications for stenting in MBO include a single, short-segment obstruction ideally located in either the proximal duodenum or the distal colon in a patient with both intermediate performance status and intermediate survival expectancy (30–60 days) [3,8].

*Venting gastrotomy*

Decompressive gastrostomy is an effective adjunct to medical therapy in patients not otherwise eligible for palliative surgery or stenting. As noted previously, NGT drainage is an effective initial intervention, providing relief from nausea, emesis, and painful abdominal distention. Unfortunately, prolonged NGT use is associated with an increased risk of aspiration, sinusitis, and ulceration [3,4,8,63]. Most investigators encourage a transition to percutaneous endoscopic or open gastrostomy tube after 48 to 76 hours of abdominal decompression if still needed. For these patients, venting gastrotomy provides symptom control in 84% to 92% of patients and may allow the resumption of comfort oral feeding [3,64]. A recent systematic review of the efficacy of venting gastrostomy in 1194 patients with MBO noted a 92% rate of symptom control and the ability to tolerate diet in 84% of patients. The rate of failed insertion was 9%. Median survival in this cohort was comparable to reported studies (14–74 days) [64].

## Surgical Palliation

Beyond the restoration of intestinal transit, surgical palliation aims to improve QOL by relieving obstructive symptoms and facilitating oral intake resumption [3–5,23,40]. For patients with MBO, however, the benefits of surgery remain controversial and should be weighed against high perioperative morbidity and mortality. With prospective data lacking, a few studies have reported effective palliation of obstructive symptoms in patients treated with surgery [6,34,65,66]. In a systematic review of 868 patients with malignant bowel obstruction from peritoneal carcinomatosis, Olson and colleagues reported resolution of obstruction in 32% to 100% of patients and postoperative diet tolerance in 45% to 75%. Reobstruction rates, although lower than those noted for nonoperative management (6%–47% vs 71%) rates, remained elevated.

Mortality and serious complications rates were similarly prohibitive, with 6% to 32% and 7% to 47%, respectively [67]. A recently updated Cochrane review by Cousins and colleagues failed to break the stalemate. The investigators conducted a pooled analysis of 4295 patients who underwent surgical intervention for MBO. Resolution of obstruction, which was poorly defined, ranged from 26.7% to 68%. The ability to tolerate diet ranged from 30% to 100%. Reflecting the absence of standardized outcome measures, reobstruction, morbidity, and 30-day mortality rates varied greatly, ranging from 0% to 63%, 5% to 86.6%, and 4% to 40%, respectively [68].

Surgical intervention is currently reserved for carefully selected patients with preserved functional status, limited peritoneal disease, and localized obstruction. Surgical approaches are determined by the nature and location of the obstruction, the patient's nutritional and overall functional status, and history of radiation exposure [8,22,40]. Proximal diversion using either an ileostomy or colostomy may be considered in patients at risk of impending bowel perforation, those deemed to be marginal surgical candidates, and those in whom shortened mesentery or impaired wound healing would preclude adequate primary anastomosis [65,66]. Resection with primary anastomosis is best suited to address single segment occlusion and obstruction occurring in the setting of localized mesenteric tumor infiltration in patients with minimal peritoneal dissemination [3,66]. Multisegment obstructions and obstruction in the setting of diffuse peritoneal dissemination may be amenable to either enteric bypass or cytoreductive surgery in highly selected patients [7,65,66]. Studies comparing outcomes between surgical modalities suggest that resection with primary anastomosis may be superior to proximal diversion and enteroenteric bypass in adequately selected patients, with reported perioperative survival twice as high for surgical resection (7.2 months compared with 3.4 and 2.7 months), respectively [66].

Although there is no consensus on what constitutes an absolute contraindication for surgical intervention, various studies have identified factors associated with poor postoperative outcome in patients with MBO. Patient factors presaging the futility of surgical intervention include involuntary weight loss greater than 9 kg or cachexia, multilevel obstruction, hypoalbuminemia, prior pelvic radiotherapy, palpable abdominal masses, malignant ascites less than 3 L, extraabdominal metastatic disease, and renal or hepatic impairment [3,7,8,34,67].

## SUMMARY

Malignant bowel obstruction is a frequent and often lethal condition affecting patients with advanced gastrointestinal cancers. Multimodal medical therapy is the treatment of choice, as it offers adequate symptom control for the lowest morbidity. Interventional and surgical palliation is indicated in carefully selected patients. Therapeutic strategies should include a multidisciplinary approach to achieving goals of care as identified by the patient and their surrogates.

## CLINICS CARE POINTS

- The foremost step in evaluating patients with MBO is the determination of individual goals of care. Advanced care planning discussions and early involvement of palliative care are essential.
- A thorough assessment of the patient's physiologic status and overall state of health using tools such as ECOG and Karnofsky scores will help identify patients who could benefit from interventional or surgical palliation.
- Nasogastric decompression and medical therapy, including antiemetics, analgesics, steroids, and antisecretory drugs, is the initial therapy and the building block around which all adjunctive therapies (interventional or surgical palliation) are built.
- Octreotide, the most effective antisecretory agent on the market, can be expensive. A reasonable alternative option is a combination of proton pump inhibitors, histamine receptor antagonist (H2), and steroids.

## DISCLOSURE

The authors have nothing to disclose.

## References

[1] Anthony T, Baron T, Mercadante S, et al. Report of the clinical protocol committee: development of randomized trials for malignant bowel obstruction. J Pain Symptom Manage 2007;34(1 Suppl):S49–59.
[2] Laval G, Marcelin-Benazech B, Guirimand F, et al. Recommendations for Bowel Obstruction With Peritoneal Carcinomatosis. J Pain Symptom Manage 2014;48(1):75–91.
[3] Tuca A, Guell E, Martinez-Losada E, et al. Malignant bowel obstruction in advanced cancer patients: epidemiology, management, and factors influencing spontaneous resolution. Cancer Manag Res 2012;4:159.
[4] Binet Q, Duck L. Management of end-stage malignant bowel obstruction: an evidence-based review for clinical practice. Belg J Med Oncol 2019;13(4):123–8.
[5] Roses RE, Folkert IW, Krouse RS. Malignant bowel obstruction: reappraising the value of surgery. Surg Oncol Clin N Am 2018;27(4):705–15.
[6] al KY et. Surgical and Conservative Management of Malignant Bowel Obstruction: Outcome and Prognostic Factors | EndNote Click. Available at: https://kopernio.com/viewer?doi=10.2147%2Fcmar.s256219&token=WzE5MjEwNjAsIjEwLjIxNDcvY21hci5zMjU2MjE5Il0.wjA3STYUls5SggsLnlz9hs80fiI. Accessed December 4, 2020.
[7] Bento JH, Bianchi ET, Tustumi F, et al. Surgical management of malignant intestinal obstruction: outcome and prognostic factors. Chirurgia (Bucur) 2019;114(3):343–51.
[8] Ripamonti CI, Easson AM, Gerdes H. Management of malignant bowel obstruction. Eur J Cancer 2008;44(8):1105–15.
[9] Ferrell BR, Temel JS, Temin S, et al. Integration of palliative care into standard oncology care: american society of clinical oncology clinical practice guideline update. J Clin Oncol 2017;35(1):96–112.
[10] Bakitas MA, Tosteson TD, Li Z, et al. Early versus delayed initiation of concurrent palliative oncology care: patient outcomes in the ENABLE III randomized controlled trial. J Clin Oncol 2015;33(13):1438–45.
[11] Haun MW, Estel S, Rücker G, et al. Early palliative care for adults with advanced cancer. Cochrane Database Syst Rev 2017;(6):CD011129.

[12] Dionne-Odom JN, Azuero A, Lyons KD, et al. Benefits of early versus delayed palliative care to informal family caregivers of patients with advanced cancer: outcomes from the ENABLE III randomized controlled trial. J Clin Oncol 2015;33(13):1446–52.
[13] Brinkman-Stoppelenburg A, Rietjens JAC, van der Heide A. The effects of advance care planning on end-of-life care: a systematic review. Palliat Med 2014;28(8):1000–25.
[14] Kubi B, Istl AC, Lee KT, et al. Advance Care Planning in Cancer: Patient Preferences for Personnel and Timing. JCO Oncol Pract 2020;16(9):e875–83.
[15] Teno JM, Gruneir A, Schwartz Z, et al. Association between advance directives and quality of end-of-life care: a national study. J Am Geriatr Soc 2007;55(2):189–94.
[16] Khandelwal N, Kross EK, Engelberg RA, et al. Estimating the effect of palliative care interventions and advance care planning on ICU utilization: a systematic review. Crit Care Med 2015;43(5):1102–11.
[17] Mor V, Laliberte L, Morris JN, et al. The Karnofsky performance status scale: An examination of its reliability and validity in a research setting. Cancer 1984;53(9):2002–7; https://doi.org/10.1002/1097-0142(19840501)53:9<2002::AID-CNCR2820530933>3.0.CO;2-W. Available at:.
[18] Allard P, Dionne A, Potvin D. Factors associated with length of survival among 1081 terminally ill cancer patients. J Palliat Care 1995;11(3):20–4.
[19] Jin H( W and JO. Performance Status in Patients With Cancer | EndNote Click. Available at: https://kopernio.com/viewer?doi=10.1001%2Fjamaoncol.2015.3113&token=WzE5MjEwNjAsIjEwLjEwMDEvamFtYW9uY29sLjIwMTUuMzExMyJd.7SSneiYesX-Rab8FPxxTNxJ-Qfik. Accessed December 22, 2020.
[20] Yates JW, Chalmer B, McKegney FP. Evaluation of patients with advanced cancer using the karnofsky performance status. Cancer 1980;45(8):2220–4; https://doi.org/10.1002/1097-0142(19800415)45:8<2220::AID-CNCR2820450835>3.0.CO;2-Q. Available at:.
[21] Hwang SS, Scott CB, Chang VT, et al. Prediction of Survival for Advanced Cancer Patients by Recursive Partitioning Analysis: Role of Karnofsky Performance Status, Quality of Life, and Symptom Distress. Cancer Invest 2004;22(5):678–87.
[22] The publication of The Art and Science of Palliative Medicine - Annals of Palliative Medicine. Available at http://apm.amegroups.com/announcement/view/101. Accessed December 7, 2020.
[23] Krouse RS, McCahill LE, Easson AM, et al. When the Sun Can Set on an Unoperated Bowel Obstruction: Management of Malignant Bowel Obstruction. J Am Coll Surg 2002;195(1):12.
[24] Miccò M, Sbarra M, Gui B, et al. Prognostic CT findings of malignant bowel obstruction in patients with advanced ovarian cancer. Tumori 2020;106(2):149–54.
[25] Filippone A, Cianci R, Storto ML. Bowel obstruction: comparison between multidetector-row CT axial and coronal planes. Abdom Imaging 2007;32(3):310–6.
[26] Maglinte DDT, Kelvin FM, Sandrasegaran K, et al. Radiology of small bowel obstruction: contemporary approach and controversies. Abdom Imaging 2005;30(2):160–78.
[27] Silva AC, Pimenta M, Guimaraes LS. Small Bowel Obstruction: What to Look For. RadioGraphics 2009;29(2):423–39.
[28] Abbas S, Bissett IP, Parry BR. Oral water soluble contrast for the management of adhesive small bowel obstruction. Cochrane Database Syst Rev 2007;2007(3); https://doi.org/10.1002/14651858.CD004651.pub3.
[29] Khasawneh MA, Eiken PW, Srvantstyan B, et al. Use of the Gastrografin challenge in patients with a history of abdominal or pelvic malignancy. Surgery 2013;154(4):769–75 [discussion: 775–6].
[30] Syrmis W, Richard R, Jenkins-Marsh S, et al. Oral water soluble contrast for malignant bowel obstruction. Cochrane Database Syst Rev 2018;2018(3); https://doi.org/10.1002/14651858.CD012014.pub2.

[31] Dolan EA. Malignant Bowel Obstruction: A Review of Current Treatment Strategies. Am J Hosp Palliat Care 2011;28(8):576–82.
[32] al NM et. Health-related quality of life in patients with inoperable malignant bowel obstruction: secondary outcome from a double-blind, parallel, placebo-controlled randomised trial of octreotide | EndNote Click. Available at: https://kopernio.com/viewer?doi=10.1186%2Fs12885-020-07549-y&token=WzE5MjEwNjAsIjEwLjExODYvczEyODg1L-TAyMC0wNzU0OS15Il0.OYH8-z-k9dyliZcfLkkGwZK3m2c. Accessed December 7, 2020.
[33] Miller G, Boman J, Shrier I, et al. Small-bowel obstruction secondary to malignant disease: an 11-year audit. Can J Surg 2000;43(5):353–8.
[34] Blair SL, Chu DZJ, Schwarz RE. Outcome of palliative operations for malignant bowel obstruction in patients with peritoneal carcinomatosis from nongynecological cancer. Ann Surg Oncol 2001;8(8):632–7.
[35] Hsu K, Prommer E, Murphy MC, et al. Pharmacologic management of malignant bowel obstruction: when surgery is not an option. J Hosp Med 2019;14(6):367–73.
[36] MacDougall MR, Sharma S. Physiology, Chemoreceptor Trigger Zone. In: StatPearls [Internet]. Treasure Island (FL): StatPearls Publishing; 2020 Jan PMID: 30725818.
[37] Babic T, Browning KN. The role of vagal neurocircuits in the regulation of nausea and vomiting. Eur J Pharmacol 2014;722:38–47.
[38] Walsh D, Davis M, Ripamonti C, et al. 2016 Updated MASCC/ESMO consensus recommendations: Management of nausea and vomiting in advanced cancer. Support Care Cancer 2017;25(1):333–40.
[39] Mercadante S, Ferrera P, Villari P, et al. Aggressive pharmacological treatment for reversing malignant bowel obstruction. J Pain Symptom Manage 2004;28(4):412–6.
[40] al AJF et. Management of Malignant Bowel Obstruction Associated With GI Cancers | EndNote Click. Available at: https://kopernio.com/viewer?doi=10.1200%2Fjop.2017.022210&token=WzE5MjEwNjAsIjEwLjEyMDAvam9wLjIwMTcuMDIyMjE-wIl0.j0TYaVnpvZtaN70pRzGWHxBX_gE. Accessed December 8, 2020.
[41] Halley A. A systematic review of the use of anti-secretory medicines for the control of gastrointestinal symptoms in patients with malignant bowel obstruction. Palliat Med 2016;30(4): S8–9.
[42] Magee C. Octreotide in the management of nausea and vomiting secondary to inoperable malignant bowel obstruction: a systematic review. Palliat Med 2014;28(6).
[43] D. C. Currow - Double-Blind, Placebo-Controlled, Randomized Trial of Octreotide in Malignant Bowel Obstruction. Available at: https://kopernio.com/viewer?doi=10.1016%2Fj.jpainsymman.2014.09.013&token=WzE5MjEwNjAsIjEwLjEwMTY-vai5qcGFpbnN5bW1hbi4yMDE0LjA5LjAxMyJd.LGcMWnkJaMm9RRdHzz7J3U3JR-8. Accessed December 19, 2020.
[44] Laval G, Rousselot H, Toussaint-Martel S, et al. SALTO: a randomized, multicenter study assessing octreotide LAR in inoperable bowel obstruction. Bull Cancer 2012;99(2):E1–9.
[45] Currow DC, Quinn S, Agar M, et al. Double-blind, placebo-controlled, randomized trial of octreotide in malignant bowel obstruction. J Pain Symptom Manage 2015;49(5):814–21.
[46] Peng X, Wang P, Li S, et al. Randomized clinical trial comparing octreotide and scopolamine butylbromide in symptom control of patients with inoperable bowel obstruction due to advanced ovarian cancer. World J Surg Oncol 2015;13:50.
[47] Clark K, Lam L, Currow D. Reducing gastric secretions—a role for histamine 2 antagonists or proton pump inhibitors in malignant bowel obstruction? Support Care Cancer 2009;17(12):1463.
[48] al GL et. Recommendations for Bowel Obstruction With Peritoneal Carcinomatosis | EndNote Click. Available at: https://kopernio.com/viewer?doi=10.1016%2Fj.jpainsymman.2013.08.022&token=WzE5MjEwNjAsIjEwLjEwMTYvai5qcGFpbnN5bW1hbi4yMDEzLjA4LjAyMiJd.Hg5MPJnjkGZsecGuQY83oagDo0A. Accessed December 22, 2020.

[49] al TM et. Practice Patterns of Medications for Patients With Malignant Bowel Obstruction Using a Nationwide Claims Database and the Association Between Treatment Outcomes and Concomitant Use of H2-Blockers/Proton Pump Inhibitors and Corticosteroids With Octreotide | EndNote Click. Available at: https://kopernio.com/viewer?doi=10.1016%2Fj.jpainsymman.2017.10.019&token=WzE5MjEwNjAsIjEwLjEwMTY-vai5qcGFpbnN5bW1hbi4yMDE3LjEwLjAxOSJd.dEe3v6_Q_OJpjzJfxHVo5i8QhTw. Accessed December 22, 2020.
[50] Vayne-Bossert P, Haywood A, Good P, et al. Corticosteroids for adult patients with advanced cancer who have nausea and vomiting (not related to chemotherapy, radiotherapy, or surgery). Cochrane Database Syst Rev 2017;7:CD012002.
[51] Gunten ER and CFV. Current concepts in malignant bowel obstruction management | EndNote Click. Available at: https://kopernio.com/viewer?doi=10.1007%2Fs11912-009-0042-2&token=WzE5MjEwNjAsIjEwLjEwMDcvczExOTEyLTAwOS0wMDQyLTIiX-Q.ishQe1sfF3iKcCP9scto7jnntqU. Accessed December 22, 2020.
[52] Feuer DJ, Broadley KE. Systematic review and meta-analysis of corticosteroids for the resolution of malignant bowel obstruction in advanced gynaecological and gastrointestinal cancers. Systematic Review Steering Committee. Ann Oncol 1999;10(9):1035–41.
[53] Cancer Pain Syndromes- ClinicalKey. Available at: https://www-clinicalkey-com.proxy-hu.wrlc.org/#!/content/playContent/1-s2.0-S0889858818300121?scrollTo=%23hl0000472. Accessed December 22, 2020.
[54] al MTG et. Quality of Cancer Pain Management: An Update of a Systematic Review of Undertreatment of Patients With Cancer | EndNote Click. Available at: https://kopernio.com/viewer?doi=10.1200%2Fjco.2014.56.0383&token=WzE5MjEwNjAsIjEwLjEyMDAvamNvLjIwMTQuNTYuMDM4MyJd.YEo781kPiGF0_uNGuvvEjf36O4U. Accessed December 22, 2020.
[55] Sun V, Borneman T, Piper B, et al. Barriers to pain assessment and management in cancer survivorship. J Cancer Surviv 2008;2(1):65–71.
[56] Available at: Barriers_Final.pdf. Accessed December 22, 2020. https://s3.amazonaws.com/rdcms-iasp/files/production/public/Content/ContentFolders/GlobalYearAgainstPain2/CancerPainFactSheets/Barriers_Final.pdf.
[57] Al-Ghabeesh SH, Bashayreh IH, Saifan AR, et al. Barriers to Effective Pain Management in Cancer Patients From the Perspective of Patients and Family Caregivers: A Qualitative Study. Pain Manag Nurs 2020;21(3):238–44.
[58] Chapman EJ, Edwards Z, Boland JW, et al. Practice review: Evidence-based and effective management of pain in patients with advanced cancer. Palliat Med 2020;34(4):444–53.
[59] Lin J, Hsieh R-K, Chen J-S, et al. Satisfaction with pain management and impact of pain on quality of life in cancer patients. Asia-Pacific J Clin Oncol 2020;16(2):e91–8.
[60] Caraceni A, Shkodra M. Cancer Pain Assessment and Classification. Cancers (Basel) 2019;11(4); https://doi.org/10.3390/cancers11040510.
[61] Jaruvongvanich V, Chesta F, Baruah A, et al. Palliative treatment for malignant gastrointestinal obstruction with peritoneal carcinomatosis: enteral stenting versus surgery. Endosc Int Open 2020;8(10):E1487–94.
[62] Boland PA, Kelly ME, Donlon NE, et al. Outcomes following colonic stenting for malignant left-sided bowel obstruction: a systematic review of randomised controlled trials. Int J Colorectal Dis 2019;34(10):1625–32.
[63] Paul Olson TJ, Pinkerton C, Brasel KJ, et al. Palliative surgery for malignant bowel obstruction from carcinomatosis: a systematic review. JAMA Surg 2014;149(4):383–92.
[64] Thampy S, Najran P, Mullan D, et al. Safety and Efficacy of Venting Gastrostomy in Malignant Bowel Obstruction: A Systematic Review. J Palliat Care 2020;35(2):93–102.
[65] Chen P-J, Wang L, Peng Y-F, et al. Surgical intervention for malignant bowel obstruction caused by gastrointestinal malignancies. World J Gastrointest Oncol 2020;12(3):323–31.
[66] Shariat-Madar B, Jayakrishnan TT, Gamblin TC, et al. Surgical management of bowel obstruction in patients with peritoneal carcinomatosis. J Surg Oncol 2014;110(6):666–9.

[67] al TJPO et. Palliative Surgery for Malignant Bowel Obstruction From Carcinomatosis | EndNote Click. Available at: https://kopernio.com/viewer?doi=10.1001%2Fjamasurg.2013.4059&token=WzE5MjEwNjAsIjEwLjEwMDEvamFtYXN1cmcuMjAxMy40MDU5Il0.7KSBrW33LNOQ9z-ivrA8eGcDj6k. Accessed December 8, 2020.
[68] Cousins SE, Tempest E, Feuer DJ. Surgery for the resolution of symptoms in malignant bowel obstruction in advanced gynaecological and gastrointestinal cancer [Systematic Review]. Cochrane Database Syst Rev 2016;(1):CD002764.

Advances in Surgery 55 (2021) 49–56

ADVANCES IN SURGERY

# Nonoperative Treatment of Diverticulitis

Matthew Symer, MD, MS[a], Heather L. Yeo, MD, MBA, MHS[b,*]

[a]Department of Surgery, New York-Presbyterian Hospital, Weill Cornell Medicine, 525 East 68th Street, PO Box 172, New York, NY 10065, USA; [b]Department of Healthcare Policy and Research, New York-Presbyterian, Weill Cornell Medicine, 525 East 68th Street, PO Box 172, New York, NY 10065, USA

**Keywords**

• Diverticulitis • Antibiotics • Colonic diseases • Laparoscopic resection • Colorectal surgery • Colon

**Key points**

- Diverticulitis is now frequently managed nonoperatively with excellent results.
- Increasing nonoperative management of diverticulitis has not increased the need for emergent colectomy.
- Colonoscopy is essential to rule out an underlying malignancy after nonoperative management of diverticulitis.

## INTRODUCTION

Diverticulitis is one of the most common gastrointestinal disorders and often primarily managed by surgeons. In 2010, there were more than 2 million office visits and approximately 262,000 emergency department visits for diverticular disease in the United States with associated health care costs totaling more than 2 billion dollars [1,2].

The prevalence of diverticula increases with age; by 60 years old, most Americans have endoscopic evidence of diverticulosis [3]. The cause of diverticulitis is likely multifactorial, with the low-fiber, high-fat Western diet a frequently cited cause [4]. Attention is now also being focused on the role of chronic inflammation and alterations in gut microbiota in the development

Conflicts-of-interest disclosure: Dr H.L. Yeo serves on the medical advisory board of Survivornet.

*Corresponding author. Department of Surgery, New-York Presbyterian, Weill Cornell Medicine, 525 East 68th Street, PO Box 172, New York, NY 10065. *E-mail address:* hey9002@med.cornell.edu

https://doi.org/10.1016/j.yasu.2021.05.004

of diverticula and subsequent diverticulitis [5,6]. Altered motility also plays a role, with segments of affected colon demonstrating increased contractility and an abnormal response to neuropeptides [7–9]. A genetic component has also been described [10].

Classification of diverticulitis is useful to help guide management, inform patient expectations, and establish a prognosis. Complicated diverticulitis is defined by clinical or radiographic signs of obstruction, perforation, bleeding, abscess or fistula formation, or the presence of diffuse peritonitis or hemodynamic instability on examination. Uncomplicated diverticulitis lacks these features. The modified Hinchey classification (Table 1) is helpful in further subcategorizing diverticulitis episodes based on radiographic and clinical features [11].

Obstruction of diverticula and resulting inflammation and infection clinically manifest as a wide spectrum of disease. Typical symptoms include left lower quadrant abdominal pain, fever, changes in bowel habits, and intolerance of oral intake [12]. The goals of treatment are to address symptoms, identify underlying malignancy when present, and avoid the need for emergency surgery with its attendant risks of morbidity and stoma creation. Over the past decade, the management of diverticulitis has shifted as insight into the natural history of diverticulitis has allowed increasing use of a nonoperative approach for many patients.

## EPIDEMIOLOGY

The incidence of diverticulitis has been increasing over that past 2 decades. In 1 population-level study in Minnesota, the incidence of diverticulitis in a large longitudinal cohort increased 50% between 1980 to 1989 and 2000 to 2007. The largest relative increase in incidence during that time was in younger patients [13]. From a population perspective, this increase appears to be related to worsening obesity, dietary habits, and aging of the population. Greater utilization of cross-sectional imaging has also increased the number of diagnoses of diverticulitis [14].

**Table 1**
Modified Hinchey classification [11]

| Classification | Radiographic or clinical findings |
|---|---|
| 0 | Mild clinical diverticulitis |
| 1a | Pericolic inflammation or phlegmon |
| 1b | Pericolic abscess |
| 2 | Pelvic, intra-abdominal, or retrocolic abscess |
| 3 | Generalized purulent peritonitis |
| 4 | Generalized feculent peritonitis |

*From* Gielens MPM, Mulder IM, van der Harst E, et al. Preoperative staging of perforated diverticulitis by computed tomography scanning. Tech Coloproctol 2012;16(5):363-368. doi: 10.1007/s10151-012-0853-2

A theoretic disadvantage of nonoperative management of diverticulitis is the potential to increase the number of colectomies performed emergently, which may have been averted with an elective procedure. However, administrative data have not borne out this concern. Ricciardi and colleagues [15] examined nationwide secular trends in hospitalization for diverticulitis and found that overall admissions for diverticulitis increased 50% from 1991 to 2005. Over that time, there was a modest decrease in the proportion of patients undergoing elective colectomy and no change in the fraction of all diverticulitis cases presenting with free perforation, which remained stable at 1.5%.

## DIVERTICULITIS RECURRENCE

Recurrence after an initial episode of diverticulitis appears to be relatively uncommon. In a large multicenter study of 2366 patients undergoing nonoperative management after a first episode requiring hospitalization, 13% had recurrent diverticulitis after 8.9 years of average follow-up. After the second episode, the risk of a third episode of diverticulitis increased to 29% [16]. Risk factors for higher likelihood of recurrence include young age and the presence of an abscess during the index episode [17].

The risk of recurrence is elevated in patients with complicated diverticulitis. In a cohort of 99 patients with complicated diverticulitis managed nonoperatively, approximately half (n = 46) developed recurrent diverticulitis during 76 months of follow-up. Twenty patients subsequently underwent elective colectomy, although none needed emergent surgery [18]. In another, similar cohort of patients with a diverticular abscess, 30% recurred at 23 months, although only 2.7% required an emergent procedure [19].

The first episode of diverticulitis is generally the most severe with subsequent episodes of similar or diminished severity. In an administrative database review from the United Kingdom, 72% of those treated for complicated diverticulitis had no history of prior episodes [20]. Similarly, the most severe presentation of free perforation is most likely in those without a history of diverticulitis. The incidence of free perforation causing peritonitis decreases with increasing number of recurrences [21]. The need for emergency surgery after nonoperative management is rare. In a Spanish cohort of 267 patients managed nonoperatively, only 5% subsequently required an emergent colectomy during 91 months of mean follow-up [22]. This was confirmed by Anaya and Flum [23], who found in a statewide administrative database that only 5.5% of patients admitted for diverticulitis managed nonoperatively would later have emergent colectomy or ostomy creation at an average follow-up of 4.3 years.

## ADVANTAGES OF THE NONOPERATIVE APPROACH

Despite the introduction of minimally invasive techniques, enhanced recovery protocols, and patient safety initiatives, there remains considerable morbidity after surgery for diverticulitis. A chief advantage of the nonoperative approach, therefore, is avoiding the morbidity of surgery. In 1 large series of elective laparoscopic sigmoid colectomies for diverticulitis, major postoperative complications occurred in 14% and increased to 20% in patients with complicated diverticulitis [24]. Complications are also more frequent after an emergency procedure, with as many as 40% experiencing a postoperative complication [25]. The avoidance of temporary or permanent fecal diversion with an ostomy is another major advantage of nonoperative management. Although one might expect that nonoperatively treated patients might have a shorter length of stay, a randomized trial comparing nonoperative management versus elective colectomy in complicated diverticulitis found a similar length of hospital admission regardless of the approach taken, largely because of the need for intravenous antibiotics in the nonoperative group [26]. Finally, although colectomy is highly effective in addressing diverticular symptoms, recurrent diverticulitis after sigmoidectomy is reported to occur in 4% of patients [27].

## UNCOMPLICATED DIVERTICULITIS

The management of uncomplicated diverticulitis has shifted not only away from surgery but also away from the use of antibiotics in select patients. Prospective and randomized studies have demonstrated that oral antibiotics are equivalent to parenteral antibiotics in uncomplicated diverticulitis [28,29]. A shorter 4-day course of antibiotic therapy has also been shown to be as efficacious as a 7-day course [30]. Several large randomized controlled trials and subsequent meta-analyses have demonstrated equivalence between antibiotic and antibiotic-sparing regimens in regard to recurrence and complications from uncomplicated diverticulitis. Notably, these trials were in selected, otherwise healthy patients with relatively mild diverticulitis (modified Hinchey classification 1a or less) [31,32]. The 2020 American Society of Colon and Rectal Surgeons clinical practice guidelines endorse this approach in select patients [33].

When to offer colectomy to a patient with recurrent bouts of uncomplicated diverticulitis is a common clinical question. Accumulating evidence clearly shows that a nonoperative approach to most patients is advantageous for the reasons noted above regarding the typically indolent and self-limited natural history of diverticulitis [34]. The authors' approach, after an informed and individualized discussion, is to offer colectomy to highly select patients with uncomplicated diverticulitis. The authors are more likely to offer colectomy to patients with an increasing frequency of attacks, which are uncomplicated but nonetheless disabling in their quality of life, to immunocompromised patients, symptoms from stricture, and those who travel frequently to remote locations without reliable medical care. The authors do not use the number of attacks of diverticulitis to guide decision making [35].

## COMPLICATED DIVERTICULITIS

Patients with diffuse peritonitis or hemodynamic instability require emergent operation. For many others, however, complicated diverticulitis can initially be managed nonoperatively. In 1 series of nearly 210 patients admitted for a diverticular abscess, only 25 (12%) failed initial nonoperative management with antibiotics with or without image-guided percutaneous drainage [36]. However, in the same series, 60% of patients recurred within 5.3 months, and recurrences were frequently as severe or more severe than the initial presentation. These data and other similar series support the use of elective, interval colectomy after resolution of the initial episode of complicated diverticulitis [33].

Because recurrence after complicated diverticulitis is frequent but not certain, select patients who desire to avoid surgery can be managed nonoperatively [33]. For example, in 1 series of patients undergoing expectant management after drainage of a diverticular abscess, approximately half recurred, but all of these recurrences were successfully managed nonoperatively [37].

The use of percutaneous drainage catheters has increased as imaging has improved and more patients are managed nonoperatively [38]. An attempt at percutaneous drainage should be made for abscesses larger than 3 cm, although the level of evidence supporting drainage catheters is weak [39,40]. Retrospective single-center series have demonstrated the safety of this approach as well as a higher likelihood of eventual surgical management with larger abscesses [41,42].

## SYMPTOMATIC UNCOMPLICATED DIVERTICULAR DISEASE AND CHRONIC ABDOMINAL PAIN

Acute abdominal pain is a hallmark of diverticulitis, but diverticular disease can also be associated with chronic pain. Symptomatic uncomplicated diverticular disease (SUDD) is a syndrome of chronic abdominal pain and diverticulosis without associated colitis [43]. Visceral hypersensitivity similar to that observed in irritable bowel syndrome has been noted in patients with SUDD, suggesting some overlap in pathophysiology [6,44]. Medical management of SUDD with mesalamine, rifaximin, probiotics, and fiber supplementation have all been studied, demonstrating efficacy in symptom control [45,46].

Surgery for chronic abdominal pain in the setting of SUDD should only be undertaken with great caution. Although many patients with overt diverticulitis report improvement of their quality of life with elective resection, chronic abdominal pain can occur after surgery in as many as 25% of patients [47,48].

## NEED FOR ENDOSCOPIC EXAMINATION

One advantage of operative management of diverticular disease is subsequent pathologic confirmation of the diagnosis. Meyer and colleagues [49] performed a meta-analysis of studies reporting colorectal cancer incidence in patients with diverticulitis. In more than 50,000 patients, the prevalence of colorectal cancer was 7.9% in patients with complicated diverticulitis and 1.3% in patients with uncomplicated diverticulitis. These data underlie the current recommendation for colonoscopy after recovery from an initial episode of diverticulitis, particularly in patients with complicated disease [33,50].

## SUMMARY

Diverticular disease is characterized by a benign, remitting course. For most patients, the first episode of diverticulitis is the most severe with recurrence being infrequent and typically less severe than the initial presentation. Recognition of the natural history of the disease has led to many more patients avoiding an operation and its attendant risks. There has not been an increase in the need for emergency surgery because of this changing approach. Operation should be reserved in the emergent setting to those with peritonitis, hemodynamic compromise, or those who fail an initial attempt at nonoperative management. In the elective setting, complicated diverticulitis will usually but not always require operation, and patients with stricture or repeated episodes that limit functionality should be offered surgery. For uncomplicated diverticulitis, a tailored approach to the individual patient is best. Patients managed nonoperatively should undergo colonoscopy to exclude the possibility of an underlying malignancy.

## CLINICS CARE POINTS

- Patients with diffuse peritonitis or hemodynamic instability require emergent operation.
- Consider omitting antibiotics in the treatment of select patients with uncomplicated diverticulitis.
- In the elective setting, avoid using the number of episodes of diverticulitis to determine the need for operation.

## References

[1] Woolhandler S, Campbell T, Himmelstein DU. Costs of health care administration in the United States and Canada. N Engl J Med 2003;349(8):768–75.

[2] Peery AF, Crockett SD, Barritt AS, et al. Burden of gastrointestinal, liver, and pancreatic diseases in the United States. Gastroenterology 2015;149(7):1731–41.e3.

[3] Peery AF, Keku TO, Martin CF, et al. Distribution and characteristics of colonic diverticula in a United States screening population. Clin Gastroenterol Hepatol 2016;14(7):980–5.e1.

[4] Von Rahden BHA, Germer C-T. Pathogenesis of colonic diverticular disease. Langenbecks Arch Surg 2012;397(7):1025–33.

[5] Daniels L, Philipszoon LE, Boermeester MA. A hypothesis: important role for gut microbiota in the etiopathogenesis of diverticular disease. Dis Colon Rectum 2014;57(4):539–43.

[6] Strate LL, Modi R, Cohen E, et al. Diverticular disease as a chronic illness: evolving epidemiologic and clinical insights. Am J Gastroenterol 2012;107(10):1486–93.

[7] Guagnini F, Valenti M, Mukenge S, et al. Neural contractions in colonic strips from patients with diverticular disease: role of endocannabinoids and substance P. Gut 2006;55(7):946–53.

[8] Maselli MA, Piepoli AL, Guerra V, et al. Colonic smooth muscle responses in patients with diverticular disease of the colon: effect of the NK2 receptor antagonist SR48968. Dig Liver Dis 2004;36(5):348–54.

[9] Golder M, Burleigh DE, Ghali L, et al. Longitudinal muscle shows abnormal relaxation responses to nitric oxide and contains altered levels of NOS1 and elastin in uncomplicated diverticular disease. Colorectal Dis 2007;9(3):218–28.

[10] Maguire LH. Genetic risk factors for diverticular disease-emerging evidence. J Gastrointest Surg 2020;24(10):2314–7.

[11] Gielens MPM, Mulder IM, van der Harst E, et al. Preoperative staging of perforated diverticulitis by computed tomography scanning. Tech Coloproctol 2012;16(5):363–8.
[12] Shahedi K, Fuller G, Bolus R, et al. Long-term risk of acute diverticulitis among patients with incidental diverticulosis found during colonoscopy. Clin Gastroenterol Hepatol 2013;11(12):1609–13.
[13] Bharucha AE, Parthasarathy G, Ditah I, et al. Temporal trends in the incidence and natural history of diverticulitis: a population-based study. Am J Gastroenterol 2015;110(11): 1589–96.
[14] Lee TH, Setty PT, Parthasarathy G, et al. Aging, obesity, and the incidence of diverticulitis: a population-based study. Mayo Clin Proc 2018;93(9):1256–65.
[15] Ricciardi R, Baxter NN, Read TE, et al. Is the decline in the surgical treatment for diverticulitis associated with an increase in complicated diverticulitis? Dis Colon Rectum 2009;52(9): 1558–63.
[16] Broderick-Villa G, Burchette RJ, Collins JC, et al. Hospitalization for acute diverticulitis does not mandate routine elective colectomy. Arch Surg 2005;140(6):576–81 [discussion: 581].
[17] Hupfeld L, Burcharth J, Pommergaard H-C, et al. Risk factors for recurrence after acute colonic diverticulitis: a systematic review. Int J Colorectal Dis 2017;32(5):611–22.
[18] Nelson RS, Ewing BM, Wengert TJ, et al. Clinical outcomes of complicated diverticulitis managed nonoperatively. Am J Surg 2008;196(6):969–72 [discussion: 973].
[19] Garfinkle R, Kugler A, Pelsser V, et al. Diverticular abscess managed with long-term definitive nonoperative intent is safe. Dis Colon Rectum 2016;59(7):648–55.
[20] Humes DJ, West J. Role of acute diverticulitis in the development of complicated colonic diverticular disease and 1-year mortality after diagnosis in the UK: population-based cohort study. Gut 2012;61(1):95–100.
[21] Ritz J-P, Lehmann KS, Frericks B, et al. Outcome of patients with acute sigmoid diverticulitis: multivariate analysis of risk factors for free perforation. Surgery 2011;149(5):606–13.
[22] Suarez Alecha J, Amoza Pais S, Batlle Marin X, et al. Safety of nonoperative management after acute diverticulitis. Ann Coloproctol 2014;30(5):216–21.
[23] Anaya DA, Flum DR. Risk of emergency colectomy and colostomy in patients with diverticular disease. Arch Surg 2005;140(7):681–5.
[24] Bhakta A, Tafen M, Glotzer O, et al. Laparoscopic sigmoid colectomy for complicated diverticulitis is safe: review of 576 consecutive colectomies. Surg Endosc 2016;30(4):1629–34.
[25] Turley RS, Barbas AS, Lidsky ME, et al. Laparoscopic versus open Hartmann procedure for the emergency treatment of diverticulitis: a propensity-matched analysis. Dis Colon Rectum 2013;56(1):72–82.
[26] You K, Bendl R, Taut C, et al. Randomized clinical trial of elective resection versus observation in diverticulitis with extraluminal air or abscess initially managed conservatively. Br J Surg 2018;105(8):971–9.
[27] Choi KK, Martinolich J, Canete JJ, et al. Elective laparoscopic sigmoid colectomy for diverticulitis-an updated look at recurrence after surgery. J Gastrointest Surg 2020;24(2): 388–95.
[28] Ridgway PF, Latif A, Shabbir J, et al. Randomized controlled trial of oral vs intravenous therapy for the clinically diagnosed acute uncomplicated diverticulitis. Colorectal Dis 2009;11(9):941–6.
[29] Moya P, Arroyo A, Pérez-Legaz J, et al. Applicability, safety and efficiency of outpatient treatment in uncomplicated diverticulitis. Tech Coloproctol 2012;16(4):301–7.
[30] Schug-Pass C, Geers P, Hügel O, et al. Prospective randomized trial comparing short-term antibiotic therapy versus standard therapy for acute uncomplicated sigmoid diverticulitis. Int J Colorectal Dis 2010;25(6):751–9.
[31] Shabanzadeh DM, Wille-Jørgensen P. Antibiotics for uncomplicated diverticulitis. Cochrane Database Syst Rev 2012;11:CD009092.

[32] Tandon A, Fretwell VL, Nunes QM, et al. Antibiotics versus no antibiotics in the treatment of acute uncomplicated diverticulitis - a systematic review and meta-analysis. Colorectal Dis 2018; https://doi.org/10.1111/codi.14013.
[33] Hall J, Hardiman K, Lee S, et al. The American Society of Colon and Rectal Surgeons clinical practice guidelines for the treatment of left-sided colonic diverticulitis. Dis Colon Rectum 2020;63(6):728–47.
[34] Morris AM, Regenbogen SE, Hardiman KM, et al. Sigmoid diverticulitis: a systematic review. JAMA 2014;311(3):287–97.
[35] Salem L, Veenstra DL, Sullivan SD, et al. The timing of elective colectomy in diverticulitis: a decision analysis. J Am Coll Surg 2004;199(6):904–12.
[36] Devaraj B, Liu W, Tatum J, et al. Medically treated diverticular abscess associated with high risk recurrence and disease complications. Dis Colon Rectum 2016;59(3):208–15.
[37] Gaertner WB, Willis DJ, Madoff RD, et al. Percutaneous drainage of colonic diverticular abscess: is colon resection necessary? Dis Colon Rectum 2013;56(5):622–6.
[38] Li D, Baxter NN, McLeod RS, et al. Evolving practice patterns in the management of acute colonic diverticulitis: a population-based analysis. Dis Colon Rectum 2014;57(12): 1397–405.
[39] Brandt D, Gervaz P, Durmishi Y, et al. Percutaneous CT scan-guided drainage vs. antibiotherapy alone for Hinchey II diverticulitis: a case-control study. Dis Colon Rectum 2006;49(10): 1533–8.
[40] Gregersen R, Mortensen LQ, Burcharth J, et al. Treatment of patients with acute colonic diverticulitis complicated by abscess formation: a systematic review. Int J Surg 2016;35: 201–8.
[41] Siewert B, Tye G, Kruskal J, et al. Impact of CT-guided drainage in the treatment of diverticular abscesses: size matters. AJR Am J Roentgenol 2006;186(3):680–6.
[42] Kumar RR, Kim JT, Haukoos JS, et al. Factors affecting the successful management of intra-abdominal abscesses with antibiotics and the need for percutaneous drainage. Dis Colon Rectum 2006;49(2):183–9.
[43] Rezapour M, Ali S, Stollman N. Diverticular disease: an update on pathogenesis and management. Gut Liver 2018;12(2):125–32.
[44] Clemens CHM, Samsom M, Roelofs J, et al. Colorectal visceral perception in diverticular disease. Gut 2004;53(5):717–22.
[45] Moniuszko A, Rydzewska G. The effect of cyclic rifaximin therapy on symptoms of diverticular disease from the perspective of the gastroenterology outpatient clinic: a "real-life" study. Prz Gastroenterol 2017;12(2):145–51.
[46] Picchio M, Elisei W, Brandimarte G, et al. Mesalazine for the treatment of symptomatic uncomplicated diverticular disease of the colon and for primary prevention of diverticulitis: a systematic review of randomized clinical trials. J Clin Gastroenterol 2016;50(Suppl 1): S64–9.
[47] Forgione A, Leroy J, Cahill RA, et al. Prospective evaluation of functional outcome after laparoscopic sigmoid colectomy. Ann Surg 2009;249(2):218–24.
[48] Egger B, Peter MK, Candinas D. Persistent symptoms after elective sigmoid resection for diverticulitis. Dis Colon Rectum 2008;51(7):1044–8.
[49] Meyer J, Orci LA, Combescure C, et al. Risk of colorectal cancer in patients with acute diverticulitis: a systematic review and meta-analysis of observational studies. Clin Gastroenterol Hepatol 2019;17(8):1448–56.e17.
[50] Sharma PV, Eglinton T, Hider P, et al. Systematic review and meta-analysis of the role of routine colonic evaluation after radiologically confirmed acute diverticulitis. Ann Surg 2014;259(2):263–72.

Advances in Surgery 55 (2021) 57–73

ADVANCES IN SURGERY

# The Current Management of Visceral Artery Aneurysms

Bara Zuhaili, MD[a], James H. Black III, MD[b,*]

[a]Michigan Vascular Center, Michigan State University, 5020 W Bristol Road, Flint, MI 48507, USA; [b]The David Goldfarb, MD Professor of Surgery, Division of Vascular Surgery and Endovascular Therapy, Johns Hopkins School of Medicine, Halsted 668, 600 North Wolfe Street, Baltimore, MD 21287, USA

**Keywords**

• Visceral • Aneurysms • Rupture • Endovascular • Abdominal

**Key points**

- Visceral artery aneurysms are rare.
- Indication to treat varies depending on the patient age, comorbidities, presentation, aneurysm location, and size.
- Most visceral artery aneurysms can be treated with endovascular methods, especially when done electively.

## BACKGROUND

An aneurysm is defined by a focal arterial dilatation 1.5 to 2.0 times greater than the diameter of a normal artery. Visceral artery aneurysm (VAA) is a rare entity. Although the true prevalence is unknown because most of VAA cases are asymptomatic, the estimated prevalence ranges between 0.01% and 2% [1].

### Anatomic distribution

Within the VAA cohort, splenic artery aneurysm is the most common entity, with a 60% prevalence. Hepatic artery (HA) has an estimated prevalence of 20%, followed by superior mesenteric artery (6%); celiac artery (4%); gastric and gastroepiploic arteries (4%); jejunal, ileal, and colic arteries (3%); pancreaticoduodenal artery (PDA) and pancreatic artery (2%); gastroduodenal artery (GDA; 1.5%); and inferior mesenteric artery (<1%) [2].

*Corresponding author: *E-mail address:* jhblack@jhmi.edu

https://doi.org/10.1016/j.yasu.2021.05.005

### Causes

The disorder that leads to VAA is yet to be established. Because of the paucity of cases, most current theories are based on small, retrospective case series. Among all possible causes, atherosclerosis is cited the most, followed by medial degeneration, and trauma [3,4]. Other possibilities are connective tissue disorders (Marfan syndrome, Ehlers-Danlos syndrome), portal hypertension, pregnancy, and antiphospholipid syndrome, with the last of these being suggested based on a single case report presentation [5]. For unknown reasons, superior mesenteric artery (SMA) aneurysms are associated with infection [6].

## CLINICAL PRESENTATION

### Nonruptured visceral artery aneurysm

Most nonruptured VAAs are asymptomatic and are usually found incidentally on abdominal imaging done for different reasons [3]. When symptomatic, nonruptured VAAs tend to have nonspecific vague abdominal pain, nausea, and/or vomiting. Rarely, SMA aneurysms can dissect, leading to typical mesenteric ischemia symptoms [7]. Within the nonruptured VAA cohort, GDA aneurysms tend to be more symptomatic than other VAAs, usually presenting with vague epigastric pain that radiates to the back. Sixty percent of GDA aneurysms are associated with pancreatitis [8].

### Ruptured visceral artery aneurysm

When ruptured, VAAs present with sudden epigastric or generalized abdominal pain. Hemodynamic instability may be present if the VAA ruptures into the peritoneum. Specific to ruptured splenic artery aneurysms, a double-rupture phenomenon has been described; the initial rupture is a contained rupture with a transient hemodynamic instability if contained in the lesser omentum. If not treated promptly, it could progress to free intraperitoneal rupture with associated persistent hemodynamic instability [9].

## PHYSICAL EXAMINATION

In general, physical examination in nonruptured VAA is nonspecific and does not yield significant positive findings. However, about half of splenic artery aneurysms present with moderate splenomegaly [10].

## WORK-UP

Broad work-up for abdominal pain usually precedes the diagnosis of VAA. This work-up includes ruling out biliary colic, pancreatitis, gastroesophageal reflux disease, and/or stomach/duodenal ulcer. Once VAA diagnosis is established, the imaging modality of choice is computed tomography angiography of the abdomen and pelvis, which establishes the anatomy and exact measurement of the aneurysm and arterial structures proximal and distal to it. The authors also recommend visceral artery duplex to establish baseline measurements and velocities of the visceral arteries for long-term follow-up.

## MEDICAL TREATMENT

Most small VAAs tend to have slow growth with small chance of rupture. Abbas and colleagues [9] published one of the largest retrospective analyses of splenic artery aneurysms. Among 217 patients, only 4% presented with rupture. The smallest ruptured aneurysm was 2.3 cm. Abbas and colleagues [9] identified pregnancy and liver cirrhosis as risk factors for rupture. Given low rates of rupture [11], there is consensus not to treat asymptomatic VAA unless it meets specific size criteria, exists in specific patient populations, and/or exists in specific anatomic locations.

Most providers recommend annual or semiannual serial imaging with a modality based on the presenting size and location. A Mayo Clinic retrospective study identified reversible/controllable risk factors associated with VAA as hypertension (50%), hypercholesterolemia (21%), and diabetes (10%). Although none of those diseases has an established causative relation with VAA, the authors recommend maximizing the medical treatment of those diseases. Unlike aortic aneurysms or dissections, there is no defined target blood pressure to achieve with VAA.

## INTERVENTIONAL TREATMENT

### Indication for intervention

The plan to intervene or observe a VAA should be tailored to each individual patient. Although this is true for any vascular disorder, it is more so in VAA management because surgical exposure of many VAAs is hazardous. The Society for Vascular Surgery (SVS) published clinical practice guidelines on the management of visceral aneurysms. Those were updated most recently in July 2020 [12]. A summary of those guidelines is provided in Table 1.

### Intervention options

Endovascular techniques have facilitated thrombosis and exclusion of VAA. The main goal in treating a visceral aneurysm is to exclude the blood flow from the aneurysm while, ideally, preserving the blood flow toward the end organ. If the end organ has other sources of circulation (whether native or collateral), then the aneurysm can be totally occluded. This exclusion can be done either open with surgical ligation or endovascular with embolization. If the end organ does not have other sources of circulation (whether native or collateral), then the aneurysmal artery must be preserved while excluding the aneurysm, either by open bypass or endovascular stent graft placement.

Thus, the functional and anatomic factors that modify treatment strategies are:

- Hemodynamic stability on presentation
- Location of the aneurysm
- Status of the native artery proximal and distal to the aneurysm
- Presence of other chronic comorbidities and/or active unrelated medical issues
- Institute and/or surgeon expertise in either modality
- Status of the abdominal cavity: virgin versus hostile abdomen

**Table 1**
Guidelines for indication for intervention according to the Society for Vascular Surgery guideline

| Location | Indication for intervention | Level of recommendation | Quality of evidence |
|---|---|---|---|
| Renal artery | >3 cm | Grade 2 (weak) | C (low) |
| | Symptomatic or ruptured | Grade 1 (strong) | B (moderate) |
| | Childbearing woman regardless of size | Grade 2 (weak) | B (moderate) |
| | Refractory hypertension regardless of size | Grade 2 (weak) | C (low) |
| Splenic artery | Ruptured | Grade 1 (strong) | A (high) |
| | Pseudoaneurysm regardless of size | Grade 1 (strong) | B (moderate) |
| | Childbearing woman regardless of size | Grade 1 (strong) | B (moderate) |
| | >3 cm | Grade 1 (strong) | C (low) |
| Celiac artery | Ruptured | Grade 1 (strong) | A (high) |
| | Pseudoaneurysm regardless of size | Grade 1 (strong) | B (moderate) |
| | >2 cm with increased in size or with symptoms | Grade 1 (strong) | C (low) |
| Gastric or gastroepiploic artery | Any size, any presentation | Grade 1 (strong) | B (moderate) |
| HA | Pseudoaneurysm regardless of size | Grade 1 (strong) | A (high) |
| | Symptomatic | Grade 1 (strong) | A (high) |
| | >2 cm, no comorbidities | Grade 1 (strong) | A (high) |
| | >5 cm, significant comorbidities | Grade 1 (strong) | B (moderate) |
| | Vasculopathy or vasculitis regardless of size | Grade 1 (strong) | C (low) |
| | Positive blood culture regardless of size | Grade 1 (strong) | C (low) |
| Superior mesenteric artery | Any size, any presentation | Grade 1 (strong) | A (high) |
| | Dissection with refractory symptoms | Grade 2 (weak) | B (moderate) |
| Jejunal, ileal, or colic artery | >2 cm: jejunal/ileal<br>Any size for colic | Grade 1 (strong) | B (moderate) |
| | Symptomatic, ruptured, any pseudoaneurysm | Grade 1 (strong) | A (high) |
| PDA or GDA | Any size, any presentation | Grade 1 (strong) | B (moderate) |

Placed in order as reported in the original article.

The SVS practice guidelines on the management of visceral aneurysms provided some guidelines on the choice of intervention, as summarized in Table 2.

## SURGICAL AND ENDOVASCULAR TECHNIQUES

### Splenic artery aneurysm

For the open approach, the traditional approach for proximal and middle portion of the splenic artery has been ligation of the artery and/or aneurysmectomy with end-to-end repair. For the distal portion of the artery or hilar

**Table 2**
Guidelines for preferred modality of intervention according to the Society for Vascular Surgery guideline

| Location/presentation | Method of intervention | Level of recommendation | Quality of evidence |
|---|---|---|---|
| Renal artery | | | |
| Good surgical candidate | Open reconstructive technique | Grade 2 (weak) | B (moderate) |
| Distal branch aneurysm | Ex vivo repair with autotransplant | Grade 2 (weak) | B (moderate) |
| Poor surgical candidate | Stent graft for main artery<br>Embolization for distal branches | Grade 2 (weak) | B (moderate) |
| Splenic artery | | | |
| Ruptured: discovered intraoperatively | Ligation, without splenectomy | Grade 2 (weak) | B (moderate) |
| Ruptured: discovered preoperatively | Open or endovascular<br>Depending on presentation | Grade 2 (weak) | B (moderate) |
| Nonruptured, elective | Endovascular primarily<br>Open splenectomy if needed later<br>No need for revascularization | Grade 2 (weak) | B (moderate) |
| Distal/hilum aneurysm | Open surgical technique with possible splenectomy | Grade 2 (weak) | C (low) |
| Pregnant women/ regardless of size | Individualized per each case | NA | NA |
| Celiac artery | | | |
| Ruptured: discovered intraoperatively | Ligation if sufficient collateral documented | Grade 2 (weak) | C (low) |
| Ruptured: discovered preoperatively | Open or endovascular<br>Depending on presentation | Grade 1 (strong) | B (moderate) |
| Nonruptured, elective | Endovascular primarily<br>Open if needed later<br>Evaluate SMA, GDA* status preoperatively | Grade 2 (weak) | B (moderate) |
| Gastric or gastroepiploic artery | | | |
| Regardless | Endovascular embolization | Grade 1 (strong) | B (moderate) |
| HA | | | |
| Extrahepatic | Endovascular or open<br>Whichever preserves liver circulation | Grade 1 (strong) | A (high) |
| Intrahepatic | Endovascular embolization | Grade 1 (strong) | B (moderate) |
| Intrahepatic, large aneurysm | Liver resection of affected lobe | Grade 1 (strong) | C (low) |
| SMA | | | |
| Regardless | Endovascular approach if feasible | Grade 1 (strong) | B (moderate) |

(*continued on next page*)

**Table 2**
***(continued)***

| Location/presentation | Method of intervention | Level of recommendation | Quality of evidence |
|---|---|---|---|
| Jejunal, ileal, or colic artery | | | |
| Abdominal hematoma or possible bowel ischemia | Open ligation or aneurysm excision | Grade 2 (weak) | B (moderate) |
| Nonruptured, elective | Endovascular embolization | Grade 2 (weak) | B (moderate) |
| Polyarteritis nodosa | Medical treatment | Grade 2 (weak) | B (moderate) |
| PDA or GDA | | | |
| Intact/ruptured | Endovascular embolization | Grade 1 (strong) | B (moderate) |
| Embolization fails | Covered stent or stent-assisted embolization | Grade 2 (weak) | C (low) |
| Concomitant stenosis or occlusion | Open celiac reconstruction | Grade 2 (weak) | B (moderate) |

Placed in order as reported in the original article.
*Abbreviation:* NA, not available.

branches, splenectomy has been the traditional approach. Reconstruction of the splenic artery is usually not warranted, especially for proximal and middle-portion aneurysms, because of the excellent collateral circulation via the short gastric arteries. Splenectomy is usually performed for ruptured aneurysms or for distal aneurysms, as mentioned earlier.

Endovascular options to address splenic aneurysms include stent grafting across the aneurysm, coil embolization of the sac, and coil embolization of both ends of the splenic artery, thus rendering the aneurysm excluded. Although arterial tortuosity can be an asset in open reconstruction, it can pose an anatomic challenge when deploying a stent graft because they are difficult to track across tortuous arterial segments. Bare mental stents can be a good alternative in this case, with good success [13]. The mechanism of bare metal stents is to alter the flow inside the aneurysm into laminal flow, resulting in thrombus formation within the aneurysm as soon as 1 month after insertion [14].

## Hepatic artery aneurysm

Both open (ligation) and endovascular (embolization) occlusion of intrahepatic artery aneurysms can be done if the portal vein is confirmed to be patent [15,16].

Similarly, for extrahepatic aneurysms, occlusion of the common HA yields no significant consequences if the GDA is patent. In contrast, occlusion of the proper HA is poorly tolerated [17]. Proper HA aneurysms require either open reconstruction or endovascular stent graft to preserve the antegrade flow (Fig. 1).

For intrahepatic aneurysms, endovascular means have been preferable, including coil embolization, glue, and/or stents (Fig. 2).

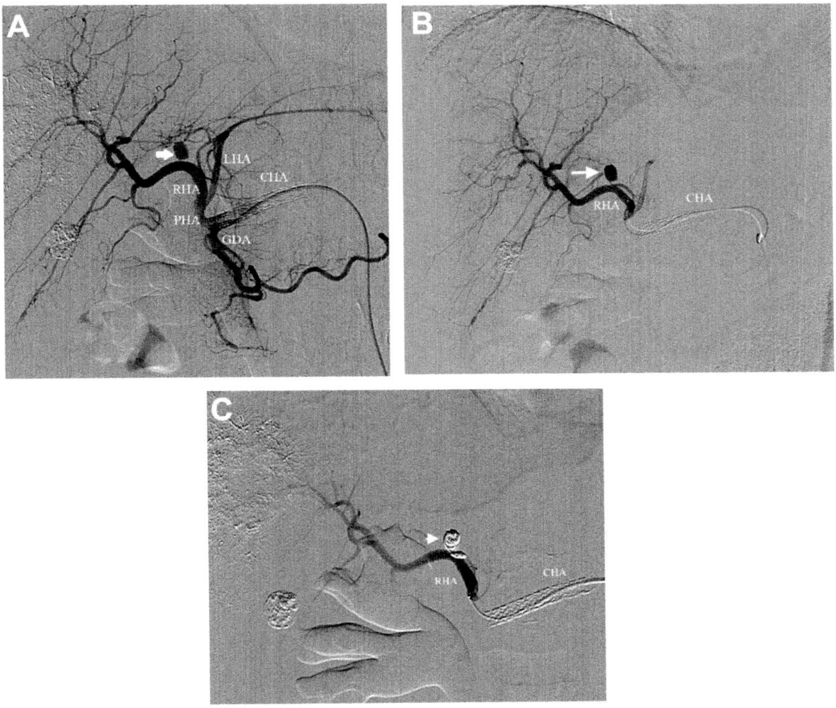


**Fig. 1.** Right HA aneurysm (*white arrow*) treated with coiling. This patient had prior common HA aneurysm that was treated with stent graft. (*A*) selective catherization of the common HA with catheter placed within the prior stent. (*B*) Selective catherization of the right HA. (*C*) Successful coiling of the aneurysm (*arrowhead*). CHA, common HA; PHA, proper HA; LHA, left HA; RHA, right HA. (Printed with permission from Husameddin El Khudari, MD, Division of Interventional Radiology, University of Alabama at Birmingham).

## Superior mesenteric artery aneurysm

Specific to the SMA aneurysm, close attention should be paid to ruling out an infectious cause and possible mycotic aneurysm. If mycotic aneurysm is suspected, open surgical reconstruction with autogenous conduit is preferable.

Endovascular methods of stent grafting are usually recommended for aneurysm or dissection of the proximal SMA, contingent on the presence of favorable anatomy of the proximal and distal native artery. If an endovascular approach is chosen for a mycotic SMA aneurysm, it is recommended to treat with broad-spectrum antibiotics before procedures [6] (Fig. 3).

If an open approach is selected based on unfavorable anatomy (such as extensive involvement of the SMA branches), the options are a simple ligation, aneurysmorrhaphy, and/or arterial bypass using a synthetic graft. If mycotic aneurysm is suspected, greater saphenous vein can be used as a conduit instead.

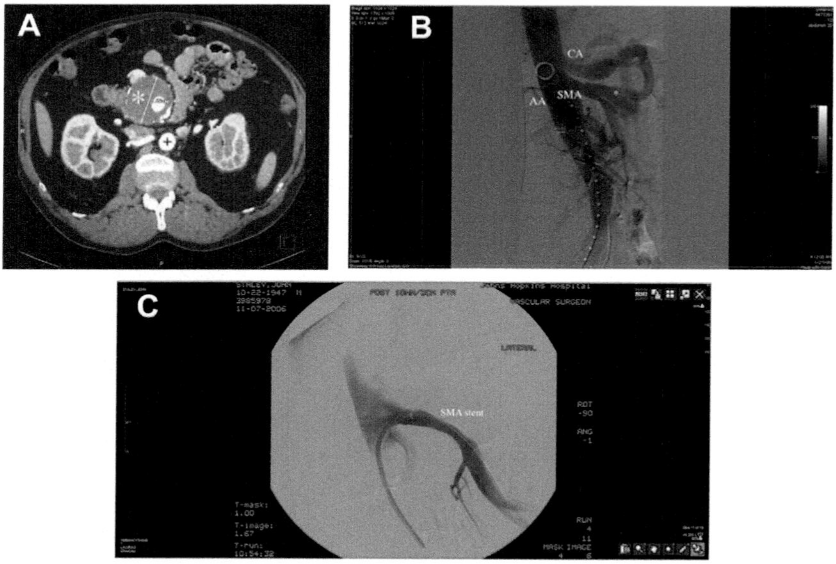


**Fig. 2.** SMA aneurysm treated with stent graft. (*A*) Preoperative cross-sectional computed tomography showing the infrarenal aorta (*black cross*) and the aneurysm sac (*white asterisk*). (*B*) Nonselective aortogram, lateral view, showing the aneurysm sac (*white asterisk*). (*C*) Selective catheterization of the SMA with deployment of stent graft. AA, abdominal aorta; CA, celiac artery. (Courtesy of James H. Black, III, MD, FACS).

*Celiac artery aneurysms*

Ligation of an aneurysmal celiac artery can be done if there are collaterals from the SMA, PDA, and/or GDA to preserve the hepatic circulation [18,19]. If ligation is determined not to be safe, the standard reconstruction is aortoceliac bypass using synthetic graft. The most common endovascular approach to aneurysm of the celiac axis is coil embolization, with stent grafting usually limited by the involvement of the celiac bifurcation and the obligate loss of the splenic artery if the distal stent extends to the common HA.

## Pancreaticoduodenal and gastroduodenal artery aneurysms

Because of the challenge to surgically expose and ligate the GDA and PDA, the endovascular approach is strongly favored for both ruptured and intact aneurysms.

Endovascular methods include coil embolization, glue embolization, and/or plugs. Close postprocedure imaging should be followed to rule out sac reperfusion. Chances of sac reperfusion are higher in this location because of the multiple feeding branches of the PDA and GDA, with some investigators advocating mandatory repeat angiography weeks to months later [15] (Fig. 4).

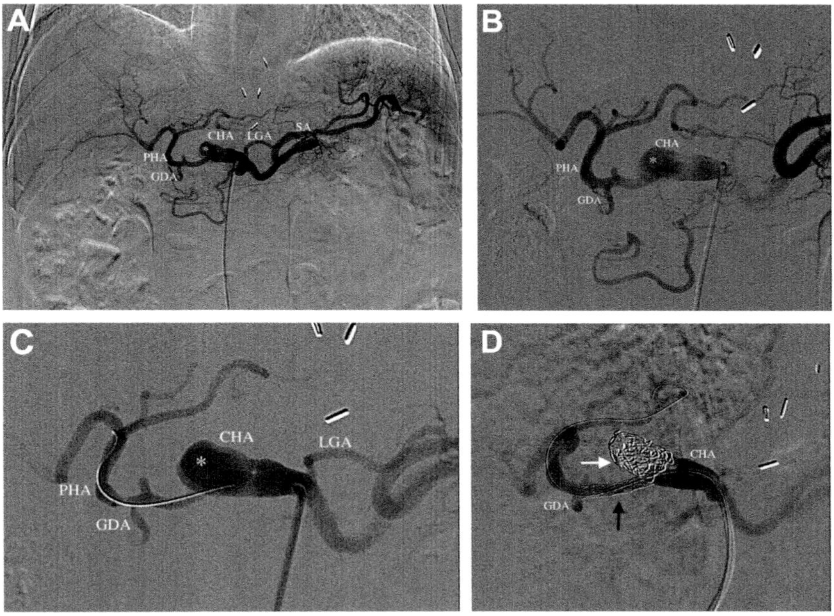


**Fig. 3.** CHA aneurysm (*white asterisk*) treated with stent-assisted coiling. (*A*) Selective catherization of the origin of the celiac artery. (*B*) Selective catherization of the CHA. (*C*) Wire positioning in the distal PHA. (*D*) Stent placed in the CHA (*black arrow*), followed by coil embolization of the aneurysm (*white arrow*). SA, splenic artery; LGA, left gastric artery. (Printed with permission from Husameddin El Khudari, MD, Division of Interventional Radiology, University of Alabama at Birmingham).

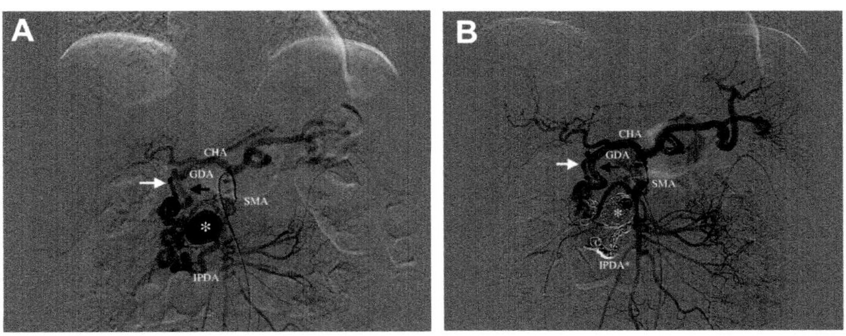


**Fig. 4.** PDA aneurysm (*white asterisk*) treated with coil embolization via the SMA. (*A*) Selective catherization of the SMA. Some of the celiac artery branches are filling contrast through extensive collaterals: anterior superior PDA (*black arrow*), posterior superior PDA (*white arrow*), and inferior PDA. (*B*) Successful coil embolization of aneurysm (*white asterisk*) and the main feeding branch. IPDA, inferior PDA; IPDA*, coiled inferior PDA. (Printed with permission from Husameddin El Khudari, MD, Division of Interventional Radiology, University of Alabama at Birmingham).

### Gastric/gastroepiploic artery aneurysms

If found electively, the preferable approach is endovascular. However, because most of those aneurysms present with rupture [20], they are usually found intraoperatively during a laparotomy. When found intraoperatively, the treatment of choice is ligation without the need for further reconstruction (Figs. 5 and 6).

### Jejunal, ileal, and colic artery aneurysms

Depending on their location and presentation, those aneurysms can either be fixed with surgical ligation or endovascular embolization. With either approach, there is slightly higher chance for subsequent small or large bowel ischemia. Segmental small bowel resection or colectomy may be needed or second-look laparotomy to ensure the distal bowel remains viable.

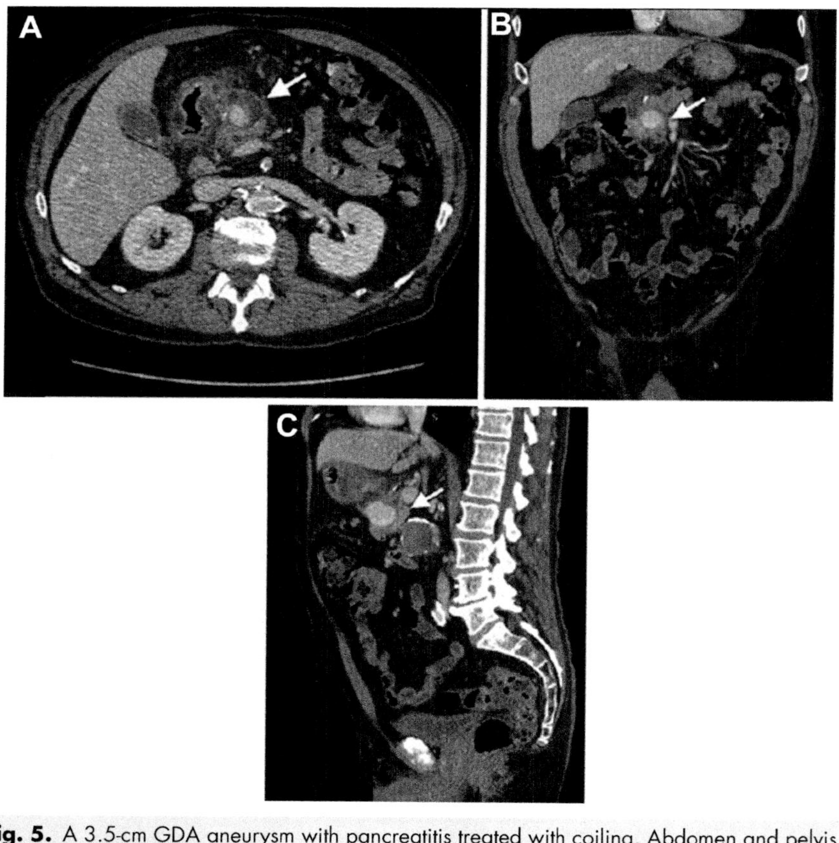


**Fig. 5.** A 3.5-cm GDA aneurysm with pancreatitis treated with coiling. Abdomen and pelvis computed tomography scan with intravenous contrast. The GDA aneurysm (*white arrow*) abutting the posterior stomach wall with significant fat stranding. (*A*) Cross-sectional plane, (*B*) coronal plane, (*C*) sagittal plane. (Reprinted with permission from Zuhaili *and colleagues* 2017).

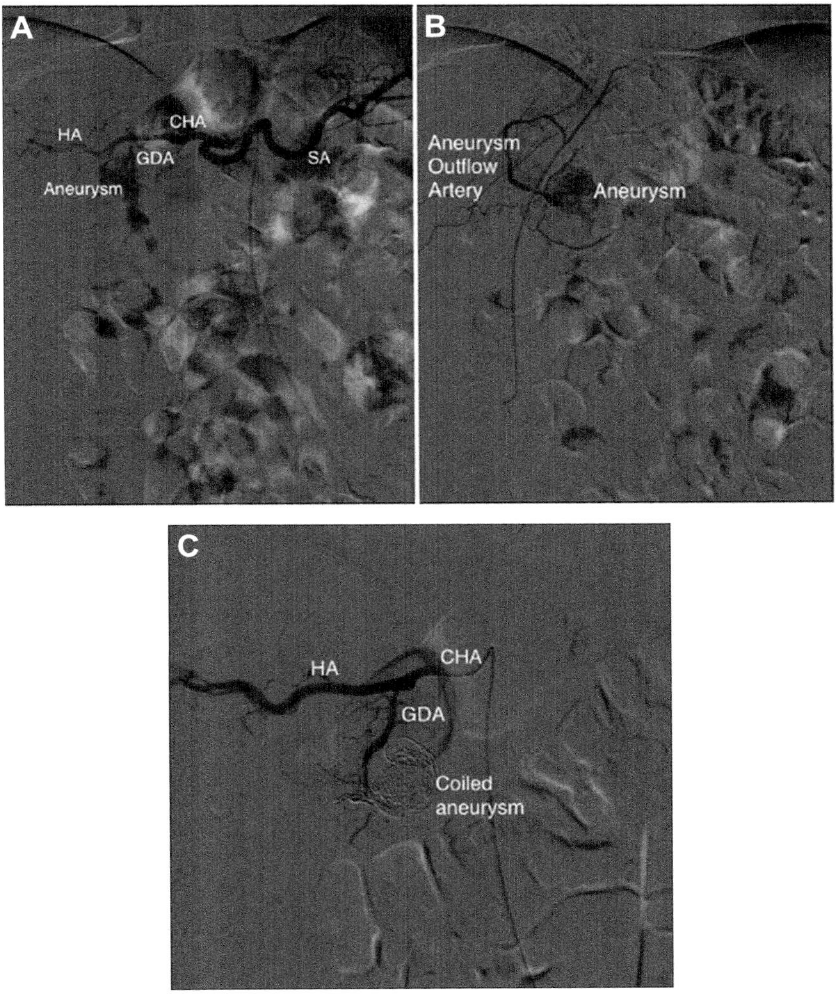


**Fig. 6.** A 3.5-cm GDA aneurysm with pancreatitis treated with coiling. Mesenteric angiogram, (*A*) precoiling selective catheterization of the celiac artery. Note the GDA filling the aneurysm. (*B*) Selective catheterization of the GDA. (*C*) Mesenteric angiogram, postcoiling. Selective catheterization of the CHA. Note absence of flow in the coiled GDA aneurysm. . (Reprinted with permission from Zuhaili *and colleagues* 2017).

## Renal artery aneurysms

For nonruptured renal aneurysms, the main factor to decide between endovascular versus open approach is the native arterial anatomy. If there is a sufficient landing zone proximally and distally, a stent graft can be used safely. For saccular aneurysm with narrow neck, coil embolization can be used. Aneurysmorrhaphy can be used for localized saccularlike aneurysms. Otherwise, bypass with either greater saphenous vein or internal iliac artery has been proved to be a durable option [21] (Figs. 7 and 8).

## COMPLICATIONS/LONG-TERM OUTCOMES

There are no statistically significant differences in mortality between endovascular and open approaches. Morbidities vary among many different reports [22]. Barrionuevo and colleagues [23] published a meta-analysis that included any study with 10 or more patients with treated VAA. A total of 80 studies are included in this quantitative analysis. Outcomes of interest include mortality, rupture of aneurysm, wound infection, need for reintervention, coil migration, target organ ischemia/infarction, myocardial infarction, stroke, pulmonary

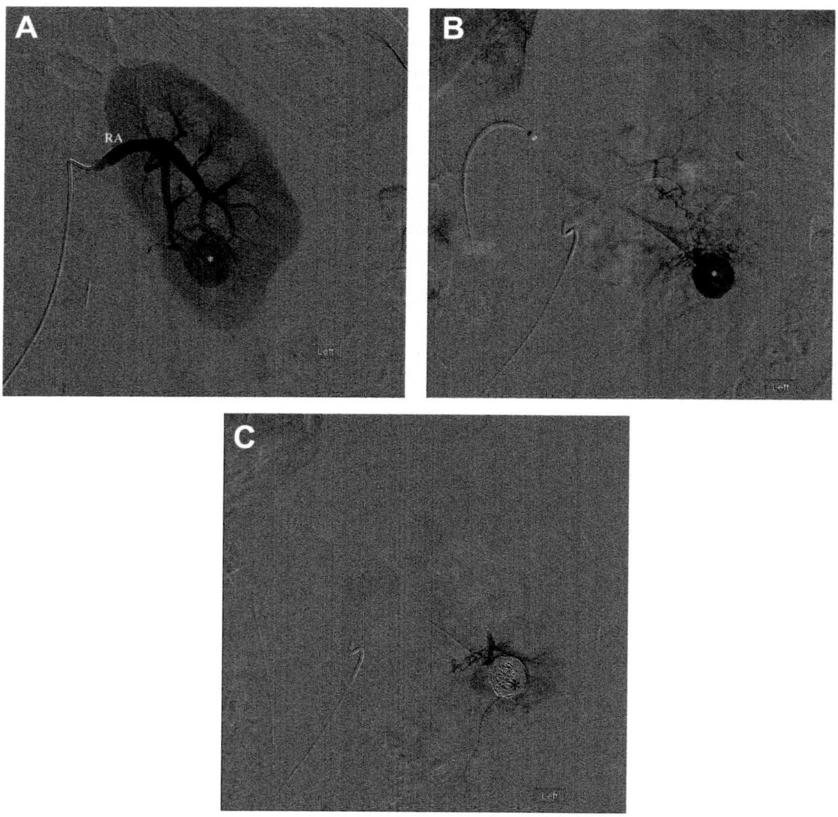


**Fig. 7.** Left renal artery aneurysm (*white asterisk*) treated with coil embolization. (*A*) Selective catherization of the left renal artery. (*B*) Selective catherization of the aneurysm. (*C*) Coil embolization of the aneurysm (*black asterisk*) with absence of flow. RA, renal artery. (Printed with permission from Husameddin El Khudari, MD, Division of Interventional Radiology, University of Alabama at Birmingham).

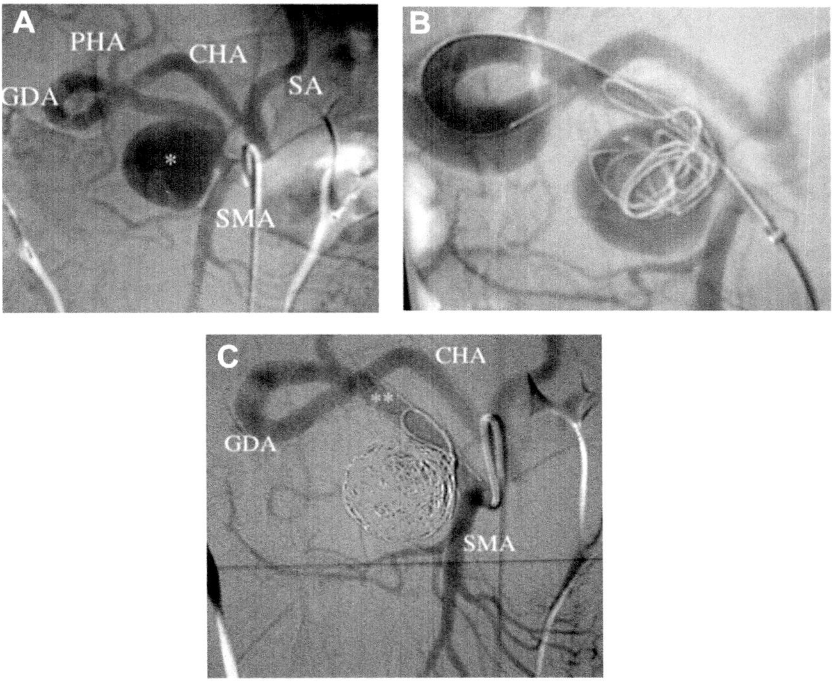


**Fig. 8.** GDA (*white asterisk*) treated with stent-assisted coiling. In this patient, the GDA was uncommonly dominant, because of the chronic celiac artery occlusion. Also note the aneurysm direct connection to the SMA versus other GDA aneurysms, which are usually supplied by both pancreaticoduodenal arcades. (*A*) Selective catheterization of the SMA with retrograde filling of the main branches of the occluded celiac trunk. (*B*) Attempted embolization of the sac resulted in the coils dislodged in the main lumen, which necessitated the deployment of stent graft. (*C*) Deployment of stent graft (*double white asterisks*) with successful coil embolization of the aneurysm. (Courtesy of James H. Black, III, MD, FACS).

embolism, deep venous thrombosis, respiratory complications, and gastrointestinal complications. Although the meta-analysis reports that "numerous complications are more likely to occur with the open approach," there is no statistically significant difference in mortality between the 2 approaches, leading to "possible equipoise" between the 2 approaches.

Endovascular methods to address splenic artery aneurysm have been very successful. Coil embolization success rates are between 90% and 100% [24]. Stent graft success rate achieved similar high rates as well [25].

The main side effect to anticipate with coil embolization is splenic infarct. Splenic infarct rates after embolization vary from 5% to 20% in certain studies [26] up to 40% in other studies [27]. Regardless, splenic infarcts are treated with pain control in almost all cases and splenectomy is rarely needed.

In treatment of HA aneurysm, endovascular methods are successful in more than 90% of nonruptured cases [28]. Even among ruptured HA aneurysm, the success rate remained around 75% [16]. Reintervention for HA aneurysm is as high as 30% to 40% [28]. The other, fairly rare, complication related to endovascular approach is liver infarction, most appreciated when either the portal vein or GDA is occluded. The open approach to HA aneurysm is associated with 20% to 30% complication rate, including graft thrombosis, bile leak, ileus, and/or postoperative abscess [15]. Similar to the splenic artery aneurysm, the meta-analysis by Barrionuevo and colleagues [23] showed no significant statistical difference in short-term and long-term mortality between the two approaches.

For SMA aneurysm with an open approach, the perioperative mortality is similar to the endovascular approach. The major exception is for the open approach for a ruptured aneurysm, in which case the mortality can be as high as 37% [29].

The endovascular approach to celiac aneurysms is successful 89% of the time [15]. Liver ischemia after coil embolization does not happen often, especially when there are enough collaterals from the SMA, PDA, and/or GDA [18,19]. Other reported complications of endovascular treatment of celiac aneurysm are liver cirrhosis deterioration, gastric ulcers, gangrenous cholecystitis, and/or liver abscess [30].

## LONG-TERM RECOMMENDATIONS

Follow-up for patients managed with observation entails annual imaging. Depending on the patient age, aneurysm size, and location, this can be spread out to every 2 to 3 years [12]. Repaired aneurysms warrant more frequent follow-up in the first 3 to 6 months, eventually extending to annual imaging, especially for visceral and renal aneurysm managed by endovascular methods. Embolized aneurysms can rupture after occult reperfusion [31]. This reperfusion is related to either incomplete thrombosis in the periprocedure period or change in the pressure dynamic transmitted through the thrombus [32]. The authors' standard protocol for both endovascular and open repair is to obtain imaging at 1 month, 6 months, 12 months, and then annually afterward.

## NEW DEVELOPMENTS

At present, most VAAs are treated with endovascular methods as the first-line modality. There have been steady advances in endovascular methods to facilitate treatment [33]:

- Balloon-assisted coiling: involves temporary inflation of a balloon while packing the aneurysm sac with coiling. This method helps by occluding the artery in case of rupture. Also, it facilitates more dense deployment of the coils inside the sac, especially in a wide-neck aneurysm [34]. Available commercial kits used for this purpose are TransForm Occlusion Balloon Catheter (Stryker Neurovascular, Fremont, CA), Scepter (Microvention, Irvine, CA), HyperForm and HyperGlide, and Ascent Balloon (Micrus Endovascular Corp, San Jose, CA).
- Stent-assisted coiling: there have been multiple new stents to assist in deployment of coils in wide-neck aneurysms. The stents can take different forms and

configurations, including T, Y, and X shapes. Examples of these include PulseRider (Pulsar Vascular, Inc, Los Gatos, CA), Low-Profile Visualized Intraluminal Support, Neuroform Atlas Stent (Stryker Neurovascular), and Barrel vascular reconstruction device (Medtronic/Covidien, Irvine, CA).

- Changes in coil characteristics: there have been significant advances in coil properties. Example include:
  - Coil length: the length has increased from the standard few centimeters to the recent addition of 60-cm coils.
  - Coil shape: this has progressed from two-dimensional helical shape to 360° or three-dimensional configurations.
  - Coil stiffness: ranging from superstiff for frame building to regular soft or supersoft, with the newest addition of Nanos, which are used to finish small residual spaces or small aneurysms.
  - Coil coating: existing coatings include polyglycolic/polylactic acid Cerecyte coil, and Matrix detachable coil. New additions have been proposed to increase the thrombotic effect of the coil within the aneurysm sac. One recent example is the second generation of Hydrogel coils containing platinum and hydrophilic acrylic copolymer. So far, they have been used with promising result in cerebral aneurysms only [35,36].

## CLINICS CARE POINTS

- Any ruptured aneurysm should be repaired emergently. The decision to repair with endovascular or open methods depends on multiple factors and is individualized to the patient.
- The following aneurysms should be repaired electively on identification regardless of size: gastric or gastroepiploic artery, SMA, colic artery, PDA, and GDA.
- The following aneurysms should be repaired electively on identification in childbearing women, regardless of size: renal artery and splenic artery.

## References

[1] Zuhaili B, Molnar RG, Malhotra NG. The endovascular management of a 3.5-cm gastroduodenal artery aneurysm presenting with gastritis and recurrent pancreatitis. Avicenna J Med 2017;7(3):130–2.

[2] Messina LM, Shanley CJ. Visceral artery aneurysms. Surg Clin North Am 1997;77(2):425–42.

[3] Ferrero E, Viazzo A, Ferri M, et al. Management and urgent repair of ruptured visceral artery aneurysms. Ann Vasc Surg 2011;25(7); https://doi.org/10.1016/j.avsg.2011.02.041.

[4] Gehlen JM, Heeren PA, Verhagen PF, et al. Visceral artery aneurysms. Vasc Endovascular Surg 2011;45(8):681–7.

[5] Ehtuish EF, Mishra A. Multiple visceral aneurysms in antiphospholipid antibody syndrome - an unusual presentation. Br J Radiol 2008;81(967):e184–7.

[6] Brown SL, Busuttil RW, Baker JD, et al. Bacteriologic and surgical determinants of survival in patients with mycotic aneurysms. J Vasc Surg 1984;1(4):541–7.

[7] Pilleul F, Beuf O. Diagnosis of splanchnic artery aneurysms and pseudoaneurysms, with special reference to contrast enhanced 3D magnetic resonance angiography: a review. Acta Radiol 2004;45(7):702–8.
[8] Eckhauser FE, Stanley JC, Zelenock GB, et al. Gastroduodenal and pancreaticoduodenal artery aneurysms: a complication of pancreatitis causing spontaneous gastrointestinal hemorrhage. Surgery 1980;88(3):335–44.
[9] Abbas MA, Stone WM, Fowl RJ, et al. Splenic artery aneurysms: two decades experience at Mayo clinic. Ann Vasc Surg 2002;16(4):442–9.
[10] Nishida O, Moriyasu F, Nakamura T, et al. Hemodynamics of splenic artery aneurysm. Gastroenterology 1986;90(4):1042–6.
[11] Carr SC, Pearce WH, Vogelzang RL, et al. Current management of visceral artery aneurysms. Surgery 1996;120(4):627–34.
[12] Chaer RA, Abularrage CJ, Coleman DM, et al. The Society for Vascular Surgery clinical practice guidelines on the management of visceral aneurysms. J Vasc Surg 2020;72(1S): 3S–39S.
[13] Cordova AC, Sumpio BE. Visceral Artery Aneurysms and Pseudoaneurysms—Should They All be Managed by Endovascular Techniques? Ann Vasc Dis 2013;6(4):687–93.
[14] Ruffino M, Rabbia C, Italian Cardiatis Registry Investigators Group. Endovascular treatment of visceral artery aneurysms with Cardiatis multilayer flow modulator: preliminary results at six-month follow-up. J Cardiovasc Surg (Torino) 2011;52(3):311–21.
[15] Sachdev U, Baril DT, Ellozy SH, et al. Management of aneurysms involving branches of the celiac and superior mesenteric arteries: a comparison of surgical and endovascular therapy. J Vasc Surg 2006;44(4):718–24.
[16] Kasirajan K, Greenberg RK, Clair D, et al. Endovascular management of visceral artery aneurysm. J Endovasc Ther 2001;8(2):150–5.
[17] Berceli SA. Hepatic and splenic artery aneurysms. Semin Vasc Surg 2005;18(4):196–201.
[18] Wagner WH, Allins AD, Treiman RL, et al. Ruptured visceral artery aneurysms. Ann Vasc Surg 1997;11(4):342–7.
[19] Graham LM, Stanley JC, Whitehouse WM Jr, et al. Celiac artery aneurysms: historic (1745-1949) versus contemporary (1950-1984) differences in etiology and clinical importance. J Vasc Surg 1985;2(5):757–64.
[20] Stanley JC, Wakefield TW, Graham LM, et al. Clinical importance and management of splanchnic artery aneurysms. J Vasc Surg 1986;3(5):836–40.
[21] Murray SP, Kent C, Salvatierra O, et al. Complex branch renovascular disease: management options and late results. J Vasc Surg 1994;20(3):338–46.
[22] Sessa C, Tinelli G, Porcu P, et al. Treatment of visceral artery aneurysms: description of a retrospective series of 42 aneurysms in 34 patients. Ann Vasc Surg 2004;18(6):695–703.
[23] Barrionuevo P, Malas MB, Nejim B, et al. A systematic review and meta-analysis of the management of visceral artery aneurysms. J Vasc Surg 2019;70(5):1694–9.
[24] Gabelmann A, Görich J, Merkle EM. Endovascular treatment of visceral artery aneurysms. J Endovasc Ther 2002;9(1):38–47.
[25] Tulsyan N, Kashyap VS, Greenberg RK, et al. The endovascular management of visceral artery aneurysms and pseudoaneurysms. J Vasc Surg 2007;45(2):276–83.
[26] Loffroy R, Guiu B, Cercueil JP, et al. Transcatheter arterial embolization of splenic artery aneurysms and pseudoaneurysms: short- and long-term results. Ann Vasc Surg 2008;22(5): 618–26.
[27] Piffaretti G, Tozzi M, Lomazzi C, et al. Splenic artery aneurysms: postembolization syndrome and surgical complications. Am J Surg 2007;193(2):166–70.
[28] Huang YK, Hsieh HC, Tsai FC, et al. Visceral artery aneurysm: risk factor analysis and therapeutic opinion. Eur J Vasc Endovasc Surg 2007;33(3):293–301.
[29] Stone WM, Abbas M, Cherry KJ, et al. Superior mesenteric artery aneurysms: is presence an indication for intervention? J Vasc Surg 2002;36(2):234–7.

[30] Leon LR Jr, Mills JL Sr, Jordan W, et al. The risks of celiac artery coverage during endoluminal repair of thoracic and thoracoabdominal aortic aneurysms. Vasc Endovascular Surg 2009;43(1):51–60.
[31] Onohara T, Okadome K, Mii S, et al. Rupture of embolised coeliac artery pseudoaneurysm into the stomach: is coil embolisation an effective treatment for coeliac anastomotic pseudoaneurysm? Eur J Vasc Surg 1992;6(3):330–2.
[32] Schwartz RA, Nichols WK, Silver D. Is thrombosis of the infrarenal abdominal aortic aneurysm an acceptable alternative? J Vasc Surg 1986;3(3):448–55.
[33] Campos JK, Lien BV, Wang AS, et al. Advances in endovascular aneurysm management: coiling and adjunctive devices. Stroke Vasc Neurol 2020;5(1):14–21.
[34] Moret J, Cognard C, Weill A, et al. The "Remodelling Technique" in the Treatment of Wide Neck Intracranial Aneurysms. Angiographic Results and Clinical Follow-up in 56 Cases. Interv Neuroradiol 1997;3(1):21–35.
[35] Abi-Aad KR, Aoun RJN, Rahme RJ, et al. New generation Hydrogel Endovascular Aneurysm Treatment Trial (HEAT): a study protocol for a multicenter randomized controlled trial. Neuroradiology 2018;60(10):1075–84.
[36] Taschner CA, Chapot R, Costalat V, et al. Second-Generation Hydrogel Coils for the Endovascular Treatment of Intracranial Aneurysms: A Randomized Controlled Trial. Stroke 2018;49(3):667–74.

Advances in Surgery 55 (2021) 75–87
ADVANCES IN SURGERY

# Mesenteric Ischemia
## When and How to Revascularize

Kristofor A. Olson, MD, PhD, Pedro G. Teixeira, MD*
Department of Surgery and Perioperative Care, The University of Texas at Austin Dell Medical School, 1500 Red River Street, Annex, Austin, TX 78701, USA

**Keywords**
• Acute mesenteric ischemia • Chronic mesenteric ischemia
• Non occlusive mesenteric ischemia (NOMI) • Mesenteric venous thrombosis
• Surgical revascularization • Endovascular techniques • Surgical bypass

**Key points**

- Mesenteric ischemia requires a high index of suspicion, and prompt surgical intervention is indicated to improve mortality.
- Revascularization should be performed early, with only frankly necrotic or perforated bowel resected.
- Open revascularization approaches remain the gold standard for the treatment of acute mesenteric ischemia, while endovascular approaches have gained favor for chronic disease.

## INTRODUCTION

Mesenteric ischemia occurs from hypoperfusion to the gut mucosa. The etiologies are multifactorial, and while progress has been made in efforts to revascularize over the past 20 years, the acute forms of the disease still portend a 30% to 70% mortality rate. As an ailment predominately of the elderly, the presence of underlying medical comorbidities often confounds and delays diagnosis, contributing to the high mortality of this disease. In this article, we discuss the diagnosis and management of acute and chronic mesenteric ischemia, recent developments in open and endovascular revascularization techniques, approach considerations, and pitfalls.

The authors have nothing to disclose.

*Corresponding author. *E-mail address:* pgteixeira@austin.utexas.edu

https://doi.org/10.1016/j.yasu.2021.05.006
0065-3411/21/

**Table 1**
The four "R's" of mesenteric ischemia management [9]

| | |
|---|---|
| Resuscitation | Fluid resuscitation to restore perfusion to bowel mucosa, crystalloid or colloid. |
| Rapid diagnosis | High index of suspicion, CT angiography |
| Early revascularization | Open vs endovascular approaches, as discussed in the following sections |
| Reassessment | Second-look laparotomy or laparoscopy depending on initial approach to evaluate bowel viability after revascularization. |



## ANATOMY

The vascular supply to the gut is derived from the aorta via the celiac artery, superior mesenteric artery (SMA), and inferior mesenteric arteries. Collateralization is dense within the arcades of the mesentery, and anastomoses between these vessels reinforce the blood supply. The major anastomoses between the celiac and SMA are via the pancreaticoduodenal arteries. The inferior and superior mesenteric arteries anastomose via the marginal artery of Drummond and the Arc of Riolan. The distal gastrointestinal tract has arterial communication between the inferior mesenteric artery and internal iliac artery via the superior and inferior hemorrhoidal arteries.

## ACUTE MESENTERIC ISCHEMIA

### Epidemiology

Acute mesenteric ischemia (AMI) presents in 0.1 to 1 in 1000 hospital admissions, with a median age at presentation of 74 years [1,2]. As a disease of predominately the elderly, patients with AMI often present with nonspecific symptoms in the setting of multiple medical comorbidities. Diagnosis, however must be prompt as mortality rates of 50% have been reported even with early identification of disease. For patients in the intensive care unit, the 30-day mortality rate is as high as 71% [3].

### Pathogenesis

The mucosal hypoperfusion injury in AMI occurs from four etiologies: arterial embolism, arterial thrombosis, mesenteric venous thrombosis (MVT), and nonocclusive mesenteric ischemia (NOMI). Arterial thromboembolism, commonly originating from the heart and occluding the SMA at variable levels depending on the size of the embolized thrombus, accounts for more than half of cases of AMI [4]. Arterial thrombosis occurs in the setting of chronic atherosclerotic disease, and when combined with arterial thromboembolism, it constitutes the vast majority of AMI. Thrombosis occurs due to dissection of the SMA, either at its ostium or via extension of aortic dissection, or from rupture of atherosclerotic plaque. MVT, specifically, thrombosis of the superior mesenteric vein, is a rare cause of mesenteric ischemia. This decreased venous outflow and subsequent congestion leads to ischemia. NOMI, hypoperfusion of the bowel despite vascular patency, most commonly occurs during critical illness with prolonged or escalating use of vasopressors [5], hypotension, and abdominal compartment syndrome. Irrespective of the etiology, injury occurs via hypoperfusion of the bowel mucosa.

## Clinical presentation

Owing to the affected patient population and baseline medical comorbidities, presenting symptoms for AMI are often nonspecific. Classically, AMI manifests as abdominal pain out of proportion to examination. Clinical suspicion should be high in patients with existing atrial fibrillation, mechanical heart valves, pre-existing peripheral vascular disease, or a history of embolic events. The onset of symptoms is often acute, severe, and rapidly progressing with embolic disease. A more subacute presentation may occur with thrombotic disease. Patients with MVT often present with vague abdominal symptoms, with slow progression over weeks as venous congestion increases. The presentation of NOMI is the most insidious, with patients ranging from asymptomatic to peritonitic [5], and often in the setting of critical illness. Laboratory tests are unreliable for the diagnosis of AMI, and a normal serum lactate does not exclude ischemia [6]. The gold standard imaging modality for diagnosis is CT angiography.

## Management of acute thrombotic or embolic mesenteric ischemia

### *Medical management*

AMI requires prompt diagnosis. Per current World Journal of Emergency Surgery guidelines, "severe abdominal pain out of proportion to physical examination findings should be assumed to be AMI until disproven" [7]. Patients should be evaluated by CT angiography to evaluate the etiology of vascular compromise, receive nasogastric decompression, and begin anticoagulation via heparin drip [8]. Fluid resuscitation should be initiated and broad-spectrum antibiotics started because of mucosal compromise and the possibility of bacterial translocation [9]. Patients with peritonitis require emergent laparotomy, and delay to the operative suite should be minimized (Table 1).

### *Indications for interventions*

The diagnosis of AMI mandates emergent surgical attention. The gold standard of treatment remains an open midline laparotomy. Revascularization should take priority. The alimentary tract should be examined from distal esophagus to rectum with only grossly necrotic or perforated bowel being resected before revascularization [10]. Questionably viable bowel may be observed until revascularization is complete, and subsequently re-evaluated at a second-look laparotomy within 48 hours [6,11].

### *Open versus endovascular revascularization*

While the open approach to revascularization via thromboembolectomy and/or bypass has traditionally been utilized, recent studies have shown some promise with endovascular approaches. No level 1 or level 2 evidence exists comparing the two approaches, however, with the best evidence coming from single-center, retrospective studies. In a review by Lim and colleagues, endovascular strategies resulted in improved short-term morbidity and mortality, decreased overall complication rates (20% vs 38%), and decreased rates and length of bowel resection [11]. These data may be confounded by the severity of patient disease, as patients with overt bowel ischemia, necrosis, or peritonitis were preferentially and appropriately treated by an open approach. Nonetheless, endovascular therapy may be preferable in a subset of patients. An algorithm proposed by Zhao and colleagues suggests that patients without peritonitis, with suitable anatomy, life expectancy less than 5 years, and poor nutritional status should be considered for endovascular therapy [12]. A hybrid algorithm for managing embolic and thrombotic AMI adapted from the studies by Zhao and Karkkainen is presented in Fig. 1. [12,13]

*Endovascular revascularization*

Anatomic considerations for endovascular treatment include the angle and tortuosity of the SMA, proximal and distal landing zones $\geq$1 cm and without main arterial branch takeoffs, and no peritonitis or intestinal necrosis [12]. In

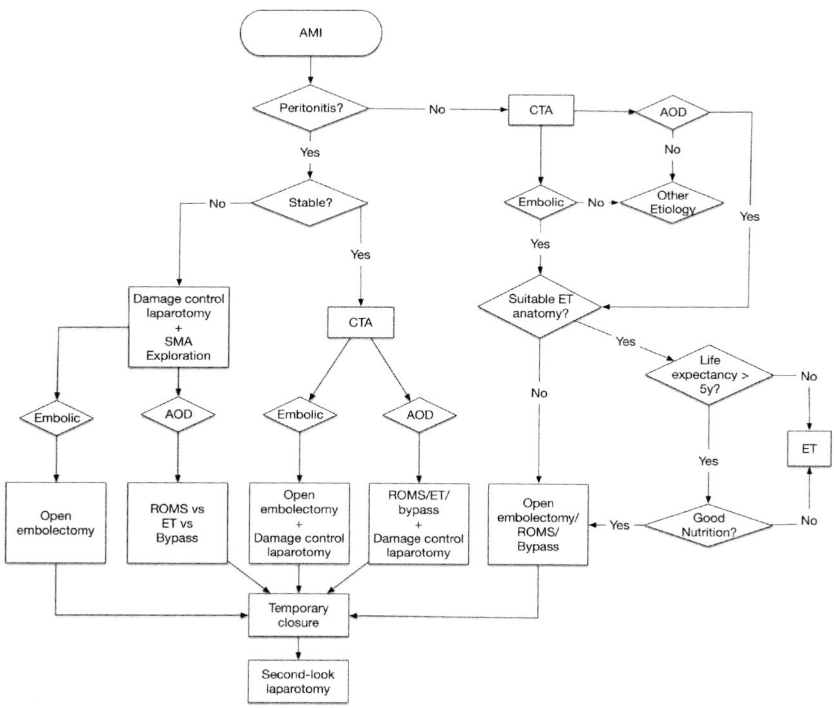


**Fig. 1.** Algorithm for management of acute embolic/thrombotic mesenteric ischemia via open versus endovascular approach [12,13]. AOD, atherosclerotic occlusive disease; CTA, CT angiography; ET, endovascular therapy.

anatomically suitable patients, endovascular access to the SMA can be obtained via either the brachial or femoral approach; however, brachial access is generally preferred owing to the steep angulation of the SMA from a retrograde approach. In general, a 6 French sheath is introduced into the descending aorta, and a guide catheter directed toward the SMA [13]. A hydrophilic guidewire is passed distal to the lesion, and recanalization can be achieved in an antegrade fashion via mechanical thrombectomy or thrombosuction, pharmacologic thrombolysis with urokinase/streptokinase, angioplasty, and stenting (Fig. 2). After initial thrombectomy, in the setting of incomplete resolution of the occlusion or distal showering of thrombus, catheter-directed thrombolysis can be considered to re-establish flow to distal branches. In a small case series, Genzel reports success in revascularization of both the main trunk SMA and its side branches with the use of a steerable sheath [14].

*Open revascularization*

In the setting of a laparotomy, owing to either bowel necrosis requiring resection, surgeon preference, or the lack of access to endovascular expertise, several options exist for revascularization. Access to the SMA is obtained by reflecting the transverse colon cephalad and the small bowel to the patient's right. After dissection through the root of the mesentery and achieving proximal and distal control, a transverse arteriotomy is made distal to the thrombus, and balloon catheters are used to remove proximal clot until pulsatile flow is returned. Smaller diameter balloon catheters are then passed distally to remove any showered clot or fragments. With restoration of pulsatile inflow, retrograde flow, and local heparinization, the arteriotomy is then closed primarily with polypropylene suture. The surgeon may then re-evaluate bowel viability and place a temporary closure device over the abdomen to facilitate further resuscitation and second look laparotomy.

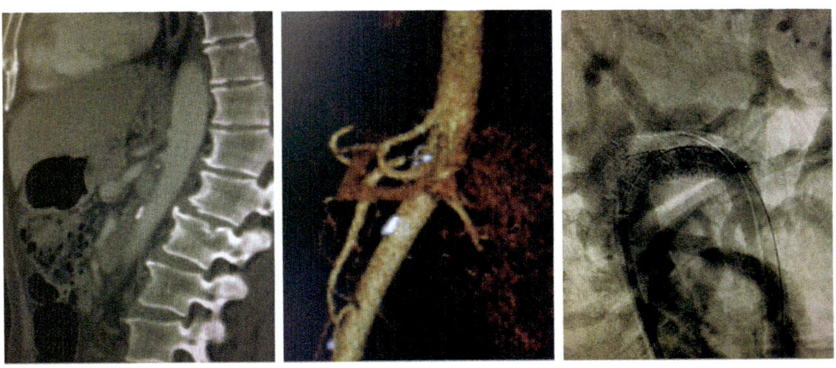

**Fig. 2.** CT angiogram and 3D reconstruction showing near-complete occlusion of the SMA, and angiogram after endovascular stent deployment.

*Open bypass*
In cases of long-segment occlusion, previous endovascular mesenteric stenting, previous bypass, or multivessel disease, open bypass may be required. Bypass may be performed in either an antegrade fashion from the supraceliac aorta or retrograde fashion from the infrarenal aorta or common iliac arteries. Much debate exists on the literature as to which approach is favorable. In the setting of multiple vessel disease such as acute SMA thrombus with both celiac and SMA arteriosclerosis, a branched polytetrafluoroethylene (PTFE) graft may be used to restore antegrade flow to both vessels; however, single-vessel revascularization is usually sufficient in the acute setting [13]. Proximal aortic control is achieved via a transcrural approach of the supraceliac or lower thoracic aorta. Supraceliac clamping and associated renal hypoperfusion may not be desirable in critically ill patients with AMI, and therefore, a retrograde approach from the infrarenal aorta or iliac arteries may be preferred. Saphenous venous conduit and PTFE grafts have both been used with success for retrograde revascularization. The desire to use autologous vein graft in the contaminated abdomen must be weighed against the increased operative time associated with vein harvest and the overall high mortality inherent to this disease process, leading some authors to default to PTFE graft irrespective of contamination [13]. In a single-center study by Scali and colleagues, 82 patients who underwent aortomesenteric bypass between 2002 and 2016 were evaluated for postoperative morbidity and mortality, with comparable outcomes for both the antegrade and retrograde bypass groups [15].

*Antegrade bypass*
Antegrade bypass is performed by mobilizing the left lobe of the liver and dividing the left crus to expose the supraceliac aorta. The SMA is exposed as previously described. After achieving proximal and distal control, an aortotomy is made in an unaffected region of the aorta, and the graft is sewn in an end-to-side fashion. The use of a side-biting clamp can facilitate antegrade aortic flow during construction of the anastomosis [15]. The graft is then tunneled in a retropancreatic plane to reach a disease-free portion of the SMA, where an end-to-side or end-to-end anastomosis is performed. In the setting of multivessel disease, as may be present with acute on chronic mesenteric ischemia, a bifurcated graft may be used with an end-to-end celiac anastomosis or end-to-side hepatic artery anastomosis.

*Retrograde bypass*
While antegrade bypass has been advocated for patients with chronic disease and requiring multivessel revascularization, studies have shown that single-vessel revascularization is sufficient in the setting of acute SMA occlusion [13]. The added complexity of supraceliac aortic exposure with the possibility of renal hypoperfusion due to supraceliac clamping lends some surgeons to prefer a retrograde bypass approach. A location for retrograde inflow is selected on the common or external iliac vessel, depending on ease of dissection and presence of atherosclerotic disease. The SMA is dissected and ligated distal

to disease. Traditionally, the use of a C-shaped graft has been described, with an end-to-side anastomosis at the iliac artery and an end-to-end or end-to-side anastomosis at the SMA.

A direct open retrograde revascularization (DORR) technique has been recently described, where autologous vein graft is anastomosed to the right common iliac in an end-to-side fashion and tunneled directly through the base of the small bowel mesentery via blunt dissection to the SMA [16]. An end-to-side or end-to-end anastomosis is performed distal to the occlusion of the SMA. In situations where both celiac and mesenteric occlusions were present, the SMA anastomosis was performed side-to-side with the vein graft continuing to the hepatic artery for an end-to-side anastomosis. When compared to the antegrade approach, the authors found a shorter operative time (282 vs 375 min) for the DORR method, with otherwise similar outcomes between the two approaches. When compared to the traditional "c-loop" retrograde approach, the DORR method carries hypothetical advantage of reducing the possibility of reintervention due to graft kinking; however, these data have not explicitly been enumerated.

*Retrograde open mesenteric stenting*

A hybrid approach has recently gained increasing traction as an alternative to open bypass in patients not amenable to endovascular therapy because of systemic risk factors, unsuitable anatomy, requirement for damage control laparotomy, or in patients with thrombosis in an area of stenosis [17]. Retrograde open mesenteric stenting (ROMS) is performed as follows. After exposing and achieving proximal and distal control of the SMA, an arteriotomy is made distal to the lesion, and a guidewire and 6 French sheath placed in a retrograde fashion. On-table angiography is performed, and a guidewire traversed proximally across the SMA lesion into the aorta. Balloon-expandable stents are deployed from the ostium to the distal extent of the lesion. With inflow confirmed via angiography, the sheath is removed, and the arteriotomy repaired with polypropylene suture.

A multicenter retrospective review of 54 patients who underwent ROMS for the treatment of acute and chronic mesenteric ischemia revealed patency rates at 2 years of 76%, similar to those of patients receiving percutaneous endovascular therapy. Unfortunately, 30-day mortality remained high in the AMI cohort, with 45% of patients not surviving their hospitalization [18]. Still, ROMS remains an attractive option for patients with atherosclerotic occlusive disease requiring laparotomy without an additional trip to the endovascular suite.

A recent study published by Andraska and colleagues compared ROMS versus open mesenteric bypass in patients with AMI from 2008 to 2019 [19]. At their center, ROMS was performed in a conventional operating room with a C-arm rather than in a hybrid endovascular suite. They found shorter operative times (189 vs 302 minutes), with similar complication, reintervention, and mortality rates to patients receiving open mesenteric bypass. To this end, they recommend ROMS be considered the initial approach to the treatment of AMI [19].

## MANAGEMENT OF MESENTERIC VENOUS THROMBOSIS

### Medical management

Therapeutic anticoagulation is the mainstay of initial treatment for patients with acute MVT [20,21]. Initial therapy with low-molecular-weight heparin bridged to warfarin or an oral anticoagulant is usually sufficient for successful treatment, with better prognosis than patients with embolic or thrombotic disease [22]. Imaging studies should be reviewed to rule out the presence of bowel ischemia. In the face of ischemia or peritonitis, the patient should be taken to the operating room for laparotomy as described for embolic and thrombotic AMI. Patients should remain on anticoagulation from 6 months to lifelong therapy depending on the underlying etiology. Fatal recurrences have been reported in up to 25% of cases [23].

### Indications for interventions

For patients with signs/symptoms of peritonitis or imaging findings concerning for ischemia, operative intervention is required for resection of necrotic bowel. As for embolic and thrombotic AMI, equivocal appearing segments should be left until revascularization is complete and reassessed at second-look laparotomy.

### Open surgical versus endovascular

Little high-quality evidence exists with regard to endovascular versus surgical approaches to MVT [24]. Catheter-directed thrombolysis via the SMA, percutaneous transhepatic thrombectomy, and open embolectomy have all been reported [25]. A small case series of 32 patients comparing postoperative catheter-directed thrombolysis versus systemic anticoagulation after open embolectomy showed improved thrombus removal and decreased 30-day mortality in the CDT group; however, massive abdominal hemorrhage was significantly more common, occurring in 20% of patients in this series [26].

More aggressive approaches to the treatment of MVT have been described. Catheter-directed thrombolysis of the superior mesenteric vein is within the armamentarium of the interventional radiologist. Transjugular intrahepatic portosystemic shunt, percutaneous transhepatic, transileocolic venous, and transplenic venous approaches have previously been described [27]. However, their necessity is rare and reserved for patients with only the most severe and progressive mesenteric venous occlusion.

## MANAGEMENT OF NON-OCCLUSIVE MESENTERIC ISCHEMIA

The hallmark of NOMI is intestinal hypoperfusion despite vascular patency [5]. Often associated with critical illness, its causes are multifactorial and may result in a spectrum of bowel injury from patchy ischemia to long-segment necrosis. Mortality rates exceed 80%. The focus of treatment should be directed at correcting the underlying cause and restoring intestinal perfusion [2,4,7]. In the setting of bowel necrosis or perforation, prompt exploration and resection should be performed.

## CHRONIC MESENTERIC ISCHEMIA

### Epidemiology and pathogenesis

Chronic mesenteric ischemia occurs in the setting of severe SMA stenosis predominately from atherosclerotic disease. The prevalence of CMI is very low, reported at 30 per 100,000 [28]. The extensive collateral circulation to the bowel and the slow progression of mesenteric artery stenosis belie the rarity of this disease. Risk factors for the development of chronic mesenteric ischemia owe to the pathophysiology of atherosclerotic disease: smoking, hyperlipidemia, hypertension, and cardiovascular disease.

### Clinical presentation

Patients with chronic mesenteric ischemia classically present with postprandial abdominal pain [2,29]. Such pain can result in weight-loss due to decreased caloric intake, frequency, and fear of eating. As expected, recurrent postprandial pain has significant impacts on patient quality of life [30]. These symptoms are often nonspecific, leading to a broad differential diagnosis. Clinically significant ischemia from chronic mesenteric atherosclerotic disease requires three factors: medical history supportive of the diagnosis; mesenteric artery stenosis of one or more vessels over 70%; and imaging, surgical, or endoscopic findings consistent with ischemia [31].

### Medical management

Owing to the impacts on quality of life, initial management of chronic mesenteric ischemia hinges on lifestyle modification. Decreased meal size and increased meal frequency may improve symptoms of postprandial pain. Treatment of underlying medical comorbidities which contribute to further atherosclerotic disease is mandatory and may be best addressed via a multidisciplinary care team.

### Indications for interventions

As previously noted, the impacts on patient quality of life cannot be understated in. To this end, symptoms refractory to medical management and lifestyle modification are a clinical indication for intervention in patients with mesenteric artery stenosis [30]. Patients must have symptoms and imaging findings consistent with the diagnosis, including single- or multi-vessel disease with greater than 70% occlusion (Fig. 3). In a study of 79 patients following revascularization via open antegrade, retrograde, or endovascular approaches, revascularization resulted in a clinically significant improvement in quality-of-life scores after revascularization [30].

### Surgical versus endovascular

Given the typical presentation and often incidental diagnosis of mesenteric stenosis on imaging, endovascular approaches are favored for revascularization.

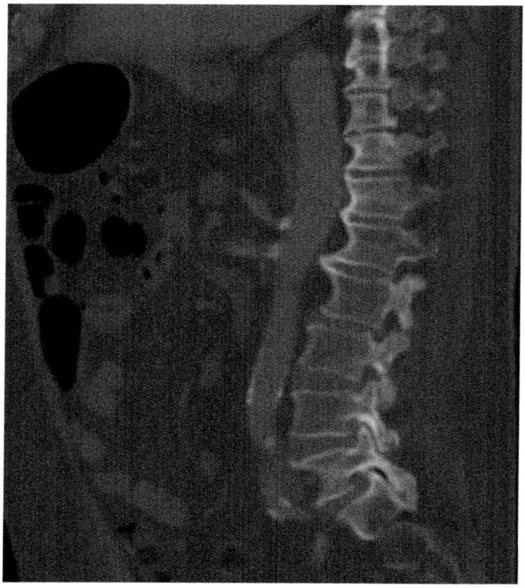

**Fig. 3.** CT showing chronic atherosclerotic disease with calcification at the ostia of the celiac and superior mesenteric arteries.

Findings suggestive of bowel infarct, such as when an acute embolus occludes a stenotic mesenteric vessel, demand laparotomy for bowel resection and revascularization as described earlier in this chapter. In these patients an open revascularization approach, such as ROMS described earlier, may be used [18]. For patients without an acute abdomen, endovascular approaches are now strongly favored over open revascularization. A systematic review and meta-analysis of 100 studies comparing endovascular versus open revascularization showed improvements in 30-day mortality and decreased in hospital complication rates with an endovascular approach [32]. However, similar to findings reported in AMI, open surgery was associated with a lower risk of 3-year symptom recurrence than endovascular stenting. There was no significant difference identified in 3-year overall survival.

## POSTOPERATIVE CARE

As a mainstay of medical management of mesenteric ischemia, patients are placed on anticoagulation at diagnosis, and should remain anticoagulated after revascularization. No level one evidence exists to suggest the duration of anticoagulation, but given the age of onset and presence of underlying comorbidities, lifetime anticoagulation is likely. Transition from heparin to vitamin K antagonists and novel oral anticoagulants have both been used for this purpose. Patients undergoing endovascular therapy should be placed on aspirin for life, with dual antiplatelet therapy for 1 to 3 months postoperatively [22]. Patients with AMI should continue to undergo further postoperative resuscitation and, in the case of bowel resection, return to the operating room for second look laparotomy in 24 to 48 hours.

## LONG-TERM FOLLOW-UP

Long-term care should be directed at addressing the patient's underlying medical comorbidities to minimize the risk of recurrent disease. Risk factor and lifestyle modification, as well as management of hyperlipidemia, hypertension, and diabetes, are necessary. Patients with bypass graft or stent placement should have surveillance imaging obtained via duplex ultrasound or CT angiography within 6 months, with frequent follow-up thereafter to enable early intervention on recurrent disease [6]. Current Society for Vascular Surgery guidelines recommend duplex ultrasonography at 1, 6, and 12 months, and then annually thereafter [33].

## SUMMARY

Mesenteric ischemia remains a relatively rare albeit high-mortality disease. In its acute form, delay in diagnosis and lack of prompt intervention contribute to the high mortality rate. Rapid diagnosis, anticoagulation, resuscitation, revascularization, and reassessment are the guiding principles in the management. In the operating room, a focus on revascularization should take priority unless frankly necrotic or perforated bowel is encountered. Classically open revascularization approaches have been used and described, owing to the frequency of concomitant damage control laparotomy and familiarity of the surgeon, but recent developments, with improvement in early diagnosis, have allowed endovascular techniques to be further explored. Much debate in the literature and little high-quality evidence exists to define the appropriate conditions and support one treatment modality over another for acute disease. However, the success of endovascular approaches for the treatment of chronic mesenteric ischemia suggests further study is warranted in this area.

## CLINICS CARE POINTS

- Mesenteric ischemia requires a high index of suspicion, and prompt surgical intervention is indicated to improve mortality.
- Revascularization should be performed early, with only frankly necrotic or perforated bowel resected.
- Open revascularization approaches remain the gold standard for the treatment of acute mesenteric ischemia, while endovascular approaches have gained favor for chronic disease.

## References


[1] Carver TW, Vora RS, Taneja A. Mesenteric ischemia. Crit Care Clin 2016;32(2):155–71.
[2] Clair DG, Beach JM. Mesenteric Ischemia. N Engl J Med 2016;374(10):959–68.
[3] Caluwaerts M, Castanares-Zapatero D, Laterre PF, et al. Prognostic factors of acute mesenteric ischemia in ICU patients. BMC Gastroenterol 2019;19(1):80.
[4] Karkkainen JM, Acosta S. Acute mesenteric ischemia (part I) - Incidence, etiologies, and how to improve early diagnosis. Best Pract Res Clin Gastroenterol 2017;31(1):15–25.
[5] Al-Diery H, Phillips A, Evennett N, et al. The pathogenesis of nonocclusive mesenteric ischemia: implications for research and clinical practice. J Intensive Care Med 2019;34(10):771–81.
[6] Tilsed JV, Casamassima A, Kurihara H, et al. ESTES guidelines: acute mesenteric ischaemia. Eur J Trauma Emerg Surg 2016;42(2):253–70.
[7] Bala M, Kashuk J, Moore EE, et al. Acute mesenteric ischemia: guidelines of the World Society of Emergency Surgery. World J Emerg Surg 2017;12:38.
[8] Luther B, Mamopoulos A, Lehmann C, et al. The ongoing challenge of acute mesenteric ischemia. Visc Med 2018;34(3):217–23.
[9] Savlania A, Tripathi RK. Acute mesenteric ischemia: current multidisciplinary approach. J Cardiovasc Surg (Torino) 2017;58(2):339–50.
[10] Ehlert BA. Acute gut ischemia. Surg Clin North Am 2018;98(5):995–1004.
[11] Lim S, Halandras PM, Bechara C, et al. Contemporary management of acute mesenteric ischemia in the endovascular era. Vasc Endovascular Surg 2019;53(1):42–50.
[12] Zhao Y, Yin H, Yao C, et al. Management of acute mesenteric ischemia: a critical review and treatment algorithm. Vasc Endovascular Surg 2016;50(3):183–92.
[13] Karkkainen JM, Acosta S. Acute mesenteric ischemia (Part II) - Vascular and endovascular surgical approaches. Best Pract Res Clin Gastroenterol 2017;31(1):27–38.
[14] Genzel P, van Dijk LC, Veger HTC, et al. Case report: direct revascularization in acute mesenteric ischemia by an endovascular approach. CVIR Endovasc 2019;2(1):31.
[15] Scali ST, Ayo D, Giles KA, et al. Outcomes of antegrade and retrograde open mesenteric bypass for acute mesenteric ischemia. J Vasc Surg 2019;69(1):129–40.
[16] Huerta CT, Orr NT, Tyagi SC, et al. Direct retrograde bypass is preferable to antegrade bypass for open mesenteric revascularization. Ann Vasc Surg 2020;66:263–71.
[17] Blauw JT, Meerwaldt R, Brusse-Keizer M, et al. Retrograde open mesenteric stenting for acute mesenteric ischemia. J Vasc Surg 2014;60(3):726–34.
[18] Oderich GS, Macedo R, Stone DH, et al. Multicenter study of retrograde open mesenteric artery stenting through laparotomy for treatment of acute and chronic mesenteric ischemia. J Vasc Surg 2018;68(2):470–80.e1.
[19] Andraska E, Haga L, Li X, et al. Retrograde open mesenteric stenting should be considered as the initial approach to acute mesenteric ischemia. J Vasc Surg 2020;72(4):1260–8.
[20] Acosta S, Bjorck M. Modern treatment of acute mesenteric ischaemia. Br J Surg 2014;101(1):e100–8.
[21] Brunaud L, Antunes L, Collinet-Adler S, et al. Acute mesenteric venous thrombosis: case for nonoperative management. J Vasc Surg 2001;34(4):673–9.
[22] Tabriziani H, Ahmad A, Narasimha D, et al. A nonsurgical approach to mesenteric vascular disease. Cardiol Rev 2018;26(2):99–106.
[23] Bergqvist D, Svensson PJ. Treatment of mesenteric vein thrombosis. Semin Vasc Surg 2010;23(1):65–8.
[24] Acosta S, Salim S. Management of acute mesenteric venous thrombosis: a systematic review of contemporary studies. Scand J Surg 2020; https://doi.org/10.1177/1457496920969084 1457496920969084.
[25] Yang S, Liu B, Ding W, et al. Acute superior mesenteric venous thrombosis: transcatheter thrombolysis and aspiration thrombectomy therapy by combined route of superior mesenteric vein and artery in eight patients. Cardiovasc Intervent Radiol 2015;38(1):88–99.

[26] Yang S, Zhang L, Liu K, et al. Postoperative catheter-directed thrombolysis versus systemic anticoagulation for acute superior mesenteric venous thrombosis. Ann Vasc Surg 2016;35:88–97.
[27] Chamarthy MR, Anderson ME, Pillai AK, et al. Thrombolysis and transjugular intrahepatic portosystemic shunt creation for acute and subacute portal vein thrombosis. Tech Vasc Interv Radiol 2016;19(1):42–51.
[28] Blauw J, Bulut T, Eenhoorn P, et al. Chronic mesenteric ischemia: when and how to intervene on patients with celiac/SMA stenosis. J Cardiovasc Surg (Torino) 2017;58(2):321–8.
[29] van Dijk LJ, van Noord D, de Vries AC, et al. Clinical management of chronic mesenteric ischemia. United Eur Gastroenterol J 2019;7(2):179–88.
[30] Blauw JTM, Pastoors HAM, Brusse-Keizer M, et al. The impact of revascularisation on quality of life in chronic mesenteric ischemia. Can J Gastroenterol Hepatol 2019;2019:7346013.
[31] Kolkman JJ, Geelkerken RH. Diagnosis and treatment of chronic mesenteric ischemia: An update. Best Pract Res Clin Gastroenterol 2017;31(1):49–57.
[32] Alahdab F, Arwani R, Pasha AK, et al. A systematic review and meta-analysis of endovascular versus open surgical revascularization for chronic mesenteric ischemia. J Vasc Surg 2018;67(5):1598–605.
[33] Zierler RE, Jordan WD, Lal BK, et al. The Society for Vascular Surgery practice guidelines on follow-up after vascular surgery arterial procedures. J Vasc Surg 2018;68(1):256–84.

Advances in Surgery 55 (2021) 89–107
ADVANCES IN SURGERY

# Watch-and-wait Management for Rectal Cancer After Clinical Complete Response to Neoadjuvant Therapy

Jonathan B. Yuval, MD, Julio Garcia-Aguilar, MD, PhD*
Colorectal Service, Department of Surgery, Memorial Sloan Kettering Cancer Center, 1275 York Avenue, New York, NY 10065, USA

**Keywords**

• Nonoperative management • Watch and wait • Rectal cancer
• Organ preservation

**Key points**

- Neoadjuvant treatment can eliminate all tumor cells in some patients with rectal cancer, but, with standard management, these patients are recognized only after rectal resection, when their specimens show pathologic complete response.
- Patients with pathologic complete response have excellent long-term oncological outcomes, and rectal resection in these patients may constitute overtreatment, causing functional impairments deleterious to patients' quality of life.
- The idea behind watch and wait is to correctly identify by the best preoperative diagnostic methods those patients whose tumors have responded completely to neoadjuvant therapy and to substitute upfront resection with strict surveillance.
- Because clinical assessment of response is not as accurate as pathologic assessment of response, strict surveillance is necessary to recognize tumor regrowth in a timely manner, when the tumor is still curable by resection.
- Although promising, most published data on watch and wait are from retrospective series. Prospectively collected data from randomized trials will soon be available.

Footnote: This article is based in part on Yuval et al. 2020. J. Gastrointest. Surg. 24:1880–1888.

*Corresponding author. *E-mail address:* garciaaj@mskcc.org

https://doi.org/10.1016/j.yasu.2021.05.007
0065-3411/21/

## INTRODUCTION

Colorectal cancer is the fourth most common cancer and second most common cause of cancer death in the United States, and nearly 30% of all newly diagnosed colorectal cancers are located in the rectum [1]. Oncological outcomes of locally advanced rectal cancer (LARC) have improved over the last 3 decades because of multidisciplinary care and standardization of diagnostic imaging, surgical technique, surgical pathology, and perioperative multimodal treatment. Accepted standard treatment of LARC includes preoperative chemoradiotherapy (CRT), total mesorectal excision (TME), and postoperative systemic chemotherapy [2]. Intensive multimodal treatment is associated with excellent local control but inadequate systemic control, with about one-third of patients succumbing to metastatic disease [3]. In addition, multimodal treatment is detrimental to patients' quality of life (QoL) because of surgical morbidity; risk of permanent stoma; and bowel, bladder, and sexual dysfunction. Two key challenges are improving survival by preventing metastases and improving patients' QoL by preventing functional impairments.

The rate of pathologic complete response (pCR) is approximately 20% in patients who undergo CRT alone, and can reach nearly 40% in patients who undergo preoperative CRT in combination with systemic chemotherapy [4]. Patients with pCR have a 5-year survival rate of 95% and a local-recurrence rate of around 1% [5] (Fig. 1). In view of these outcomes, surgical removal of the rectum in patients with pCR may constitute overtreatment, and the risk of sequelae from surgery may outweigh the risk of tumor progression during observation. In this context, avoiding surgery may provide important benefits such as lower morbidity, lower health care costs, and better QoL.

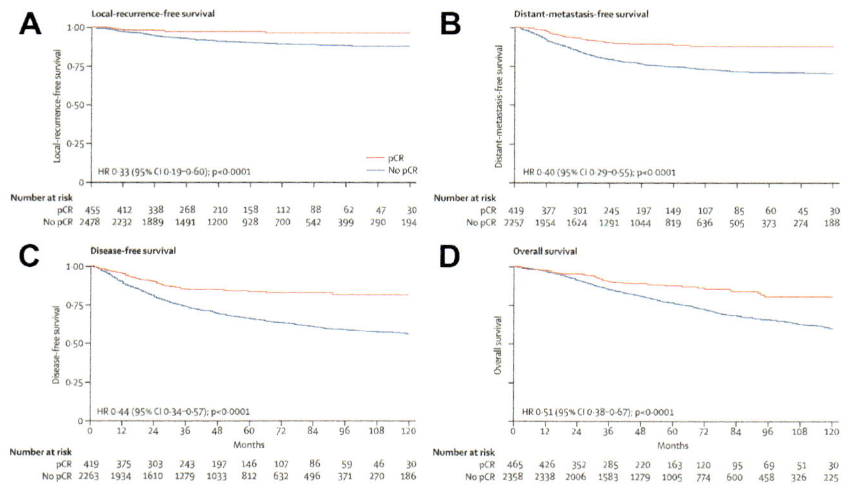


**Fig. 1.** Kaplan-Meier survival curves for patients with or without pCR. Local-recurrence-free survival (A); Distant-metastases-free survival (B); Disease-free survival (C); Overall survival (D). P values were determined by the log-rank test. CI, confidence interval; HR, hazard ratio. (*From* Maas et al. 2010, Lancet Oncol. 11:835–44; with permission.)

Acceptance is growing for watch and wait (WW) as an alternative nonstandard strategy for preserving the rectum in patients with LARC with clinical complete response (cCR), based on favorable retrospective studies conducted at specialized cancer centers. Prospective data from the phase II trial Organ Preservation in Rectal Adenocarcinoma (OPRA; NCT02008656), which is evaluating 3-year disease-free survival in patients who receive CRT plus induction or consolidation chemotherapy and then undergo WW management or TME depending on response, have been collected [6] and will soon be reported.

## TERMINOLOGY

The nonstandard approach of WW also has some nonstandard language. Although a pCR is an objective determination that no tumor cells are present in the surgical specimen, a cCR is a subjective assessment by treating physicians that no viable tumor remains in the rectum following neoadjuvant therapy (NAT). Because the decision to proceed with WW is based on this subjective assessment, some patients with cCR have clinically obscure remnants of the tumor that eventually become clinically evident.

WW is a management strategy for patients with cCR following NAT, whereas organ preservation is the desired outcome of this approach. The term nonoperative management is often used interchangeably with WW, but, because operative local excision can be a part of a strategy for organ preservation, the use of this term is potentially confusing.

Reappearance of neoplasia at the site of a treated tumor is called regrowth. Regrowth is considered salvageable when it can be cured by TME. Tumor recurrence in the context of WW is nonsalvageable regrowth or presence of cancer in the pelvis following a curative resection. The term recurrence should not be used for the presence of salvageable regrowth in patients with cCR.

NAT is administered before surgery and adjuvant therapy is administered after surgery. Systemic chemotherapy can be added to CRT in the neoadjuvant period. When chemotherapy is administered before CRT, it is called induction chemotherapy; when it is administered after CRT (but before surgery), it is called consolidation chemotherapy. A full course of induction or consolidation chemotherapy along with CRT is called total NAT (TNT).

## HISTORY OF WATCH AND WAIT

Although reports of radiotherapy curing rectal cancer without surgery appeared as early as 1920 [7], A. Habr-Gama's group pioneered WW of rectal cancer in modern times, as described in their report on 265 patients with surgically curable rectal cancer assessed for response 8 weeks after CRT [8]. Patients with incomplete response underwent surgical resection, and 71 patients with cCR (27%) entered a strict surveillance program.

With a mean follow-up of 57.3 months for patients with a cCR, 3 patients developed distant metastases. Two patients developed regrowth, which was salvaged with local therapy. Overall survival and disease-free survival did not differ significantly between patients with cCR and patients with pCR. These results showed that, with structured surveillance, deferral of surgery is safe, regrowth can be effectively treated, and sustained cCR can be comparable with a cure. Additional reports from other specialized cancer centers have provided support of the efficacy and safety of WW [9–16]. However, many surgeons are reluctant to adopt WW [17] because of the lack of standardization in response assessment and the lack of randomized prospective data.

## PATIENT PERSPECTIVES ON WATCH AND WAIT

Patients are interested in treatment strategies that preserve the rectum, and they are willing to make oncological compromises for this goal. In a study by Gani and colleagues [18], in which questionnaires were collected from patients awaiting multimodal treatment, 83% of the patients said that they would consider WW in case of cCR; 94% were willing to accept a 2-year regrowth rate of 25%, and 95% were willing to accept an intensive follow-up protocol. Although 55% of the patients would enter WW only if this approach was associated with equivalent cure rates, 30% of patients were willing to accept a 2% absolute reduction in the long-term cure rate, and 11% were willing to accept a 10% reduction. Another study [19], in which questionnaires were collected from patients with LARC following multimodal treatment, found that the median respondent would accept an absolute increase of 20% in recurrence risk with WW and would need an additional 2 years of life and an absolute increase of 10% in the likelihood of surviving 7 years to prefer TME.

## PATIENT EVALUATION

### Work-up

The decision to proceed with WW is made during response assessment following NAT, and all patients who are candidates for NAT are also potential candidates for organ preservation. The initial work-up should be the standard rectal cancer work-up based on the guidelines of the National Comprehensive Cancer Network. Documentation of the endoscopic characteristics of the tumor at baseline, ideally with endoscopic images, is important for comparison in subsequent response evaluations. Following NAT, patients with a cCR (or with a significant response that does not meet all criteria of cCR) can enter a WW protocol after the patient, the surgeon, and the disease management team agree to proceed with this nonstandard approach.

### Selection of patients based on tumor stage

Several studies on WW have reported outcomes for patients with LARC who received multimodal NAT as part of standard care. WW offers considerable potential benefit for patients with LARC, given the unsatisfactory QoL for these patients after CRT and TME. Most patients with LARC treated by both modalities have long-term bowel dysfunction, also known as low anterior resection syndrome [20]. A potential disadvantage of WW for patients with LARC is withholding a treatment modality when the risk of disease progression is not negligible. Characteristics that have been associated with risk of local recurrence include less than or equal to 1-mm distance of the tumor from the mesorectal fascia, extramural venous invasion, and extensive nodal disease or lateral pelvic nodal metastasis [21,22]. Although the presence of these features is not a contraindication for WW, a cCR in patients with advanced tumors is less probable, and assessment of response may be challenging. Ulcerated circumferential tumors may scar in a way that narrows the rectal lumen and prevents proper endoscopic evaluation. Patients with these tumors may not be appropriate candidates for WW.

Some studies have focused on WW for patients with early-stage (cT2N0M0) low rectal cancer [23,24], for which TME without NAT is the standard of care. A distal cT2N0M0 tumor can be adequately resected only by abdominoperineal resection, and the prospect of avoiding a permanent stoma is highly desirable for patients. In addition, early-stage tumors are more sensitive to NAT than more advanced tumors, and rates of organ preservation of cT2N0M0 tumors following NAT can reach 67% at 5 years [23]. However, for patients who end up with an incomplete clinical response (iCR) to NAT, NAT carries the potential disadvantage of the synergistic sequelae of radiation and surgery, compared with the option of surgery alone.

### Selection of patients based on tumor location

Patients receiving NAT for rectal cancer in any location are potential candidates for WW, but patients with distal tumors requiring a low anastomosis or abdominoperineal resection are likely to benefit the most. In addition to the prospect of avoiding a permanent stoma and poor QoL (as a consequence of a very low anastomosis in a previously irradiated rectum), patients with a distal tumor who undergo WW can benefit from distal tumors being easily evaluable by a digital rectal examination (DRE) and respond better to NAT than proximal tumors [25].

### Baseline characteristics associated with response to neoadjuvant therapy

A meta-analysis of nearly 1200 patients found that characteristics associated with pCR include older age, smaller tumor size, shorter distance from the anal verge, and negative lymph node status [26]. A large retrospective study showed that response is inversely associated with the circumferential extent of the tumor, level of carcinoembryonic antigen, and distance from the anal verge [25].

Response to NAT is also associated with certain common genomic alterations. Mutations in p53 and KRAS, found in about 70% and 40% of rectal tumors, respectively [27,28], are associated with poor response to NAT. In contrast, mismatch repair deficiency and microsatellite instability, found in less than 5% of rectal tumors, are associated with good response to radiation [29].

## RADIOTHERAPY REGIMENS

The ability of preoperative radiotherapy to prevent locoregional recurrence in patients with LARC has been well established for both short-course radiation therapy (SCRT), consisting of 5 fractions of 5 Gy (total, 25 Gy), and long-course CRT combined with a sensitizing fluoropyrimidine, consisting of multiple fractions of 1.8 to 2 Gy (total, 40–50.4 Gy) [2,30]. The interval to surgery after CRT is usually 6 to 8 weeks, whereas the interval to surgery after SCRT can be short (1 week) or extended (4–8 weeks) [2,4]. CRT is the approach most commonly used in WW protocols [8–13,15,16].

Although data on the use of SCRT in WW are limited, the incorporation of SCRT into TNT has shown promising results [31–35] and has been described in the context of WW [31,36]. In addition, SCRT has been increasingly used during the COVID-19 (coronavirus disease 2019) pandemic because of its efficiency in resource use and few patient visits needed [37,38]. This change in practice may help elucidate the effectiveness of SCRT-based TNT in organ preservation strategy.

Results of the Rectal cancer And Preoperative Induction therapy followed by Dedicated Operation (RAPIDO) trial (NCT01558921) [39], in which patients were randomized to standard CRT followed by TME and optional adjuvant chemotherapy or to SCRT and 6 cycles of capecitabine-oxaliplatin consolidation therapy followed by TME, may also provide indirect data on the value of SCRT in WW. Early reports from the trial indicate a higher pCR rate (28% vs 14%; $P<.001$) with SCRT-consolidation chemotherapy and lower rates of distant metastases [40], but raise 2 questions: (1) is SCRT consolidation more effective than CRT-consolidation, and (2) how toxic is SCRT consolidation if the rectum is not removed?

## ENHANCING THE RESPONSE TO NEOADJUVANT THERAPY

Response to NAT can be enhanced by (1) increasing the time interval to assessment, (2) increasing the radiation dose, (3) adding systemic chemotherapy to radiotherapy in the neoadjuvant setting, and/or (4) administering consolidation chemotherapy rather than induction chemotherapy.

### Interval to assessment

Tumor regression following radiation therapy is time dependent, and maximal tumor response can take months. A retrospective analysis of National Cancer Database data from more than 17,000 patients who underwent neoadjuvant CRT and TME found that intervals of more than 8 weeks from CRT to resection were associated with higher rates of pCR [41]. The rates of pCR were around 0% at 1 week and around 11% at 14 weeks, after which they remained nearly constant (Fig. 2). Longer intervals were also associated with lower rates of readmission after surgery.

In the Stockholm III trial (NCT00904813), patients who underwent SCRT with delayed surgery had a higher rate of pCR and tumor regression grade than patients who underwent surgery immediately after SCRT [42,43]. Survival did not differ between the two groups, but SCRT with delayed surgery was associated with fewer postoperative complications. In another trial [44] (NCT03287843), patients were randomized to TME either within 8 weeks after CRT or more than 8 weeks after CRT. The rate of pCR was significantly higher in the latter group (18.6% vs 10%; $P = .03$), with no difference in surgical morbidity or in the quality of resection.

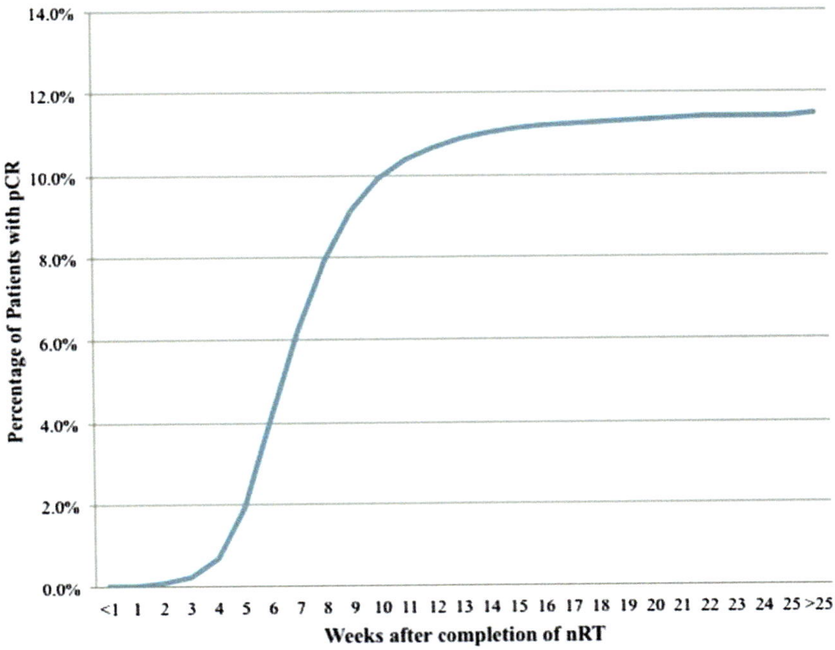


**Fig. 2.** Cumulative percentage of patients with pCR at different time points after completion of neoadjuvant radiotherapy (nRT). (*From* Probst et al. 2015, J. Am. Coll. Surg. 221:430–40; with permission.)

## Radiation dose

Higher radiation doses have been reported to be associated with higher rates of tumor response. Patients with early-stage rectal cancer treated with 54 Gy have higher rates of initial cCR and higher rates of organ preservation at 5 years than patients treated with 50.4 Gy [23]. One study found histologic evidence of a dose-response relationship in vitro with radiation doses of 50.4 to 70 Gy [45]. This range is higher than what is commonly used for LARC, and the investigators of that study concluded that the higher doses may have potential for use in WW protocols. A subsequent study by the same group investigated high-dose CRT in patients with T2 to T3 N0 to N1 disease considered for WW [12]. At 6 weeks following treatment, a remarkable 78% of patients had a cCR. Approximately a third of the patients had early-stage rectal cancer, which may have contributed to the high response rate.

## Addition of neoadjuvant systemic chemotherapy

Adding neoadjuvant systemic chemotherapy either before or after CRT can improve response rates. In a retrospective study with 628 patients [46], complete response was observed in 37% of patients who received TNT and only 21% of patients who received CRT. In a nonrandomized clinical trial [4] comparing the rate of pCR between 4 sequential groups of patients who received CRT alone or in combination with 2, 4, or 6 cycles of FOLFOX (leucovorin, fluorouracil, oxaliplatin), the pCR rate increased with each addition of 2 cycles of FOLFOX: no FOLFOX, 18%; 2 cycles, 25%; 4 cycles, 30%; 6 cycles, 38%. The rate of serious adverse events did not differ between the groups. Extension of the time interval to resection with each addition of FOLFOX cycles may have contributed to the higher pCR rates. In the Partenariat de Recherche en Oncologie Digestive (PRODIGE) 23 phase III randomized trial (NCT01804790), patients who received 6 cycles of FOLFORINOX (leucovorin, fluorouracil, irinotecan, oxaliplatin) followed by CRT, TME, and 3 months of adjuvant systemic chemotherapy had a significantly higher pCR rate (28% vs 12%; $P<.001$) and higher 3-year rates of disease-free and metastasis-free survival than patients who underwent CRT, TME, and 6 months of adjuvant systemic chemotherapy [47].

### Induction versus consolidation chemotherapy in total neoadjuvant therapy

TNT using consolidation chemotherapy is associated with higher rates of response and organ preservation than TNT using induction chemotherapy. Fokas and colleagues [48], who randomized 311 patients with stage II or III rectal cancer to either induction or consolidation TNT followed by TME, found that consolidation was associated with a higher rate of pCR (25% vs 17%; $P<.001$). The preliminary results of the OPRA trial (NCT02008656), in which patients were randomized to induction or consolidation TNT and then proceeded to surgery or WW depending on response, showed higher rates of organ preservation in the consolidation arm (58% vs 43%; $P = .01$), with no difference in disease-free survival or distant-metastasis-free survival [6]. Based on the results of these 2 trials, patients with LARC who are candidates for TNT and potentially for WW may benefit more from consolidation-based TNT than from induction-based TNT.

## COMPLICATIONS OF NEOADJUVANT THERAPY

Although NAT helps reduce the likelihood of local recurrence and facilitates organ preservation, it is associated with severe acute and chronic adverse events, including death. In the seminal randomized control trial comparing preoperative and postoperative CRT for LARC, preoperative CRT was associated with much lower toxicity than postoperative CRT, but acute grade 3 to 4 toxic effects were still seen in 27% of patients who received preoperative CRT (27% vs 40%; $P<.001$) [2]. Higher rates of toxicities can be observed with the addition of systemic chemotherapy to CRT, without a benefit in survival; grade 3 to 5 toxicities can be seen in as many as 42% of patients, and deaths attributable to NAT can be seen in as many as 1.5% of patients [49]. These rates may be even higher in elderly patients, who should receive individualized treatment, based on their overall health and frailty assessment.

## ASSESSMENT OF RESPONSE

Selection of patients for WW remains a challenge. Ideally, patients for whom a pCR would likely be identified were they to undergo resection should be selected for WW. However, the decision to manage a patient's rectal cancer with WW must be based on clinical findings, even though the correlation between clinical assessment of response and pathologic assessment of response is imperfect. In the first 2 years following NAT, regrowth occurs in up to 25% of patients with a cCR [50]. In contrast, up to 15% of patients with an iCR who undergo TME end up having a pCR [8,51]. Overly strict criteria of cCR result in some patients undergoing surgery needlessly, and overly loose criteria result in missing some cases of residual tumor.

Three modalities are routinely used to assess response: DRE, MRI, and endoscopy. Each is imperfect, but combining modalities increases accuracy. The accuracy is 98% when all 3 modalities indicate that the tumor is gone [51].

Classic endoscopic features of cCR include a flat white scar, telangiectasia, and absence of both ulcer and nodularity. Typical MRI features of cCR include a scar not thicker than the rectal wall, only dark T2 signal, no visible lymph nodes, no restricted diffusion, and lack of or low signal on apparent diffusion coefficient (ADC) map. Optimally, a DRE of a cCR should be normal, but sometimes minor mucosal abnormalities can be palpated.

One of the hurdles to widespread implementation of WW is the lack of uniform and reproducible criteria for tumor response and patient selection that also take into account borderline cases. Patients with a significant response that does not meet all criteria of cCR, called near-complete clinical response (ncCR), can enter WW if the tumor continues showing signs of response until it meets the full criteria of cCR. In some atypical cases, a cCR can take up to a year. A 3-tiered response assessment schema, which includes the gray area of ncCR, is currently being tested in the OPRA trial (Fig. 3, Table 1). Patients with iCR undergo immediate TME, whereas patients with cCR or ncCR enter WW management.

## LONG-TERM MONITORING OF RESPONSE

Surveillance protocols for patients entering WW vary but typically include measurement of the level of carcinoembryonic antigen in serum; clinical examination; DRE, endoscopy, and MRI for assessment of local recurrence; and computed tomography (CT) of the chest, abdomen, and pelvis for assessment of distant metastases. Surveillance should be most intensive in the first 2 years after treatment, because that is when most cases of regrowth occur. In years 3 to 5 following treatment, monitoring can be less frequent; after year 5, patients can enter survivorship surveillance [52]. The long-term surveillance protocol used in the OPRA trial is shown in Table 2.

## LONG-TERM OUTCOMES

### Oncological outcomes

Oncological outcomes in WW patients are similar to outcomes in TME patients, with the exception of regrowth and rectum preservation. The data for

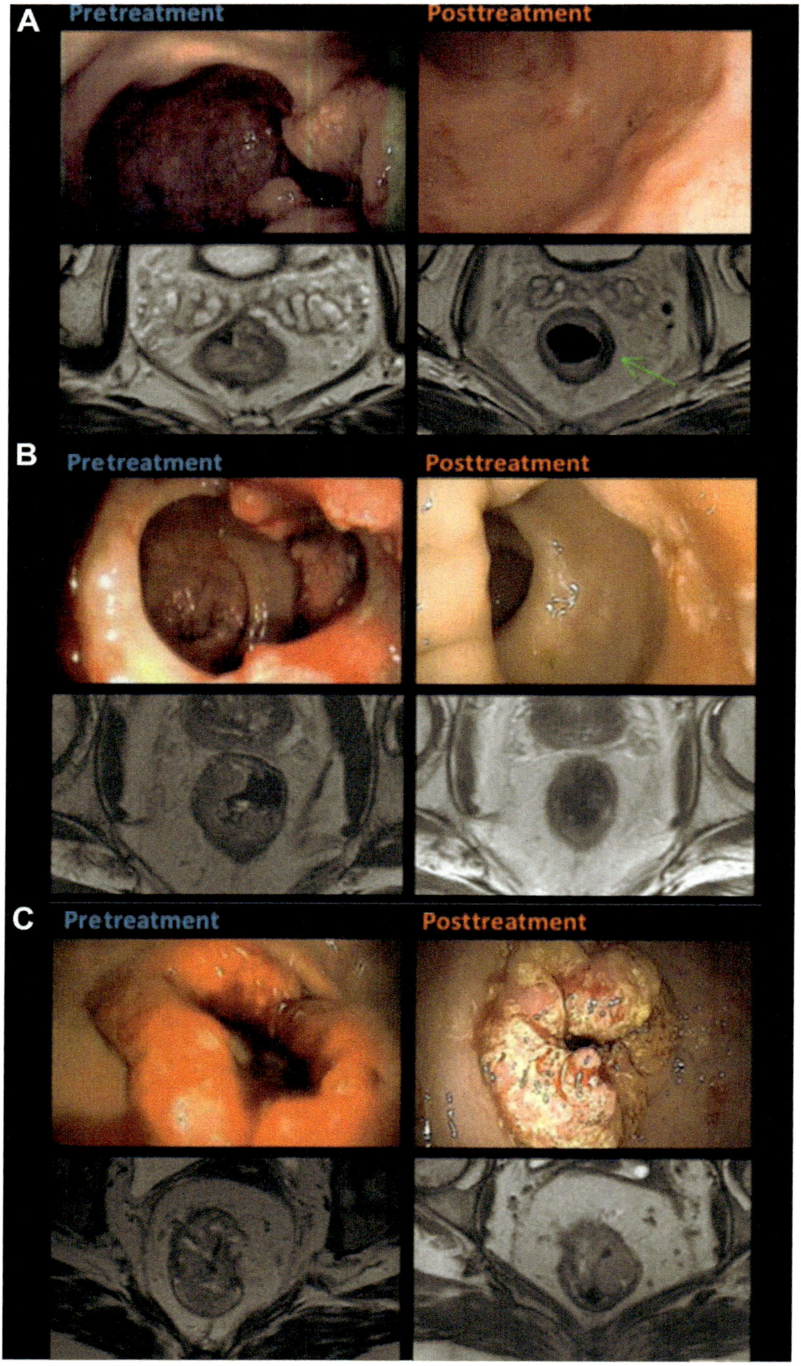


**Fig. 3.** Endoscopic and T2-weighted MRI examples of cCR (*A*), ncCR (*B*), and iCR (*C*). (*Adapted from* Smith et al. 2015, BMC Cancer 15:767; with permission.)

**Table 1**
Criteria for clinical assessment of response to neoadjuvant therapy in the Organ Preservation in Rectal Adenocarcinoma trial

| | Criteria | | |
|---|---|---|---|
| Modality | Complete response | Near-complete response | Incomplete response |
| Endoscopy | Flat white scar, telangiectasia, no ulcer, no nodularity | Irregular mucosa, small mucosal nodules or minor mucosal abnormality, superficial ulceration, mild persisting erythema of scar | Visible tumor |
| Digital rectal examination | Normal | Smooth induration or minor mucosal abnormalities | Palpable tumor nodules |
| MRI | | | |
| T2 weighted | Only dark T2 signal, no intermediate T2 signal, no visible lymph nodes | Mostly dark T2 signal, some remaining intermediate signal, or partial regression of lymph nodes | More intermediate than dark T2 signal, no T2 scar, or no regression of lymph nodes |
| Diffusion weighted | No visible tumor on B800–B1000 signal or lack of or low signal on ADC map[a] | Significant regression of B800–B1000 signal or minimal residual signal on ADC map | Insignificant regression of B800–B1000 signal or obvious low signal on ADC map |

[a]Uniform linear signal in wall above the tumor is acceptable.
*From* Yuval et al. 2020, J. Gastrointest. Surg. 24:1880–1888; with permission.

WW are largely retrospective, and interpreting oncological outcomes based on retrospective series can be tricky because of differences in treatment regimens and indications and lack of uniform criteria for staging and patient selection. The interval from completion of radiotherapy to assessment can also vary,

**Table 2**
Long-term surveillance in the OPRA Organ Preservation in Rectal Adenocarcinoma

| | Months after treatment | | | | | | | | | |
|---|---|---|---|---|---|---|---|---|---|---|
| Examination or measure | 3–6 | 9–12 | 15–18 | 21–24 | 30[a] | 36[a] | 42[a] | 48[a] | 54[a] | 60[a] |
| History and physical | √ | √ | √ | √ | √ | √ | √ | √ | √ | √ |
| Endoscopy | √ | √ | √ | √ | √ | √ | √ | √ | √ | √ |
| MRI rectum | √ | √ | — | √ | — | √ | — | √ | — | √ |
| CT CAP | — | √ | — | √ | — | √ | — | √ | — | √ |
| CEA | √ | √ | √ | √ | √ | √ | √ | √ | √ | √ |

*Abbreviations:* CAP, chest, abdomen, pelvis; CEA, carcinoembryonic antigen.
[a]±30 d.
*From* Yuval et al. 2020, J. Gastrointest. Surg. 24:1880–1888; with permission.

and the denominator is often unclear because studies begin with a cohort of patients with cCR and not with a cohort of patients starting NAT.

In the only prospective study reported to date, which investigated 40 patients with cCR in Denmark, the rate of regrowth was 25% at 2 and 3 years and 31% at 5 years following NAT [12,53]. All but 1 case of regrowth were salvaged by TME (92%). Overall survival at 2, 3, and 5 years was 100%, 95%, and 85%, respectively, and distant-metastasis-free survival at 5 years was 83%.

In a 2018 analysis of International Watch & Wait Database data from 880 patients with cCR who underwent WW at 47 medical centers in various countries [50], the rate of regrowth at 2 years was 25% (Fig. 4A); 77% of the regrowth cases were salvaged by TME. Distant metastases developed in 8% of patients (Fig. 4B). Five-year overall survival and disease-specific survival were 85% and 94%, respectively (Fig. 5).

### Rates of organ preservation

The rate of rectum preservation in patients with cCR who enter WW ranges between 70% and 82% [11,12,15,16]. However, this rate can be misleading because it misses the true denominator of patients by excluding those with an iCR. The rate of rectum preservation for all patients with LARC undergoing TNT with selective organ preservation in the OPRA trial (median follow-up, 2.1 years) was 43% in the induction chemotherapy arm and 58% in the consolidation chemotherapy arm [6].

### Functional outcomes

A few studies have investigated patient-reported functional outcomes in WW patients without a comparison with patients who underwent TME. Appelt and colleagues [12] reported good functional outcomes in WW patients 2 years after NAT, with 69% of patients reporting no fecal incontinence (median Jorge-Wexner score, 0). According to a subsequent report by the same group [53], no patients had symptoms of incontinence at 4 and 5 years following NAT. QoL scores showed little variation over time, but the overall score at 5 years was better than at baseline. The rates of selected patient-reported symptoms in that study are shown in Fig. 6.

In another study, Martens and colleagues [11] reported that, at 3 years after NAT, 14% of patients who underwent WW management reported major incontinence. A subset of patients with iCR at restaging underwent local excision. These patients had worse functional outcomes, with 43% experiencing major incontinence, in contrast with 4.5% of patients who did not require local excision.

In a 2020 study, Quezada-Diaz and colleagues [54] retrospectively compared patient-reported bowel function between patients who underwent WW and a matched cohort of patients who underwent sphincter-preserving TME. With median follow-up of 5 months, WW patients had better functional scores for diet, urgency/soilage, frequency, and overall bowel function than TME patients. Although intriguing, the findings should be reproduced in a larger prospective study with longer follow-up.

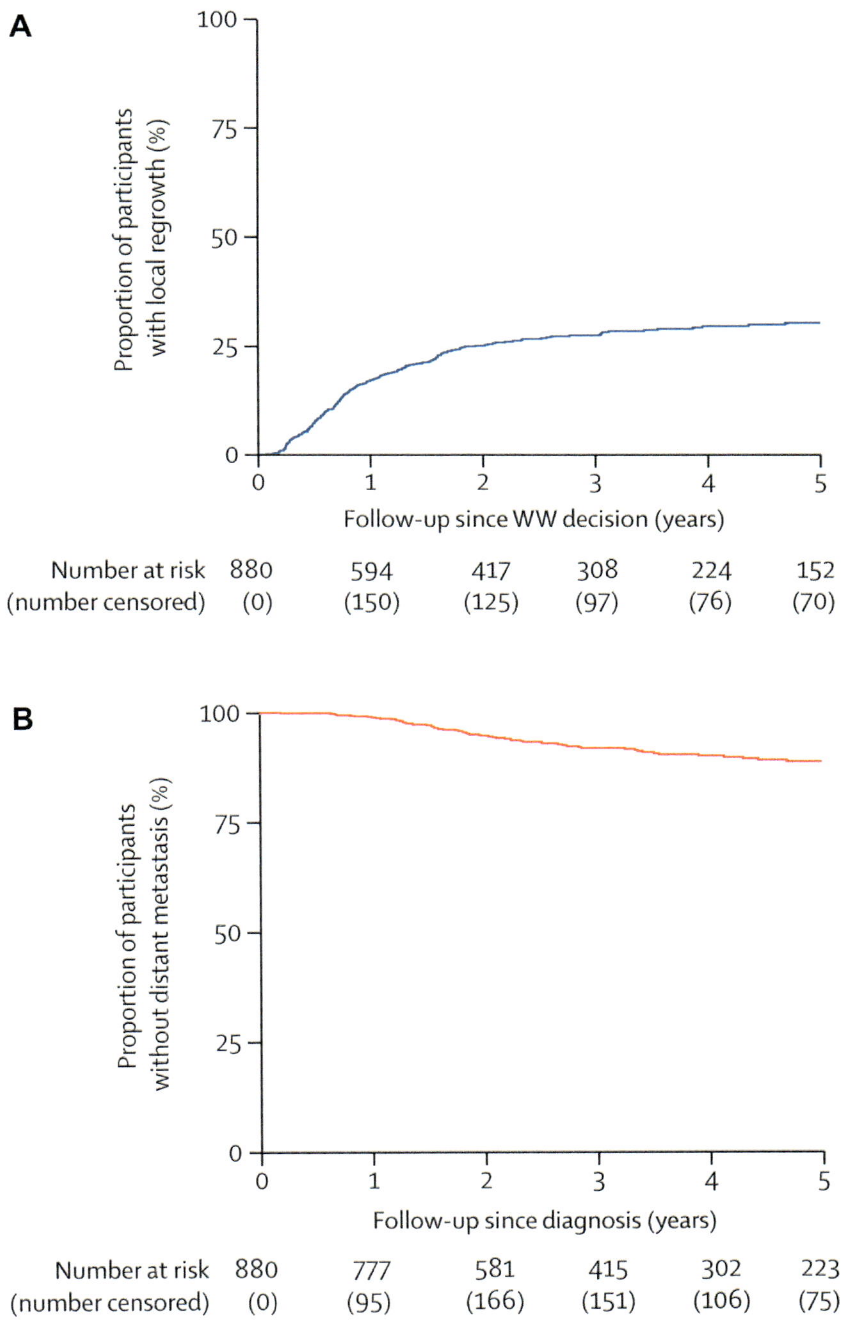


**Fig. 4.** Local tumor regrowth (A) and distant-metastasis-free survival (B) in patients with cCR. (*From* van der Valk et al. 2018, Lancet 391:2537–45; with permission.)

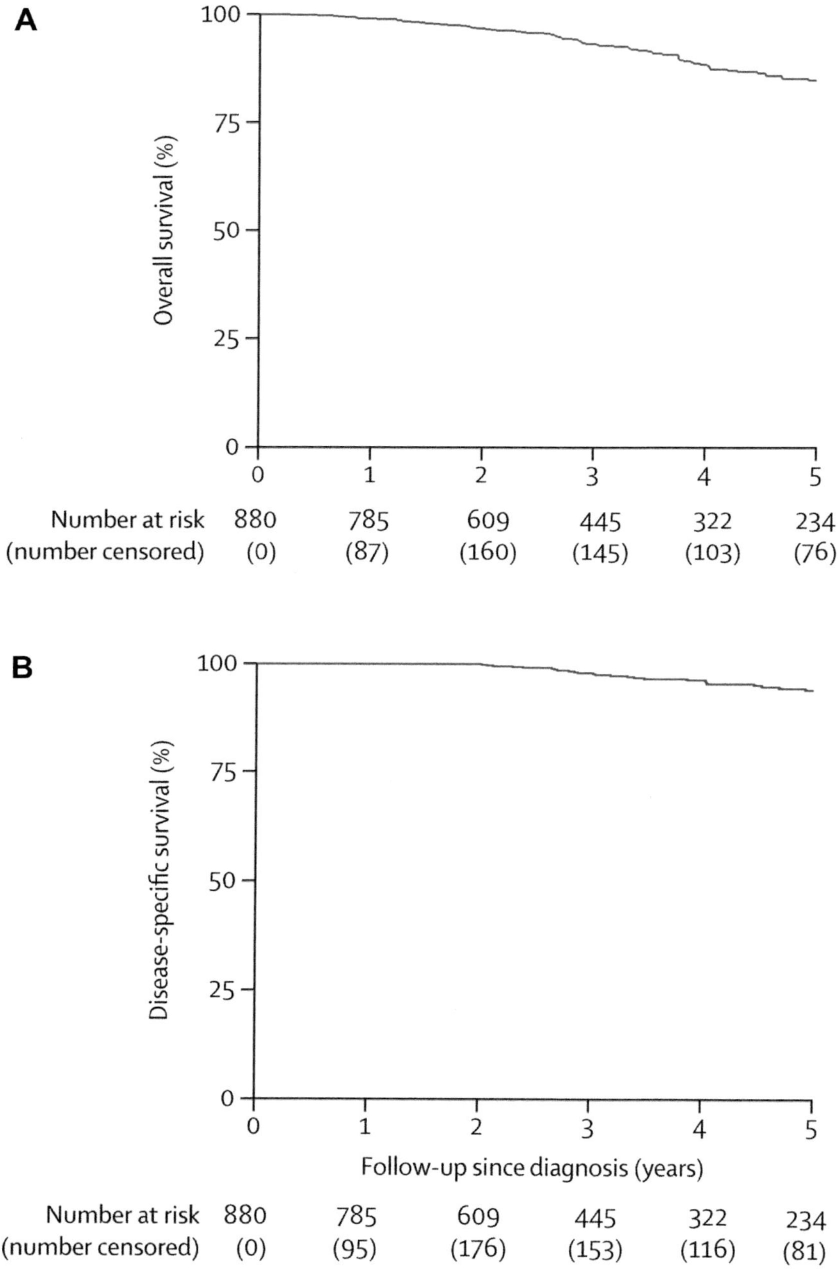


**Fig. 5.** Five-year overall survival (A) and disease-specific survival (B) in patients with cCR. (*From* van der Valk et al. 2018, Lancet 391:2537–45; with permission.)

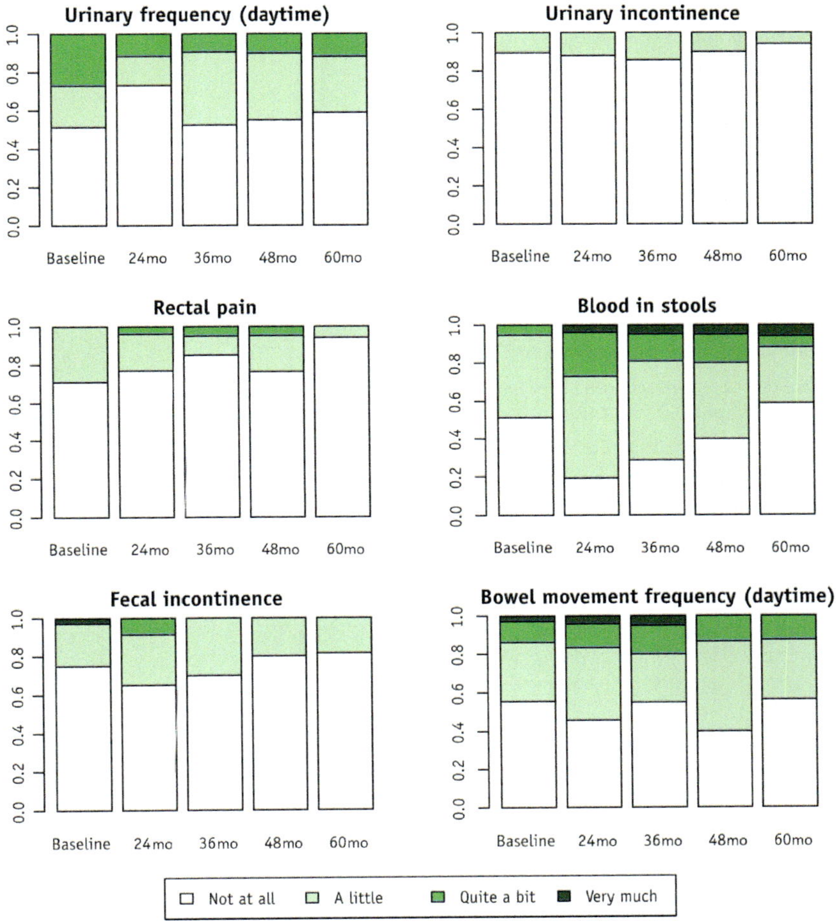


**Fig. 6.** Selected patient-reported symptoms at baseline and during follow-up. The data are proportions of WW patients with reports available at each time point. mo, months. (*From* Dizdarevic et al. 2020, Int. J. Radiat. Oncol. Biol. Phys. 106:556–63; with permission.)

## SUMMARY, DISCUSSION, AND FUTURE DIRECTIONS

Patients with a complete response to NAT may not benefit from TME, but identifying true responders by clinical assessment remains a challenge. Evidence supporting WW is largely retrospective, and prospectively collected data will be of great value. Because WW is acceptable to patients with rectal cancer who are even willing to make an oncological compromise for the prospect of organ preservation, WW should be part of the treatment discussion. Patients entering WW must have a cCR or ncCR, be well informed, and be willing to undergo intensive surveillance. At present, the best setting for patients to undergo WW may be a prospective trial with a strict protocol and objective assessment standards. Uniform and reproducible criteria for response assessment will help WW gain wider acceptance.

## CLINICS CARE POINTS

- Only patients with a cCR or ncCR can be managed by WW; all other patients should undergo treatment according to standard management guidelines.
- WW is suitable for patients who are willing to undergo strict surveillance, can manage uncertainties regarding their disease course, and have streamlined access to appropriate health care services.
- Documentation of tumors by endoscopic images at different time points helps clinicians assess response and detect regrowth.
- NAT is associated with adverse events, toxicities, and even death; management of LARC should be tailored to the patient's health and functional status.
- TNT with consolidation systemic chemotherapy may offer the best chance of rectum preservation for patients with LARC.
- Tumor response to NAT is time dependent and can take months. Patients with ncCR can proceed with WW as long as tumor response continues to improve.
- Regrowth appears in the first 2 years following NAT in about 25% of WW patients; surveillance should be most intensive during this period.
- Five-year overall survival for patients with cCR or ncCR entering WW is approximately 85%, which is comparable with 5-year overall survival for patients who undergo standard treatment including TME and who have similar tumor biology.
- Many patients are willing to make survival compromises for the potential improvement in QoL associated with organ preservation.

## DISCLOSURE

J. Garcia-Aguilar has received honoraria from Intuitive Inc, Medtronic, and Johnson & Johnson.

## FINANCIAL SUPPORT

Research at Memorial Sloan Kettering is funded in part by grant P30 CA008748 from the National Cancer Institute. J.B. Yuval's research fellowship at Memorial Sloan Kettering was funded in part by grant T32 CA009501 from the National Cancer Institute.

## References

[1] Siegel RL, Miller KD, Goding Sauer A, et al. Colorectal cancer statistics, 2020. CA Cancer J Clin 2020;70:145–64.
[2] Sauer R, Becker H, Hohenberger W, et al. Preoperative versus postoperative chemoradiotherapy for rectal cancer. N Engl J Med 2004;351:1731–40.
[3] Cunningham D, Atkin W, Lenz HJ, et al. Colorectal cancer. Lancet 2010;375:1030–47.

[4] Garcia-Aguilar J, Chow OS, Smith DD, et al. Effect of adding mFOLFOX6 after neoadjuvant chemoradiation in locally advanced rectal cancer: a multicentre, phase 2 trial. Lancet Oncol 2015;16:957–66.
[5] Maas M, Nelemans PJ, Valentini V, et al. Long-term outcome in patients with a pathological complete response after chemoradiation for rectal cancer: a pooled analysis of individual patient data. Lancet Oncol 2010;11:835–44.
[6] Garcia-Aguilar J, Patil S, Kim JK, et al. Preliminary results of the organ preservation of rectal adenocarcinoma (OPRA) trial. J Clin Oncol 2020;38:4008.
[7] Janeway H. Treatment of cancer, particularly of the tongue, tonsil and rectum, by buried emanation. Am J Roentgenol 1920;7:92.
[8] Habr-Gama A, Perez RO, Nadalin W, et al. Operative versus nonoperative treatment for stage 0 distal rectal cancer following chemoradiation therapy: long-term results. Ann Surg 2004;240:711–7 [discussion: 717–8].
[9] Maas M, Beets-Tan RG, Lambregts DM, et al. Wait-and-see policy for clinical complete responders after chemoradiation for rectal cancer. J Clin Oncol 2011;29:4633–40.
[10] Araujo RO, Valadao M, Borges D, et al. Nonoperative management of rectal cancer after chemoradiation opposed to resection after complete clinical response. A comparative study. Eur J Surg Oncol 2015;41:1456–63.
[11] Martens MH, Maas M, Heijnen LA, et al. Long-term outcome of an organ preservation program after neoadjuvant treatment for rectal cancer. J Natl Cancer Inst 2016;108:djw171.
[12] Appelt AL, Ploen J, Harling H, et al. High-dose chemoradiotherapy and watchful waiting for distal rectal cancer: a prospective observational study. Lancet Oncol 2015;16:919–27.
[13] Smith JD, Ruby JA, Goodman KA, et al. Nonoperative management of rectal cancer with complete clinical response after neoadjuvant therapy. Ann Surg 2012;256:965–72.
[14] Ayloor Seshadri R, Kondaveeti SS, Jayanand SB, et al. Complete clinical response to neoadjuvant chemoradiation in rectal cancers: can surgery be avoided? Hepatogastroenterology 2013;60:410–4.
[15] Renehan AG, Malcomson L, Emsley R, et al. Watch-and-wait approach versus surgical resection after chemoradiotherapy for patients with rectal cancer (the OnCoRe project): a propensity-score matched cohort analysis. Lancet Oncol 2016;17:174–83.
[16] Smith JJ, Strombom P, Chow OS, et al. Assessment of a Watch-and-Wait Strategy for Rectal Cancer in Patients With a Complete Response After Neoadjuvant Therapy. JAMA Oncol 2019;5:e185896.
[17] Caycedo-Marulanda A, Patel SV, Verschoor CP, et al. A snapshot of the international views of the treatment of rectal cancer patients, a multi-regional survey: international tendencies in rectal cancer. World J Surg 2020;45(1):302–12.
[18] Gani C, Gani N, Zschaeck S, et al. Organ Preservation in Rectal Cancer: The Patients' Perspective. Front Oncol 2019;9:318.
[19] Gunjur A, Chazan G, Newnham G, et al. Pilot study of patients' preferences for immediate resection versus a watch and wait approach after neoadjuvant chemoradiation for locally advanced rectal cancer. JCO Oncol Pract 2020;17(2):e149–57.
[20] Chen TY, Wiltink LM, Nout RA, et al. Bowel function 14 years after preoperative short-course radiotherapy and total mesorectal excision for rectal cancer: report of a multicenter randomized trial. Clin Colorectal Cancer 2015;14:106–14.
[21] Smith N, Brown G. Preoperative staging of rectal cancer. Acta Oncol 2008;47:20–31.
[22] Kim YI, Jang JK, Park IJ, et al. Lateral lymph node and its association with distant recurrence in rectal cancer: A clue of systemic disease. Surg Oncol 2020;35:174–81.
[23] Habr-Gama A, Sao Juliao GP, Vailati BB, et al. Organ Preservation in cT2N0 Rectal Cancer After Neoadjuvant Chemoradiation Therapy: The Impact of Radiation Therapy Dose-escalation and Consolidation Chemotherapy. Ann Surg 2019;269:102–7.
[24] Lezoche E, Baldarelli M, Lezoche G, et al. Randomized clinical trial of endoluminal locoregional resection versus laparoscopic total mesorectal excision for T2 rectal cancer after neoadjuvant therapy. Br J Surg 2012;99:1211–8.

[25] Das P, Skibber JM, Rodriguez-Bigas MA, et al. Predictors of tumor response and downstaging in patients who receive preoperative chemoradiation for rectal cancer. Cancer 2007;109:1750–5.
[26] Huang Y, Lee D, Young C. Predictors for complete pathological response for stage II and III rectal cancer following neoadjuvant therapy - A systematic review and meta-analysis. Am J Surg 2020;220(2):300–8.
[27] Chen MB, Wu XY, Yu R, et al. P53 status as a predictive biomarker for patients receiving neoadjuvant radiation-based treatment: a meta-analysis in rectal cancer. PLoS One 2012;7: e45388.
[28] Garcia-Aguilar J, Chen Z, Smith DD, et al. Identification of a biomarker profile associated with resistance to neoadjuvant chemoradiation therapy in rectal cancer. Ann Surg 2011;254:486–92 [discussion: 492–3].
[29] de Rosa N, Rodriguez-Bigas MA, Chang GJ, et al. DNA mismatch repair deficiency in rectal cancer: benchmarking its impact on prognosis, neoadjuvant response prediction, and clinical cancer genetics. J Clin Oncol 2016;34:3039–46.
[30] Swedish Rectal Cancer T, Cedermark B, Dahlberg M, et al. Improved survival with preoperative radiotherapy in resectable rectal cancer. N Engl J Med 1997;336:980–7.
[31] Jia AY, Narang A, Safar B, et al. Sequential short-course radiation therapy and chemotherapy in the neoadjuvant treatment of rectal adenocarcinoma. Radiat Oncol 2019;14: 147.
[32] Bujko K, Nowacki MP, Nasierowska-Guttmejer A, et al. Long-term results of a randomized trial comparing preoperative short-course radiotherapy with preoperative conventionally fractionated chemoradiation for rectal cancer. Br J Surg 2006;93:1215–23.
[33] Markovina S, Youssef F, Roy A, et al. Improved Metastasis- and Disease-Free Survival With Preoperative Sequential Short-Course Radiation Therapy and FOLFOX Chemotherapy for Rectal Cancer Compared With Neoadjuvant Long-Course Chemoradiotherapy: Results of a Matched Pair Analysis. Int J Radiat Oncol Biol Phys 2017;99:417–26.
[34] Myerson RJ, Tan B, Hunt S, et al. Five fractions of radiation therapy followed by 4 cycles of FOLFOX chemotherapy as preoperative treatment for rectal cancer. Int J Radiat Oncol Biol Phys 2014;88:829–36.
[35] van der Valk MJM, Marijnen CAM, van Etten B, et al. Compliance and tolerability of short-course radiotherapy followed by preoperative chemotherapy and surgery for high-risk rectal cancer - Results of the international randomized RAPIDO-trial. Radiother Oncol 2020;147:75–83.
[36] Jin J, Liu S, Zhu Y, et al. The Updated Results for the Phase 3 Study of 5×5 Gy Followed By Chemotherapy in Locally Advanced Rectal Cancer (STELLAR trial). Int J Radiat Oncol Biol Phys 2017;99:E157.
[37] Romesser PB, Wu AJ, Cercek A, et al. Management of Locally Advanced Rectal Cancer During The COVID-19 Pandemic: A Necessary Paradigm Change at Memorial Sloan Kettering Cancer Center. Adv Radiat Oncol 2020;5:687–9.
[38] Raj Kumar B, Pandey D, Rohila J, et al. An observational study of the demographic and treatment changes in a tertiary colorectal cancer center during the COVID-19 pandemic. J Surg Oncol 2020;122(7):1271–5.
[39] Nilsson PJ, van Etten B, Hospers GA, et al. Short-course radiotherapy followed by neoadjuvant chemotherapy in locally advanced rectal cancer–the RAPIDO trial. BMC Cancer 2013;13:279.
[40] Hospers G, Bahadoer RR, Dijkstra EA, et al. Short-course radiotherapy followed by chemotherapy before TME in locally advanced rectal cancer: The randomized RAPIDO trial. J Clin Oncol 2020;38:4006.
[41] Probst CP, Becerra AZ, Aquina CT, et al. Extended Intervals after Neoadjuvant Therapy in Locally Advanced Rectal Cancer: The Key to Improved Tumor Response and Potential Organ Preservation. J Am Coll Surg 2015;221:430–40.

[42] Erlandsson J, Holm T, Pettersson D, et al. Optimal fractionation of preoperative radiotherapy and timing to surgery for rectal cancer (Stockholm III): a multicentre, randomised, non-blinded, phase 3, non-inferiority trial. Lancet Oncol 2017;18:336–46.
[43] Pettersson D, Lorinc E, Holm T, et al. Tumour regression in the randomized Stockholm III Trial of radiotherapy regimens for rectal cancer. Br J Surg 2015;102:972–8 [discussion: 978].
[44] Akgun E, Caliskan C, Bozbiyik O, et al. Randomized clinical trial of short or long interval between neoadjuvant chemoradiotherapy and surgery for rectal cancer. Br J Surg 2018;105:1417–25.
[45] Appelt AL, Ploen J, Vogelius IR, et al. Radiation dose-response model for locally advanced rectal cancer after preoperative chemoradiation therapy. Int J Radiat Oncol Biol Phys 2013;85:74–80.
[46] Cercek A, Roxburgh CSD, Strombom P, et al. Adoption of Total Neoadjuvant Therapy for Locally Advanced Rectal Cancer. JAMA Oncol 2018;4:e180071.
[47] Conroy T, Lamfichekh N, Etienne P-L, et al. Total neoadjuvant therapy with mFOLFIRINOX versus preoperative chemoradiation in patients with locally advanced rectal cancer: Final results of PRODIGE 23 phase III trial, a UNICANCER GI trial. J Clin Oncol 2020;38:4007.
[48] Fokas E, Allgauer M, Polat B, et al. Randomized Phase II Trial of Chemoradiotherapy Plus Induction or Consolidation Chemotherapy as Total Neoadjuvant Therapy for Locally Advanced Rectal Cancer: CAO/ARO/AIO-12. J Clin Oncol 2019;37:3212–22.
[49] Allegra CJ, Yothers G, O'Connell MJ, et al. Neoadjuvant 5-FU or capecitabine plus radiation with or without oxaliplatin in rectal cancer patients: a phase iii randomized clinical trial. J Natl Cancer Inst 2015;107:djv248.
[50] van der Valk MJM, Hilling DE, Bastiaannet E, et al. Long-term outcomes of clinical complete responders after neoadjuvant treatment for rectal cancer in the International Watch & Wait Database (IWWD): an international multicentre registry study. Lancet 2018;391:2537–45.
[51] Maas M, Lambregts DM, Nelemans PJ, et al. Assessment of Clinical Complete Response After Chemoradiation for Rectal Cancer with Digital Rectal Examination, Endoscopy, and MRI: Selection for Organ-Saving Treatment. Ann Surg Oncol 2015;22:3873–80.
[52] Yuval JB, Thompson HM, Garcia-Aguilar J. Organ Preservation in Rectal Cancer. J Gastrointest Surg 2020;24:1880–8.
[53] Dizdarevic E, Frostrup Hansen T, Ploen J, et al. Long-Term Patient-Reported Outcomes After High-Dose Chemoradiation Therapy for Nonsurgical Management of Distal Rectal Cancer. Int J Radiat Oncol Biol Phys 2020;106:556–63.
[54] Quezada-Diaz FF, Smith JJ, Jimenez-Rodriguez RM, et al. Patient-Reported Bowel Function in Patients With Rectal Cancer Managed by a Watch-and-Wait Strategy After Neoadjuvant Therapy: A Case-Control Study. Dis Colon Rectum 2020;63:897–902.

Advances in Surgery 55 (2021) 109–122
ADVANCES IN SURGERY
ELSEVIER
MOSBY

# Paraesophageal Hernia

## Current Management

Laura Mazer, MD, MHPE, Dana A. Telem, MD, MPH*

Department of Surgery, Division of Minimally Invasive Surgery, University of Michigan, 1500 E. Medical Center Dr., Ann Arbor, MI 48109, USA

**Keywords**

• Paraesophageal hernia • Hiatal hernia • Fundoplication • Gastric volvulus

**Key points**

- Paraesophageal hernias represent 5% to 15% of all hiatal hernias.
- Watchful waiting is appropriate for selected asymptomatic patients; symptomatic patients should be referred for elective repair.
- Acute gastric volvulus is a surgical emergency and should be treated with gastric decompression followed by surgical repair within the same hospital stay.
- Several controversies exist in the ideal surgical treatment of paraesophageal hernia, including surgical approach, role of mesh, esophageal lengthening procedure, and the type of fundoplication.

## INTRODUCTION

First described in 1853 by Henry Bowditch as a "very curious dilation of the esophageal opening," hiatal hernia is present in up to 50% of the population [1]. These hernias are classified into four types based primarily on the location of the gastroesophageal junction (GEJ) (Fig. 1):

- Type 1: Sliding hernias, the GEJ slides through the hiatus into the thoracic cavity. Approximately 95% of hiatal hernias are of type I. Frequently associated with gastroesophageal reflux disease (GERD)
- Type II: "True" paraesophageal hernias, occur when the posterolateral phrenoesophageal attachments are preserved. The GEJ remains below the diaphragm and the gastric fundus herniates anteriorly
- Type III: Mixed type, where both the GEJ and the gastric fundus herniate into the mediastinum

*Corresponding author. *E-mail address:* dtelem@med.umich.edu

https://doi.org/10.1016/j.yasu.2021.05.008
0065-3411/21/

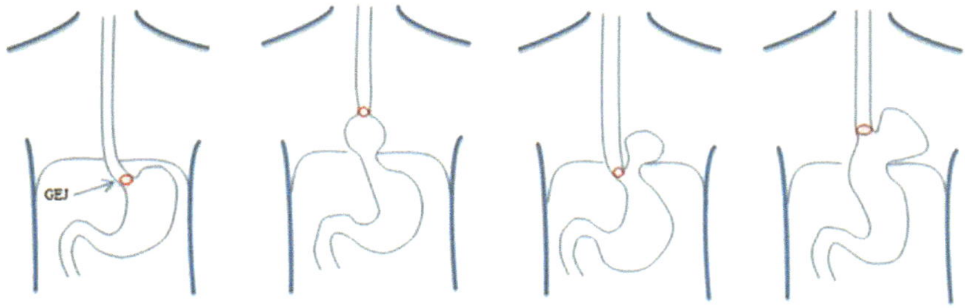


| Normal esophagus and stomach | Hiatal Hernia Type I ("*sliding*") | Hiatal Hernia Type 2 ("*rolling*") | Hiatal Hernia Type 3 ("*mixed*") |
|---|---|---|---|

**Fig. 1.** Types of hiatal hernia. (taken from Treatment and controversies in paraesophageal hernia repair by Lebenthal and colleagues, Front Surg, 2015)

- Type IV: Type III features *plus* additional viscera (eg, colon, spleen, pancreas) migrates into the hernia sac

Types II-IV are considered *paraesophageal hernias* (*PEH*), comprising between 5% and 15% of all hiatal hernias. The vast majority of these are mixed type III, and over time, a greater portion of the stomach becomes drawn into the left chest [2]. While surgical repair is similar for all types of hiatal hernias, the PEH have a distinct presentation, preoperative workup, and risk of acute presentation that sets them apart from the more common sliding hernias.

## Presentation

Sliding hernias most commonly present with symptoms of GERD, but this is a less common presentation for PEH. The presentation ranges from an incidental finding in an asymptomatic patient to an acute presentation with gastric volvulus and impending ischemia (Table 1). The typical patient is an elderly woman beyond the 6th decade of life, and the condition is more common in Western populations [3]. Symptoms for PEH are classified as obstructive or nonobstructive. Nonobstructive symptoms include GERD, esophagitis, or chronic anemia from Cameron's lesions (mucosal ulceration at the level of the diaphragm). Obstructive symptoms include dysphagia, regurgitation, epigastric pain, early satiety, postprandial fullness, chest pain, or shortness of breath. Shortness of breath can be mechanical, especially if it is postprandial, or a sequelae of repeated lung injury from microaspirations. It is common for patients to present with chest pain or shortness of breath and undergo a workup for cardiac or pulmonary disease with eventual discovery of a PEH as the cause of the symptoms.

*Acute presentation* with PEH is a true surgical emergency: acute incarceration or strangulation of the stomach or other contents or gastric volvulus. Gastric

**Table 1**
Presentation of paraesophageal hernia

| | Asymptomatic | Symptomatic | Acute |
|---|---|---|---|
| Presentation | Incidentally discovered on imaging | Obstructive (dysphagia, regurgitation, early satiety, chest pain, nausea/emesis)<br>Nonobstructive (GERD, erosive esophagitis, chronic anemia) | Borchardt's Triad:<br>1) Unproductive retching<br>2)Severe epigastric pain<br>3) Inability to pass NGT |
| Diagnosis | Incidental finding on imaging | Esophagram<br>EGD<br>Manometry<br>Imaging | Chest x-ray<br>Computed tomography (CT)<br>Esophagogastroduodenoscopy (EGD) |
| Treatment | Watchful waiting if truly asymptomatic vs elective repair, patient preference | Elective minimally invasive repair | Fluoroscopic or endoscopic NGT for decompression<br>If septic, emergent surgical exploration and possible gastrostomy tube and gastropexy ± crural repair<br>If stable, resuscitate and operate within the index hospitalization |

volvulus is a rare condition, but the most common cause in adults is a large PEH in which the stomach rotates more than 180°, causing a closed loop obstruction [4]. The twist can occur in the organoaxial direction, around the cardio-pylorus longitudinal axis, or transversely, mesenteroaxial volvulus. The two types can be distinguished on an upper gastrointestinal series (UGIS), but the distinction is not prognostic and should not impact treatment decisions [4,5]. *Borchardt's Triad*, first described by the German physician in 1904, is still considered clinically diagnostic of gastric volvulus: (1) unproductive retching, (2) severe epigastric pain, and (3) inability to pass a nasogastric tube (NGT) [4]. Until the volvulus is released, the stomach is at high risk for ischemia and perforation.

## Diagnosis

Diagnosis for patients referred for antireflux surgery focuses in large part on confirming the diagnosis of GERD and ruling out other etiologies for the patient's symptoms. These considerations are less important in PEH, where symptoms are frequently related to the hernia itself rather than acid reflux. The main goal of preoperative testing is to define the anatomy and confirm the location of the GEJ and fundus.

*Defining the anatomy*

1) Chest x-ray: especially in an acute setting, an air-fluid level above the diaphragm should raise suspicion for PEH
2) CT scan: helpful in operative planning in cases of a very large hernia, to rule out other pathology, or in suspected type IV hernia to determine what other abdominal contents are present in the hernia sac
3) UGIS: double-contrast barium esophagram followed by video fluoroscopy, this is the preferred diagnostic test and can identify the size and location of the esophagus, stomach, and GEJ. This is the best radiographic test for differentiating type I, II, and III hernias. Because it is a dynamic test, it can also help identify reflux or motility disorders and identify and define gastric volvulus if present [5]. In a patient with acute obstruction, this may be the only test necessary before surgery.
4) Esophagogastroduodenoscopy (EGD): useful for examining the gastric mucosa, diagnosing ulcerations in the chronic patient, or suspected ischemia in the acute setting. A type II PEH is seen by retroflexing the scope to demonstrate the GEJ at the diaphragmatic pinch, but with a separate large orifice adjacent to it. Large sliding type I and mixed type III hernias can be difficult to differentiate on EGD and are better evaluated with UGIS [6].

*Functional studies*

1) Twenty-four-hour pH monitoring: While recommended for most sliding hiatal hernias, this is less essential for PEH where the indications for operation are not necessarily related to GERD. In addition, anatomic derangements in a giant PEH may make the test difficult to perform accurately, and false-negatives are more likely [6].
2) Esophageal manometry: Similarly, manometry is challenging in giant PEH, and probe placement less likely to be accurate. Wirsching and colleagues performed high-resolution manometry (HRM) in 212 patients undergoing PEH repair and found abnormal motility in 53%; however, postoperative outcomes after repair were similar to those with normal motility [7]. The reliability of HRM to provide an accurate assessment of esophageal motility in the setting of giant PEH has been questioned, as has the role of manometry results in helping to determine the ideal type of fundoplication [8].

## Indications for repair

Historically, all PEHs were recommended for surgical treatment based on studies in the 1960s and 1970s showing an up to 30% mortality rate for an acute gastric volvulus [9,10]. This has changed over time, as newer studies have shown a less than 1% per year risk of acute presentation, and the mortality of surgical repair has dramatically decreased [2]. Overall, there are no large randomized trials comparing elective surgery to watchful waiting (WW) in this population. The best data come from a statistical model using the Markov Monte Carlo decision analysis by Stylopoulos and colleagues in 2002, concluding that 83% of cases would be better off with a WW approach [11]. In the two decades since that article, laparoscopic repair became the procedure of choice, and perioperative outcomes dramatically improved [12,13]. The same group repeated the analysis in 2018, simulating hypothetical patients' clinical course through a surgical and nonsurgical state, and found that despite the improved surgical options, 82% of hypothetical patients would still benefit from WW [14]. This represents a dramatic departure from the traditional wisdom on PEH and indicates that WW is a safe choice for the right patient.

Despite the relatively low annual risk of acute presentation, emergent surgery still carries a higher morbidity and mortality than elective repair, with a higher likelihood of open surgery and intensive care unit (ICU) admission. In addition, the risk of incarceration and the risk of postoperative complication increases with patient age. The risks and benefits of WW should be discussed with patients in detail before deciding on this approach, which should be tailored to individual patient risk factors. Ballian and colleagues developed a clinical prediction model to estimate which asymptomatic patients are at higher risk for acute presentation; large hernia size (defined as >75% intrathoracic stomach) was an independent predictor of urgent repair [15]. Patients, even when asymptomatic, with greater than 75% intrathoracic stomach should be considered for elective repair. A good history is also essential, as many "incidentally" discovered PEH patients will give a history of postprandial pain, shortness of breath, or nausea [6].

### Management of acute presentation

Acute presentation of PEH includes gastric volvulus or acutely incarcerated or strangulated viscera. This is a true surgical emergency, and prompt recognition and treatment is absolutely necessary to minimize morbidity and mortality. For patients presenting with signs and symptoms of gastric volvulus, rapid decompression and detorsion is essential. NGT placement for decompression is successful in most patients, although the tube must be placed with image or endoscopic guidance. Inability to place a tube at bedside is a diagnostic feature of gastric volvulus, and repeated attempts at blind NGT placement in the setting of volvulized stomach can result in GEJ perforation [7]. Upon suspicion of gastric volvulus, the following steps should be taken to ensure stability and detorse the stomach:

1) NGT placement can be attempted under fluoroscopic guidance.
2) If unsuccessful, immediate EGD with gastric decompression, assessment of the mucosa for signs of ischemia, and endoscopic NGT insertion should be performed. If the mucosa appears threatened, the patient is taken directly to the operating room.
3) Once the stomach is decompressed and a tube placed, the patient is admitted for fluid resuscitation and UGIS.
4) Urgent/semielective surgical repair can then be planned.

All patients with suspected volvulus must be treated as a potential emergency, and evidence of necrotic stomach on EGD or sepsis physiology is a clear indication for emergent operation. The ideal timing of repair in patients who present acutely but are able to have successful endoscopic or fluoroscopic detorsion is more controversial. Polomsky and colleagues performed a population-based analysis of emergent admissions for intrathoracic stomach in New York hospitals and found that 66% of acute presentations with PEH were discharged without any surgical intervention [16]. In an National Health Serivice database of over 12,000 admissions over 16 years for acute PEH presentation causing obstruction or gangrene, only 12.8% underwent urgent surgery at the initial hospitalization. Emergency surgery was *less* likely in high-volume centers and carried significantly higher 30- and 90-day mortality rates [17]. Of course, those patients undergoing emergency surgery were more likely to have actual gastric necrosis on presentation, confounding any conclusion regarding the optimal timing of repair. In a single-center retrospective review of acute PEH presentation, only 8% of patients went for emergent repair, and 35% were delayed more than 30 days. The semielective approach increased the likelihood of successful laparoscopic repair and decreased the likelihood of gastrostomy tube placement. Conversely, 30% of patients delayed more than a month re-presented to the emergency room (ER) in that timeframe with a subsequent episode [7]. Bhavani and colleagues looked at 224 patients in the National Surgical Quality Improvement Program (NSQIP) database with PEH and obstruction and compared emergent (within the day of admission) to semielective (>1 d) repair and found that delayed repair had a significantly higher rate of postoperative sepsis and a longer length of stay, but without mortality differences [18]. Overall, the optimal timing of repair after successful detorsion is unclear. Delay for resuscitation and patient optimization is likely safe, but significant delay should be avoided given the high risk of recurrence and representation to the ER. If possible, repair should be performed during the index hospitalization.

## Surgical repair

PEHs can be repaired in a variety of approaches, including open transabdominal, laparoscopic, open transthoracic, and thoracoscopic. The following steps describe a standard laparoscopic repair; the indications to choose a different approach are described in the following points.

1) Set up and port placement
   a. Patient is placed supine; some surgeons prefer split-leg positioning with the surgeon on the patient's right side or between the legs. The patient is placed in a steep reverse Trendelenburg position with laparoscopy towers at the head.
   b. Access to the abdomen is gained either through a Veress needle at Palmer's point or an open Hasson cutdown at the 10-mm supraumbilical port. Remaining ports are placed as seen in Fig. 2.
2) Dissection of the crura and reduction of the hiatal hernia
   a. Dissection is usually started on the right by opening the pars flaccida (gastrohepatic ligament); this may contain an accessory or replaced left hepatic artery that should be avoided if possible and sacrificed if necessary. Dissection can also be started on the left.
   b. The right crus is identified, and the phrenoesophageal ligament opened. The right crus is mobilized away from the esophagus, moving circumferentially anteriorly and posteriorly to identify the left crus. Care is taken to identify and preserve the anterior and posterior vagus nerves. The dissection plane should

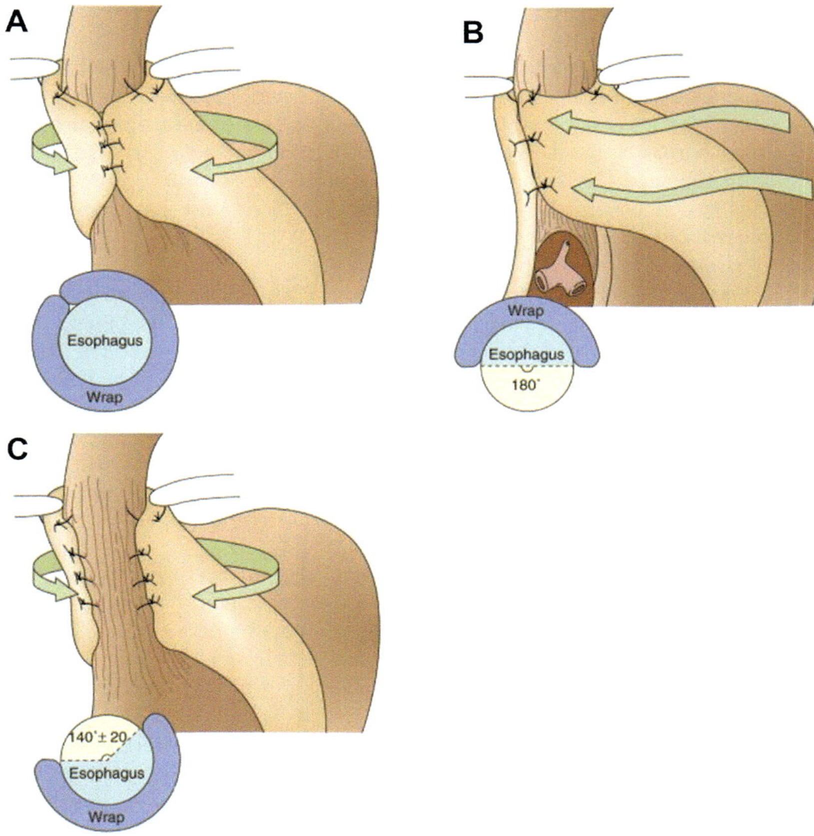


**Fig. 2.** Types of fundoplication. (*A*) 360° Nissen fundoplication, (*B*) 180° anterior Dor fundoplication, (*C*) 180 to 270 posterior Toupet fundoplication. Source: Sabiston Textbook of Surgery. Yates, Robert B.; Oelschlager, Brant K; Pelligrini Carlos A. Published January 1, 2017. Gastroesophageal Reflux Disease and Hiatal Hernia. Pages 1043 to 1064. Figure 42–15

leave the peritoneum on the muscle of the crura, as stripping the peritoneum can weaken the cruroplasty.

3) Mobilize the esophagus to ensure 3 cm of intra-abdominal length
   a. After finishing crural dissection, place a quarter-inch penrose drain around the esophagus to provide retraction.
   b. Dissection is now carried up into the mediastinum, working circumferentially with blunt and bipolar-type energy dissection for any small vessels. This dissection should be carried cephalad until the inferior pulmonary veins are visualized, 3 cm of esophagus is present below the diaphragm when the penrose is relaxed, and there is no tension on the stomach.
4) Divide the short gastrics and mobilize the fundus

a. The lesser sac is entered at around the bottom of the spleen, dividing the short gastric vessels with an energy device along the greater curve.
b. Confirm adequate mobilization of the stomach including division of any posterior attachments by passing the fundus posterior to the GE junction; the stomach should remain in place on the hepatic side of the esophagus. If the stomach retracts back after placement, it is an indication of inadequate mobilization. A "shoeshine" maneuver can be performed by grasping both sides of the fundus and pulling back and forth around the esophagus to demonstrate adequate mobility.

5) Crural closure
   a. The stomach is released back into its anatomic position and retracted laterally with the penrose drain. The crural stitches are then placed, beginning at the most inferior portion. Note that the right crus tends to be more vertical than the left, which runs at an angle; crural stitches should be placed at an angle that slants downward to the patient's left to avoid unnecessary tension on the left crus. (Figure)
   b. The crura are reapproximated with 3 to 4 nonabsorbable 0 sutures. Options at this point include the use of small polytetrafluoroethylene (PTFE) pledgets, especially if the peritoneum has been stripped off the crura.
6) Fundoplication
   a. The fundoplication is then performed. Critical steps at this point are being sure that the stomach is not twisted in any way, incorporating the fundus, not the body of the stomach, in the wrap, and making sure that the wrap sits on the esophagus itself.
   b. A bougie can be used to prevent overtightening of either the crural repair or the fundoplication, but is not necessary.
   c. The wrap of choice is then created with 2 to 0 braided nonabsorbable sutures. With any of the wrap options, the goal is to create a short, floppy wrap of no more than 3 cm in length to reduce the incidence of postoperative dysphagia.

*Surgical approach: minimally invasive, thoracoscopic, open*

The first laparoscopic hiatal hernia repair was reported by Cuschieri and colleagues in 1992 [19], and even in early comparisons, the laparoscopic approach carried a lower morbidity, less blood loss, and reduced ICU stay [20]. In the early 2000s, longer term outcomes began to show a recurrence rate of nearly 50% on routine esophagram, compared with only 15% in an open surgery cohort [21]. Most recurrences were asymptomatic and did not require surgical intervention. A decade later, the same group published new data showing a laparoscopic recurrence rate of 18%, with a change in practice to include a high rate of Collis gastroplasty (40%) and mesh reinforcement (84%) [22]. While the high, but generally asymptomatic, recurrence rate remains a concern, the minimally invasive approach carries a dramatic reduction in postoperative morbidity and mortality with similar improvements in quality-of-life outcomes and is the standard of care for PEH repair [23–25].

Both transthoracic and transabdominal approaches have been described. The transthoracic approach offers better visualization of the esophagus and potentially improved mobilization, which can lead to greater intra-abdominal length in a shortened esophagus. Early comparisons balanced these advantages against the higher morbidity and mortality of an open thoracic repair than a minimally invasive transabdominal approach [26]. More recently, thoracoscopic repairs have been described, although direct comparisons of the thoracoscopic Belsey-Mark IV fundoplication and a laparoscopic fundoplication are lacking. In giant PEHs and severely foreshortened esophagus, a combined thoracoscopic and laparoscopic approach may be beneficial [27,28]. Transthoracic repair can also be considered in the setting of a hostile abdomen, or recurrent hernia.

*Type of fundoplication*

The ideal type of fundoplication remains a topic of debate. The first modern antireflux procedure was performed by Allison and Barrett in London in the 1950s, combining a transthoracic reduction of the herniated stomach with fixation to the diaphragm and reapproximation of the crura. Rudolph Nissen described wrapping the stomach around the esophagus in the late 1950s; Dor later described the first anterior fundoplication in 1962, and Toupet proposed a posterior wrap in 1963 [1]. All these techniques are still widely used: the 360-degree complete wrap (Nissen), the 180° anterior wrap (Dor), and the 270° posterior wrap (Toupet) (Fig. 2). Other less common options include the Hill procedure, which involves a posterior gastropexy, or the thoracic Belsey Mark IV.

Fundoplication during repair of a sliding hiatal hernia is considered mandatory, as it is primarily an antireflux procedure. The 2013 SAGES guidelines for management of hiatal hernia recommend that "a fundoplication is also important during paraesophageal hernia repair" but considered the level of evidence to be weak [29]. Case reports and small single-center series have investigated hernia reduction and crural closure without fundoplication for PEH, but the results are mixed; in general, reflux symptoms are higher without fundoplication, and dysphagia is higher with fundoplication [29]. This presents a more challenging dilemma for PEH, where dysphagia may be a more prevalent presenting symptom than heartburn. The data to support 360-degree Nissen fundoplication versus partial Toupet fundoplication are similarly mixed. In general, the complete wrap has a higher incidence of dysphagia, and the partial wrap carries a higher incidence of reflux. In the PEH cohort, where manometry is likely unreliable and preoperative GERD less common, this can be an argument for routinely performing a partial wrap.

*Utility of mesh*

The role of mesh reinforcement of the crural repair is also controversial. Proponents of routine mesh usage argue that reinforcement results in decreased recurrence rates. A 2002 prospective randomized controlled trial compared cruroplasty alone with suture repair plus PTFE reinforcement; they found 22% recurrence at 1 year with primary closure versus zero recurrences in the mesh group [30]. A 2009 study of 297 patients compared sutures alone, mesh alone, and mesh-reinforced cruroplasty; they found that both mesh groups had significantly lower recurrence rates than the suture alone group [31]. Despite promising early results in single-center trials, a 2016 meta-analysis found that while mesh decreased the odds of recurrence, it did not impact the odds of reoperation. Furthermore, most studies did not provide sufficient data to differentiate symptomatic from asymptomatic recurrence [32].

The argument against mesh is the potential for complications, including erosion, stricture, and dysphagia from wrapping a foreign body around the esophagus. The true incidence of erosion and fibrosis is unknown, as many studies to not include complications, and long-term follow up is lacking [33,34]. Biologic mesh has been proposed as an alternative to synthetic, in an attempt to provide similar recurrence benefits with a lower risk of mesh complications. Small single-center studies have shown a decrease in short-term recurrence rates with biologic mesh placement versus suture repair alone [35,36], but the difference disappeared when follow-up was extended to 5 years [37]. There is overall insufficient evidence to recommend routine mesh placement, but the ideal role for mesh, including type of mesh and configuration, is still controversial.

### Need for esophageal lengthening procedure

Large type III hiatal hernias have a higher risk of shortened esophagus, making adequate intraabdominal length a challenge in these patients. An insufficient dissection with less than 3 cm of tension-free esophagus below the diaphragm is a risk factor for early recurrence. The Collis gastroplasty is an option to increase intraabdominal length, by performing a wedge gastrectomy to create 3-5 cm of neoesophagus around which the fundoplication is performed. The procedure was initially described by Collis in 1957 with mobilization of the esophagus to the level of the aortic arch and required a thoracoabdominal incision [38]. Swanstrom and colleagues described the first minimally invasive Collis gastroplasty in 1996, although the original approach still required a combination of laparoscopic and thoracoscopic access [39]. The first completely transabdominal approach was described by Johnson and colleagues in 1998, made possible in part by the development of an articulating endoscopic linear stapler. This has since become the approach of choice for transabdominal hiatal hernia repair with shortened esophagus [40].

The benefit of the Collis procedure is a reduction in recurrence rates, and failure to adequately identify and treat a shortened esophagus is thought to contribute to the high recurrence rates after laparoscopic repair [40]. The potential complications include staple line leak, dysphagia due to abnormal peristalsis in the neoesophagus, and persistent parietal cells above the wrap leading to recurrent GERD. As with many controversies in the treatment of PEH, conclusions are difficult to make in part because of the varied techniques, lack of randomization, and short-term follow-up of the literature. Nason and colleagues found a significantly higher rate of postoperative leak (2.7% vs 0.6%) after the Collis procedure versus Nissen alone [41], whereas Houghton and colleagues in a similar cohort found no difference [42]. The quality-of-life outcomes, including incidence of gas bloat and GERD resolution, are generally equivalent or better after Collis procedure than with fundoplication alone [41–43]. Other options for short esophagus include deliberate transection of one or both vagus nerves, but this is not routinely performed [44].

### Need for gastropexy

In high-risk patients, anterior gastropexy with a gastrostomy tube can be performed as a stand-alone procedure that allows for reduction of the stomach and provides both gastric decompression and feeding access. Although this procedure has a high recurrence rate, it is a reasonable choice for a patient who would not likely tolerate a long anesthetic [29]. The role for suture gastropexy combined with hiatal hernia repair, performed by tacking the stomach with either intracorporeal stitches or transfacial sutures to the abdominal wall, is less clear. For PEH in particular, the Lower esophageal sphincter (LES) is more likely to be competent than in a sliding hiatal hernia. Daigle and colleagues reported on 101 patients with PEH treated with crural repair and gastropexy alone, without fundoplication; they found that 70% of patients were reflux-free, and a 17% recurrence rate at 1 year [45].

## SUMMARY

PEHs represent a small subset of hiatal hernia, with a relative preservation of the LES and a higher incidence of acute presentation with gastric volvulus or incarceration. WW is a reasonable option for truly asymptomatic patients, but a careful discussion of risks and benefits is essential. Acute gastric volvulus is a surgical emergency and should be recognized and treated promptly. Several controversies still exist regarding the ideal surgical management of these hernias, including the best surgical approach, the role for mesh, the type of fundoplication, and the role for gastropexy or esophageal lengthening procedure.

## DISCLOSURE

The authors have nothing to disclose.

### References

[1] Stylopoulos N, Rattner DW. The history of hiatal hernia surgery: From Bowditch to laparoscopy. Ann Surg 2005; https://doi.org/10.1097/01.sla.0000149430.83220.7f.
[2] Siegal SR, Dolan JP, Hunter JG. Modern diagnosis and treatment of hiatal hernias. Langenbeck's Arch Surg 2017; https://doi.org/10.1007/s00423-017-1606-5.
[3] Oleynikov D, Jolley JM. Paraesophageal Hernia. Surg Clin North Am 2015; https://doi.org/10.1016/j.suc.2015.02.008.
[4] Cardile AP, Heppner DS. Gastric volvulus, Borchardt's Triad, and Endoscopy: A Rare Twist. Hawaii Med J 2011.
[5] Baker ME, Rice TW. Radiologic evaluation of the esophagus: Methods and value in motility disorders and GERD. Semin Thorac Cardiovasc Surg 2001; https://doi.org/10.1053/stcs.2001.26581.
[6] Oddsdóttir M. Paraesophageal hernia. Surg Clin North Am 2000; https://doi.org/10.1016/S0039-6109(05)70222-X.

[7] Wirsching A, El Lakis MA, Mohiuddin K, et al. Acute Vs. Elective Paraesophageal Hernia Repair: Endoscopic Gastric Decompression Allows Semi-Elective Surgery in a Majority of Acute Patients. J Gastrointest Surg 2018; https://doi.org/10.1007/s11605-017-3495-x.
[8] Siboni S, Sozzi M, Bonavina L. What Is the Value of Preoperative Esophageal Manometry in Patients with Giant Paraesophageal Hernia? J Am Coll Surg 2019; https://doi.org/10.1016/j.jamcollsurg.2018.11.010.
[9] Skinner D, Belsey R. Surgical management of esophageal reflux and hiatal hernia: long-term results with 1030 patients. J Thorac Cardiovasc Surg 1967;53:33–54.
[10] Hill LD. Incarcerated paraesophageal hernia: A surgical emergency. Am J Surg 1973; https://doi.org/10.1016/S0002-9610(73)80165-5.
[11] Stylopoulos N, Gazelle GS, Rattner DW. Paraesophageal hernias: Operation or observation? Ann Surg 2002; https://doi.org/10.1097/00000658-200210000-00012.
[12] Mungo B, Molena D, Stem M, et al. Thirty-day outcomes of paraesophageal hernia repair using the NSQIP database: Should laparoscopy be the standard of care? J Am Coll Surg 2014; https://doi.org/10.1016/j.jamcollsurg.2014.02.030.
[13] Jassim H, Seligman JT, Frelich M, et al. A population-based analysis of emergent versus elective paraesophageal hernia repair using the Nationwide Inpatient Sample. Surg Endosc 2014; https://doi.org/10.1007/s00464-014-3626-3.
[14] Jung JJ, Naimark DM, Behman R, et al. Approach to asymptomatic paraesophageal hernia: watchful waiting or elective laparoscopic hernia repair? Surg Endosc 2018; https://doi.org/10.1007/s00464-017-5755-y.
[15] Ballian N, Luketich JD, Levy RM, et al. A clinical prediction rule for perioperative mortality and major morbidity after laparoscopic giant paraesophageal hernia repair. J Thorac Cardiovasc Surg 2013; https://doi.org/10.1016/j.jtcvs.2012.12.026.
[16] Polomsky M, Hu R, Sepesi B, et al. A population-based analysis of emergent vs. elective hospital admissions for an intrathoracic stomach. Surg Endosc 2010; https://doi.org/10.1007/s00464-009-0755-1.
[17] Markar SR, Mackenzie H, Huddy JR, et al. Practice patterns and outcomes after hospital admission with acute para-esophageal hernia in England. Ann Surg 2016; https://doi.org/10.1097/SLA.0000000000001877.
[18] Bhayani NH, Kurian AA, Sharata AM, et al. Wait only to resuscitate: Early surgery for acutely presenting paraesophageal hernias yields better outcomes. Surg Endosc 2013; https://doi.org/10.1007/s00464-012-2436-8.
[19] Cuschieri A, Shimi S, Nathanson LK. Laparoscopic reduction, crural repair, and fundoplication of large hiatal hernia. Am J Surg 1992; https://doi.org/10.1016/0002-9610(92)90046-T.
[20] Schauer PR, Ikramuddin S, McLaughlin RH, et al. Comparison of laparoscopic versus open repair of paraesophageal hernia. Am J Surg 1998; https://doi.org/10.1016/S0002-9610(98)00272-4.
[21] Hashemi M, Peters JH, DeMeester TR, et al. Laparoscopic repair of large type III hiatal hernia: Objective followup reveals high recurrence rate. J Am Coll Surg 2000; https://doi.org/10.1016/s1072-7515(00)00260-x.
[22] Zehetner J, DeMeester SR, Ayazi S, et al. Laparoscopic versus open repair of paraesophageal hernia: The second decade. J Am Coll Surg 2011; https://doi.org/10.1016/j.jamcollsurg.2011.01.060.
[23] Lidor AO, Chang DC, Feinberg RL, et al. Morbidity and mortality associated with antireflux surgery with or without paraesophogeal hernia: A large ACS NSQIP analysis. Surg Endosc 2011; https://doi.org/10.1007/s00464-011-1676-3.
[24] Lidor AO, Steele KE, Stem M, et al. Long-term quality of life and risk factors for recurrence after laparoscopic repair of paraesophageal hernia. JAMA Surg 2015; https://doi.org/10.1001/jamasurg.2015.25.

[25] Schlottmann F, Strassle PD, Farrell TM, et al. Minimally Invasive Surgery Should Be the Standard of Care for Paraesophageal Hernia Repair. J Gastrointest Surg 2017; https://doi.org/10.1007/s11605-016-3345-2.
[26] Zaman JA, Lidor AO. The Optimal Approach to Symptomatic Paraesophageal Hernia Repair: Important Technical Considerations. Curr Gastroenterol Rep 2016; https://doi.org/10.1007/s11894-016-0529-6.
[27] Lugaresi M, Mattioli B, Perrone O, et al. Results of left thoracoscopic Collis gastroplasty with laparoscopic Nissen fundoplication for the surgical treatment of true short oesophagus in gastro-oesophageal reflux disease and Type III-IV hiatal hernia. Eur J Cardio-thoracic Surg 2016; https://doi.org/10.1093/ejcts/ezv381.
[28] Molena D, Mungo B, Stem M, et al. Novel combined VATS/laparoscopic approach for giant and complicated paraesophageal hernia repair: description of technique and early results. Surg Endosc 2015; https://doi.org/10.1007/s00464-014-3662-z.
[29] Kohn GP, Price RR, Demeester SR, et al. Guidelines for the management of hiatal hernia. Surg Endosc 2013; https://doi.org/10.1007/s00464-013-3173-3.
[30] Frantzides CT, Madan AK, Carlson MA, et al. A prospective, randomized trial of laparoscopic polytetrafluoroethylene (PTFE) patch repair vs simple cruroplasty for large hiatal hernia. Arch Surg 2002; https://doi.org/10.1001/archsurg.137.6.649.
[31] Soricelli E, Basso N, Genco A, et al. Long-term results of hiatal hernia mesh repair and antireflux laparoscopic surgery. Surg Endosc 2009; https://doi.org/10.1007/s00464-009-0425-3.
[32] Tam V, Winger DG, Nason KS. A systematic review and meta-analysis of mesh vs suture cruroplasty in laparoscopic large hiatal hernia repair. Am J Surg 2016; https://doi.org/10.1016/j.amjsurg.2015.07.007.
[33] Furnée E, Hazebroek E. Mesh in laparoscopic large hiatal hernia repair: A systematic review of the literature. Surg Endosc 2013; https://doi.org/10.1007/s00464-013-3036-y.
[34] Li J, Cheng T. Mesh erosion after hiatal hernia repair: the tip of the iceberg? Hernia 2019; https://doi.org/10.1007/s10029-019-02011-w.
[35] Massullo JM, Singh TP, Dunnican WJ, et al. Preliminary study of hiatal hernia repair using polyglycolic acid: Trimethylene carbonate mesh. J Soc Laparoendosc Surg 2012; https://doi.org/10.4293/108680812X13291597715943.
[36] Oelschlager BK, Pellegrini CA, Hunter J, et al. Biologic prosthesis reduces recurrence after laparoscopic paraesophageal hernia repair: A multicenter, prospective, randomized trial. Ann Surg 2006; https://doi.org/10.1097/01.sla.0000237759.42831.03.
[37] Oelschlager BK, Pellegrini CA, Hunter JG, et al. Biologic prosthesis to prevent recurrence after laparoscopic paraesophageal hernia repair: Long-term follow-up from a multicenter, prospective, randomized trial. J Am Coll Surg 2011; https://doi.org/10.1016/j.jamcollsurg.2011.05.017.
[38] COLLIS JL. An operation for hiatus hernia with short oesophagus. Thorax 1957; https://doi.org/10.1136/thx.12.3.181.
[39] Swanstrom LL, Marcus DR, Galloway GQ. Laparoscopic Collis gastroplasty is the treatment of choice for the shortened esophagus. Am J Surg 1996; https://doi.org/10.1016/S0002-9610(96)00008-6.
[40] Kunio NR, Dolan JP, Hunter JG. Short Esophagus. Surg Clin North Am 2015; https://doi.org/10.1016/j.suc.2015.02.015.
[41] Nason KS, Luketich JD, Awais O, et al. Quality of life after Collis gastroplasty for short esophagus in patients with paraesophageal hernia. Ann Thorac Surg 2011; https://doi.org/10.1016/j.athoracsur.2011.06.030.
[42] Houghton SG, Deschamps C, Cassivi SD, et al. Combined Transabdominal Gastroplasty and Fundoplication for Shortened Esophagus: Impact on Reflux-Related and Overall Quality of Life. Ann Thorac Surg 2008; https://doi.org/10.1016/j.athoracsur.2008.02.080.

[43] Garg N, Yano F, Filipi CJ, et al. Long-term symptomatic outcomes after Collis gastroplasty with fundoplication. Dis Esophagus 2009; https://doi.org/10.1111/j.1442-2050.2009.00943.x.
[44] Oelschlager BK, Yamamoto K, Woltman T, et al. Vagotomy during hiatal hernia repair: A benign esophageal lengthening procedure. J Gastrointest Surg 2008; https://doi.org/10.1007/s11605-008-0520-0.
[45] Daigle CR, Funch-Jensen P, Calatayud D, et al. Laparoscopic repair of paraesophageal hernia with anterior gastropexy: a multicenter study. Surg Endosc 2015; https://doi.org/10.1007/s00464-014-3877-z.

Advances in Surgery 55 (2021) 123–130

ADVANCES IN SURGERY

ELSEVIER
MOSBY

# Surgery During a Pandemic
## Guidelines

Cole S. Brown[a], Andrew M. Cameron, MD, PhD[b,*]

[a]The University of North Carolina, 115 E Longview Street, Chapel Hill, NC 27516, USA; [b]Department of Surgery, The Johns Hopkins University School of Medicine, 720 Rutland Avenue, Ross 765, Baltimore, MD 21205, USA

**Keywords**

• COVID-19 • Pandemic • Health care systems • Elective surgery • Triage

**Key points**

- COVID-19 presented an unexpected and catastrophic burden to many hospitals and health care systems.
- Immediate government-mandated cessation of elective care had widespread ramifications.
- Resumption of elective care as the pandemic receded required guidelines for operationalization.

## INTRODUCTION: COVID-19S IMPACT ON HEALTH CARE SYSTEMS: SHUTDOWN OF ELECTIVE PROCEDURES

As Covid19 spread throughout Asia and Europe, the United States observed in some countries the deadly results of heath care systems overwhelmed [1]. As a result, the strategy to "flatten the curve" through social distancing was effectuated largely to prevent resource shortages that would catastrophically stress the health care system to its limit, that is, resources such as personal protective equipment, mechanical ventilators, and frontline health care providers. Along with attention to preservation of equipment most hospitals and states declared a pause to "elective" surgeries, although there was latitude allowed for continued performance of "urgent surgeries," the definition of which was left to hospitals [2]. Hospitals, Departments of Surgery within, and individual doctors were left to decide if certain surgeries, such as esophagectomies, prostatectomies, and pancreatic resections for cancer or organ transplants for heart or kidney failure, were truly "elective"

*Corresponding author. *E-mail address:* Acamero5@jhmi.edu

https://doi.org/10.1016/j.yasu.2021.05.009

or were more rightly considered life-saving and thus urgent. In the case of almost all hospitals, surgeries that could be delayed without imminent loss of life or limb were postponed [3]. The cost or risk of a poor outcome for those patients already scheduled for surgery but now postponed was thus made subservient to the concern for incoming patients with COVID-19, their caregivers, and the health care system as a whole that was assumed to be soon reaching a crisis situation [4]. Elective surgeries and care were suspended by the state until further notice. What follows are guidelines that speak to returning to elective care as the threat of the pandemic begins to reside.

## AFTER THE SHUTDOWN: GUIDELINES FOR RAMPING BACK UP SAFELY

### Overview

In response to governmental relaxation of the moratorium on nonessential surgery and procedures, our center began planning to resume such cases as the COVID-19 pandemic evolved. Patients with COVID-19 placed a high demand on overall capacity within the system, making available surgical acute care and intensive care unit (ICU) beds a scarce resource. As a result, the entire system of surgical/procedural postings and cases required attention to judiciously allocate such scarce resources. The scope of these guidelines includes activities performed in inpatient and outpatient hospital-based settings for cases and procedures classified into 4 tiers: (1) urgent/emergent, (2) semi-urgent, (3) elective requiring inpatient admission (includes same-day admission and extended stay), and (4) elective outpatient (ambulatory). All patients were to be screened for COVID-19 symptoms and it was highly recommended that patients are also tested for the presence of SARS-CoV-2. That screening test is ideally obtained within the 48 hours but not more than 72 hours before surgery and evidenced by laboratory results documented in the medical record. Testing was highly recommended but not mandatory for asymptomatic patients (patients without symptoms of COVID-19). At this time, patients classified in Tiers 2, 3, and 4 must be clinically asymptomatic and COVID-19 negative. Patients in Tier 1, regardless of COVID-19 status, still undergo procedure or surgery as scheduled, with appropriate precautions taken. In addition, hospital employees must be free of COVID-19-related symptoms as determined by daily self-report.

What follows is guidance to prioritize and coordinate the backlogged inpatient and outpatient hospital-based procedures accrued across a hospital system. Such cases are first classified into tiers based on their time sensitivity. Next, cases are prioritized into a queue considering their urgency in the context of local site-specific and overall health system's current capacity. Lastly, a mechanism for oversight and a transparent appeals process is outlined to help operationalize the ramp-up.

### Priorities

These guidelines seek to consider and balance the following: (1) monitoring and maintenance of overall hospital capacity and critical supplies (personal protective equipment [PPE]) to remain prepared to safely respond to surge in patients with COVID-19, (2) desire to resume procedures for patients who have had their medical/surgical care deferred, (3) understanding that health care systems may represent a heterogeneous group of sites that will have differing clinical backlog and differing capacity to ramp back up, (4) a need for transparency and consistency in hospital policy while recognizing urgency and heterogeneity of situations across system sites and even within sites, recognition, and consistency with published position statements from relevant bodies (American College of Surgery/American Heart Association (ACS/AHA) Joint Statement https://www.facs.org/covid-19/clinical-guidance/roadmap-elective-surgery), and (5) a desire to optimize the operating room (OR)/procedural schedule with maximal utilization of the OR/procedure blocks while minimizing holds in the ORs/procedure rooms and postanesthesia care units (PACUs), optimally matching surgical demand to non-COVID capacity. Realizing the complexity of the system, modeling tools and simulations should guide decisions, whenever available [5].

The key operational questions to consider when posting a case include the following: (1) how many resources will this case use? (2) can we safely perform this surgery/procedure? (3) is there any specific resource we will not be able to provide that will harm the patient? (4) will doing this case severely reduce our ability to help other patients? (5) are we optimally using our resources available to us so we can help the most people, in the safest way, and in the timeliest fashion? In order to operationalize application of the aforementioned framework the authors developed clear definitions and triage criteria for each case. Triage of each case is based on (1) acuity of the procedure (tier system), (2) availability of supplies (PPE, blood products, medications), and (3) demand on capacity (perioperative and inpatient). These variables are further described in the following section.

### Acuity

Suspension of elective procedures and surgery clearly specified that urgent or emergent procedures and surgery should continue during the COVID-19 pandemic–these are the essential services hospitals provide to the community. These cases have continued at our center throughout the pandemic and are considered here as "Tier 1." To facilitate stratification of cases that have been deferred, we now specify "Tier 2" cases as "semi-urgent" defined as procedures that have a time-sensitive nature and cannot be delayed more than 3 months without adverse effect on patient care. "Tier 3" cases are those that are considered elective and can be delayed 3 months or longer without adverse effect on patient outcomes and require inpatient admission (includes same-day admission and extended stay). Lastly, we have designated elective outpatient procedures as "Tier 4" cases that can occur in parallel to Tier 1 in inpatient settings to fill in OR time when predicted inpatient capacity is exceeded for Tier 2 and 3 cases, as long as they do not consume supplies excessively relative to available stocks (Table 1).

All Tier 2 and 3 cases that have been deferred over the past weeks due to the moratorium during COVID-19 pandemic are to be entered into a queue or

**Table 1**
The 4-tier system to categorize acuity of surgery cases

| Surgical urgency | Tier 1: *urgent/emergent* | Tier 2: *semi-urgent* | Tier 3: *elective* | Tier 4: *ambulatory* |
|---|---|---|---|---|
| Note: | Still currently doing in our system | Should not wait >3 mo | Could be delayed >3 mo | N/A |

"depot" for stratification to be scheduled and completed, as scenarios allow for resumption of activity. Initially, as elective procedures and surgery resume, capacity will not be at pre-COVID-19 levels. Block time for elective cases is to be granted based on caseload (both number and time required to complete cases) represented in the depot of waiting cases. Decisions regarding ordering of elective cases within assigned block time should be made at the divisional level after evaluation of capacity.

## Supplies

Availability of supplies should be assessed on a regular basis at both health system and entity levels. A red-yellow-green light system is used (red = do not proceed; yellow = proceed with caution; green = proceed as usual) based on the following: (1) PPE supply assessment ($\geq$3 or more weeks = green, 2–3 weeks = yellow, and $\leq$1 week = red–only Tier 1 cases proceed). (2) Blood product availability is assessed based on institutional supply and case requirements. Use of blood order schedule is encouraged. Communication with blood bank for any case requiring 15+ units of packed red blood cells is required ahead of time. (3) Similar to blood products, medications availability is assessed based on institutional supply and case requirements. Critical shortages are regularly reported.

## Capacity

Capacity is defined by the ability to provide services to the patient and consists of perioperative and inpatient capacity. *Perioperative capacity* describes the ability to provide care in preoperative areas, operating rooms/procedural rooms, and PACUs. *Inpatient capacity* describes the ability to provide care to patients requiring admission to acute care units (same-day admissions and extended stay) or ICU.

COVID burden has direct impact on institutional capacity and overall proceeding with cases other than Tier 1. Although all cases in Tiers 2 to 4 are affected, limited numbers of cases in Tier 4 may proceed based on their lack of need in inpatient capacity. Under conditions of high COVID-19 burden, capacity should be considered interchangeable across service lines with notable exceptions (eg, cardiac surgery, craniotomy patients, liver transplant, etc. requiring care in specialized environment). To further optimize utilization, bed capacity should be considered across all health care system locations whenever possible for surgical patients, similar to what happens currently with patients with COVID-19.

Procedural services (endoscopy, interventional radiology [IR], neuroIR, Cardiovascular Interventional Laboratory (CVIL), etc.) should follow the same algorithms as surgery.

## AN UNPREDICTABLE PANDEMIC: GUIDELINES FOR RAMPING BACK DOWN AS NEEDED

Given that the course of the pandemic is unpredictable and heterogeneous across the country, it is assumed that spikes of disease outbreak are inevitable. Hospitals and health care systems need to be prepared to ramp back down in terms of elective activity should local conditions worsen. A plethora of measures are available for monitoring COVID-19 status and impact at global, national, state, county, and organizational levels. Among these data, there are a few key metrics that serve as leading indicators to resurgence and foretell the need to adjust care delivery operations: early indicators (1–2 week lead); external indicators, which include increase in asymptomatic rate (week to week comparison), confirmed doubling (if <2%–on alert), absolute asymptomatic rate of greater than or equal to 5% (implies sustained community spread), COVID-19 positive rate in state, and statewide hospitalizations and ICU admissions; and internal indicators, which include hospitalizations and ICU admissions by entity, capacity (defined as available space, staffed beds, and staffing), patient populations with COVID-19 positive status (if available, by alpha/beta trauma patients admitted in the emergency department), and admissions with non-COVID-19 reasons but COVID-19 positive test results in course of patient's hospital stay.

The initial response to COVID-19 occurred in a state of crisis. Our center broadly closed operations across clinical sites within 72 hours of the declaration of the state of emergency. Going forward, it is the goal of our system to be able to maintain and build on the operations recovery that has occurred since May 2020. Some differences with a resurgence, in comparison to the initial surge, is that people requiring care for non-COVID-19 medical reasons will not wait at home as happened before, and our non-COVID-19 medical operations will be in full demand. Another difference is that many patients in surgical Tier 1 and 2 waited for their procedures for too long, and further wait will affect their outcomes disproportionately to the initial surge. However, should the resurgence cause an untenable strain on critical resources (ie, staffing, beds, medications/blood supply, PPE), ramp down will occur in a step wise, rather than an all or nothing, manner. Thus, ramp down may be specific to local entities, and the approach is to reduce non-COVID-19 volumes by unit, depending on local constraints, such as PPE, staffing, capacity, etc. For hospital transfers, specific consideration is needed for patients with the most severe cases and require advanced care.

Because the critical resources for caring for patients with COVID-19 (critical care providers and staff, beds, ventilators, high-risk PPE, blood supply) are hospital-centric, the first areas to ramp down non-COVID-19 volumes will be inpatient and extended stay surgeries/procedures. Should the resurgence continue to escalate, ramp down will next occur for hospital outpatient-based surgeries. Lastly, in the event of dramatic levels of resurgence, our system will ramp down ambulatory surgery centers and ambulatory clinics.

## GUIDELINES ON OTHER IMPORTANT CONSIDERATIONS

### Patient placement and bed management

Bed placement across system facilities should be managed centrally by the Patient Placement and Transfer Command, which should be housed in some type of Capacity Command Center. Given the continued coexistence of COVID-19 and non-COVID-19 care, the use of space across our system for the care of patients with COVID-19, and the constriction of medical ICU beds in the near future, centralized bed management authority allows for the greatest degrees of freedom and maximum efficiency.

### Infection prevention obligations and social distancing

Continue current clinical and nonclinical PPE per system HEIC policy, as described using the link found at https://intranet.insidehopkinsmedicine.org/heic/novel_coronavirus/clinical_resources.html. PPE utilization within the surgical environment is determined by high-risk and low-risk procedures. High-risk procedures are those likely aerosol-generating procedures. A current listing of high-risk procedures can be found at the HEIC link https://intranet.insidehopkinsmedicine.org/heic/_docs/2019-nCoV_agp.pdf.

PPE will be donned and doffed according to HEIC regulations and monitored by the Safety Officers. HEIC link to day of procedure PPE use (scroll to page 2):

https://intranet.insidehopkinsmedicine.org/heic/_docs/2019-nCoV_asymptomatic_testing_patients_needing_surgery_procedure.pdf.

Low-risk procedures require standard PPE and infection control precautions. N95s and modified face shields may be provided for cases requiring the surgeon to wear loupes such as ophthalmology cases. In addition, both phase 1 and phase 2 of patient recovery are considered to be low risk. PPE will be used accordingly. Weekly retrospective and prospective monitoring of PPE consumption will be necessary for safe operations.

All employees must be screened on a daily basis for symptoms related to COVID-19 per protocol. Employees who attest to having any of the aforementioned symptoms must be tested and negative for COVID-19 as well as afebrile for 72 hours to return to work, or, after a positive test, must be cleared for return to duty by occupational health. Attestation occurs via Kronos or on sign-in to a clinical workstation. Employees experiencing any symptoms consistent with COVID-19 should contact the Employee Covid Call Center. Maintain aggressive environment of care procedures adopted for COVID-19 including, but not limited to, the following areas: eliminating patient food areas, frequent cleaning of high touch surfaces in community spaces (eg, waiting rooms, door handles, elevators, etc.), restricting internal waiting rooms, and visitor restrictions. Continue appropriate infection prevention guidance including universal masking, social distancing of at least 6 feet between people whenever possible, and surgical/procedural masks with eye protection for all health care workers interacting with patients.

### Patient and visitor flow

Limit facility entrances with appropriate screening and PPE (universal masking/ COVID-19 questions) at all portals of entry for staff and visitors. Registration desk staff and patients must wear a face mask and maintain a physical distance from other people of 6 feet at all times. Limit one parent/guardian per patient. For same-day surgery patients, one visitor will be permitted and staff will escort them to the family lounge. The visitor will provide their phone number for updates and leave the building once the patient is taken to the prep area. Ensure appropriate terminal cleaning processes in clinical spaces.

### Preoperative screening

In an effort to ensure the safety of patients and staff, all preoperative patients will be symptom screened and, ideally, tested for COVID-19 in addition to the standard preoperative assessment. Screening test is ideally obtained within the 48 hours before procedure or surgery but not more than 72 hours before surgery. Testing is highly recommended but not mandatory for asymptomatic patients (patients without symptoms of COVID-19). A surgery or procedure can proceed if the clinical team and patient agree to do so without a test or if the test result occurred more than 72 hours before the surgery or procedure.

For elective procedures, the patient will be symptom screened and, ideally, tested at the designated ambulatory testing station (strongly preferred) or other location. This requires providers to place the order for COVID-19 testing before the surgery/procedure using appropriate epic criteria for tent (routine, future, clinic collect). On resulting, members of CART will call patients to communicate their test results. If a prospective ASC patient has a positive COVID-19 test, providers will contact the patient, discuss the results, and make decisions accordingly. Patients with positive COVID-19 tests will be postponed and/or considered for treatment at a hospital-based outpatient facility. Patients should be referred back to their primary care physician for management of their COVID symptoms.

### Staff safety and well-being

Ensuring the safety, health, and well-being of our staff is a priority. Physicians and other frontline health care professionals are particularly vulnerable to negative mental health effects, as they strive to balance the duty of caring for patients with concerns about their own well-being and that of their family and friends. As the hospitals ramps up to normal clinical volumes, the approach taken by the hospitals will be aligned with strategies developed by the hospital Office of Well-being. A support structure that encompasses safety, spiritual support, emotional support, mental health, and physical health ideas is valuable for management to deploy.

## SUMMARY ON GUIDELINES FOR SURGERY IN THE TIME OF PANDEMIC

COVID-19 has called on all of us to change our lives in ways both trivial and important. In the case of delaying planned medical care, the decision to delay life-saving surgeries became an ethical quandary that was quickly made irrelevant by mandates from the government. As the pandemic ebbed, at least temporarily, hospitals and health care systems were able to resume elective surgeries and care and required guidelines to help them do so in an orderly and logical manner. Ours are presented here. Likewise, hospitals must retain the ability to toggle back and forth between ramping up and down as local conditions change. Such flexibility may be the "new normal" until there is effective vaccine development and distribution and maybe beyond.

## DISCLOSURE

Neither author has any commercial or financial conflicts of interest to disclose. No external funds were used to support this manuscript.

### Reference

[1] Livingston E, Bucher K. Coronavirus disease 2019 (COVID-19) in Italy. J Am Med Assoc 2020;323(14):1335.

[2] Knezevich A. Most Baltimore-are hospitals halt elective surgeries to ease strain on resources amid coronavirus outbreak. Baltimore Sun; 2020. Available at: http://www.baltimoresun.-com/coronavirus/bs-md-coronavirus-surgeries-20200315-3ojwc7ylgrczbaqqockh5qg3fa-story.html.

[3] Evans M, Mathews AW. Hospitals push off surgeries to make room for Coronavirus patients. Wall Street J 2020. Available at: https://www.wsj.com/articles/hospitals-push-off-surgeries-to-make-room-for-coronavirus-patients-11584298575%20.

[4] Rosenbaum L. The untold toll-the pandemic's effect on patients without Covid-19. N Engl J Med 2020;382(24):2368–71.

[5] Prachand V, Milner R, Angelos P, et al. Medically-necessary, time-sensitive procedures: a scoring system to ethically and efficiently manage resource scarcity and provider risk during the COVID-19 pandemic. J Am Coll Surg 2020;231(2):281–8.

Advances in Surgery 55 (2021) 131–145

ADVANCES IN SURGERY

# The Role of Node Dissection for Thyroid Cancer

Reese W. Randle, MD[a], Susan C. Pitt, MD, MPHS[b,*]

[a]Department of Surgery, Wake Forest Baptist Health, 1 Medical Center Boulevard, Winston-Salem, NC 27157, USA; [b]Department of Surgery, University of Wisconsin, 600 Highland Avenue, Madison, WI 53792, USA

**Keywords**

• Thyroid cancer • Lymph node dissection • Thyroidectomy • Lymphadenectomy

**Key points**

- Regional lymph node metastases are common in patients with thyroid cancer.
- Thorough assessment of regional lymph nodes should be included in the evaluation of any thyroid nodule, and ultrasound is both sensitive and specific in identifying lymph node metastases.
- Complications are uncommon for high-volume surgeons.
- Lymph node dissections for thyroid cancer should be compartment-based to help lower the ratio of positive to total lymph nodes removed.
- Lymph node metastases are associated with a higher risk of thyroid cancer recurrence, but, lymph node dissections are able to provide biochemical remission in most patients.

## BACKGROUND

Well-differentiated thyroid cancer includes the most common type of thyroid cancer, papillary, as well as follicular and Hürthle cell cancers. Other thyroid cancers include medullary thyroid cancer, which derives from the parafollicular c cells, and anaplastic thyroid cancer. Although the frequency of regional lymph node metastases varies depending on the type of thyroid cancer, nodal involvement is generally common. Although the utility of a node dissection for low-risk tumors with micrometastatic disease is questionable, macroscopic nodal disease is easily identified preoperatively and should be addressed.

The authors have nothing to disclose.

*Corresponding author. *E-mail address:* pitt@surgery.wisc.edu
Twitter: @ReeseRandle (R.W.R.); @susieQP8 (S.C.P.)

https://doi.org/10.1016/j.yasu.2021.05.010

Therefore, it is important to include a thorough assessment of the cervical lymph nodes during the evaluation of thyroid nodules for potential malignancy. Similarly, attention to these regional lymph nodes is a vital part of monitoring patients with thyroid cancer for recurrence.

## EPIDEMIOLOGY

Thyroid cancer is the most common endocrine malignancy, and the observed increase in incidence in recent years is not fully attributable to earlier detection [1]. Current estimates indicate that nearly 2% of women in the United States will be diagnosed during their lifetime, and thyroid cancer accounts for approximately 3% of all new cancer diagnoses each year [2]. Papillary is the most common type of thyroid cancer accounting for nearly 90% of cases [3], and regional nodal disease is present in about a third of patients [1,4]. Nodal metastases are much less common for patients with follicular or Hürthle cell cancer as these tend to spread hematogenously. Although medullary thyroid cancer accounts for a much smaller proportion of thyroid malignancies than well-differentiated types [3], over a third will have nodal metastases at diagnosis [5], and because of its more aggressive biology, lymph node dissection is recommended regardless of the tumor size [6]. Therefore, clinicians treating thyroid cancer should be familiar with the management of nodal metastases and the role of lymph node dissection for patients with thyroid cancer.

## PATIENT EVALUATION OVERVIEW

### Initial evaluation

When a patient presents with a thyroid nodule, the history should include discussion of risk factors for thyroid cancer including a family history, prior neck radiation exposure, and obesity [7,8]. In addition to palpation of the thyroid and nodule itself, palpation of the central and lateral neck for evidence of lymphadenopathy is also important. All patients presenting with a thyroid nodule should receive an ultrasound to characterize the nodule and thoroughly evaluate cervical lymph nodes. Many high-volume surgeons prefer to perform their own preoperative ultrasound to evaluate the surrounding lymph nodes. High-resolution ultrasound in skilled hands detects nonpalpable lymph node metastases from thyroid cancer in up to a third of patients presenting with papillary thyroid cancer [4]. In addition, population-based data indicate the proportion of patients with medullary thyroid cancer presenting with regional lymph node metastases is increasing making a thorough evaluation at presentation vital [5].

### Evaluation for recurrence

Attention to the cervical lymph nodes during postoperative surveillance allows clinicians to detect early recurrence, which will often present as regional nodal metastases in the central or lateral neck. Many early recurrences reflect persistent often microscopic disease missed at the initial operation, underscoring the importance of a thorough initial evaluation [9,10]. If the thyroid was entirely removed, unstimulated thyroglobulin levels can be a sensitive indicator of persistent or recurrent disease [11]. In the case of medullary thyroid cancer, calcitonin and CEA levels can indicate the presence or absence of disease even if the initial operation was less extensive than recommended by guidelines [12]. Although tumor markers help detect recurrence, imaging is necessary even if markers are reassuring.

## Lymph node imaging

Ultrasound is the primary modality supported by American Thyroid Association (ATA) to image lymph nodes in patients with suspected or confirmed thyroid cancer and provides actionable information during the initial evaluation and follow-up [13]. Specific ultrasound findings associated with thyroid metastases are listed in Table 1 [14,15]. Unfortunately, in practice, over a third of thyroid nodule ultrasound reports do not even mention a lymph node evaluation [16]. When ultrasound does evaluate the central and lateral neck for evidence of lymphadenopathy, the sensitivity for detecting disease is 0.33 in the central neck and 0.70 in the lateral neck [17]. When high-volume surgeons perform their own ultrasound, the sensitivity for detecting disease in the lateral neck is as high as 0.88 with a negative predictive value of 0.97 [18]. Taken together, these findings indicate that ultrasound quality and results vary substantially based on where the ultrasound is performed and who performs it. Importantly, ultrasound helps guide the extent of surgery and alters the planned operation in more than 40% of thyroid cancer operations and reoperations [4].

Cross-sectional imaging with computed tomography (CT) or magnetic resonance imaging is recommended for patients with suspected advanced disease and not part of the routine initial evaluation [13]. Although ultrasound tends to be more sensitive than CT in detecting lateral neck metastases [19], the combination of CT with ultrasound is more sensitive in the central and lateral neck than ultrasound alone [20]. CT also characterizes disease in areas otherwise inaccessible with ultrasound such as the superior mediastinum (Fig. 1). Similar to ultrasonography, detection of metastatic disease on preoperative CT depends on who is reading the CT. In one report, more than half of the patients with persistent cancer after the initial resection had evidence of the missed disease on preoperative CT [10].

**Table 1**
Ultrasound findings associated with thyroid cancer lymph node metastases [14,15]

| Ultrasound finding | Prevalence in involved nodes | Sensitivity | Specificity |
|---|---|---|---|
| Hyperechoic relative to muscle | 8% | 86% | 96% |
| Cystic component | 21% | 20% | 100% |
| Calcifications | 5% | 50% | 100% |
| Loss of a fatty hilum | 99% | 88% | 90% |
| Rounded shape[a] | 34% | 80% | 71% |

[a]Short to long axis ratio 0.5 or greater.

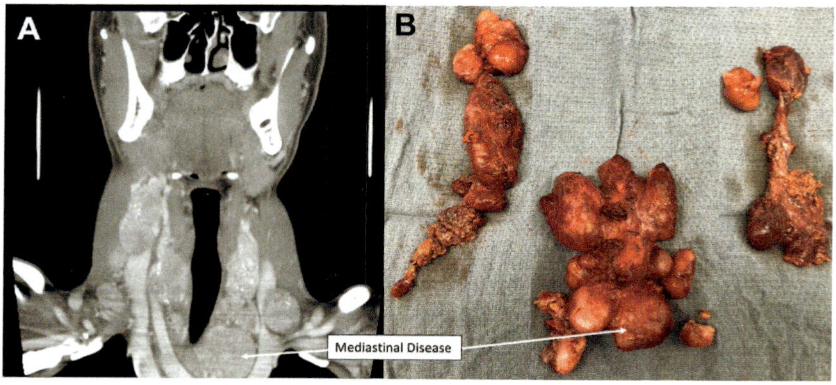


**Fig. 1.** Coronal neck CT imaging depicting significant nodal disease extending into the superior mediastinum not fully evaluated with preoperative ultrasound (*A*). The specimen that correlates with the nodal disease seen on preoperative CT (*B*).

### Functional imaging

Although functional imaging is not routinely used before the initial resection of thyroid cancer, it may play a role in recurrent nodal evaluations. For patients who receive a total thyroidectomy, a radioactive iodine whole-body scan typically alerts clinicians to persistent or recurrent disease in the cervical lymph nodes. However, in cases where thyroid cancer is not iodine avid, PET scan may help characterize the location and extent of nodal involvement.

### Lymph node biopsy

Once a suspicious lymph node is identified in the central or lateral neck, fine needle aspiration (FNA) biopsy should be performed to confirm disease and planning of the extent of the operation (Fig. 2) [13,21]. The exception to this practice is the unexpected presence of pathologic appearing central neck nodes at the time of the initial thyroidectomy. In this case, a frozen section could be performed, but it is also acceptable to perform a central neck dissection to remove the suspicious nodes without pathologic confirmation. FNA is also useful to confirm the recurrent or persistent disease in the central or lateral neck before planning excision in a reoperative field. In addition to cytologic evaluation, a thyroglobulin washout can help identify well-differentiated thyroid cancer metastases with high sensitivity and specificity [22].

## TREATMENT OPTIONS

Node dissections play an important role in the treatment and staging of thyroid cancer. When performed, a node dissection should be compartment-based and not "berry-picking" as the latter is associated with a higher risk of recurrence. Cervical lymph nodes are divided into 7 levels, or compartments, based on their location (Fig. 3). Levels 6 and 7 are considered to be in the central

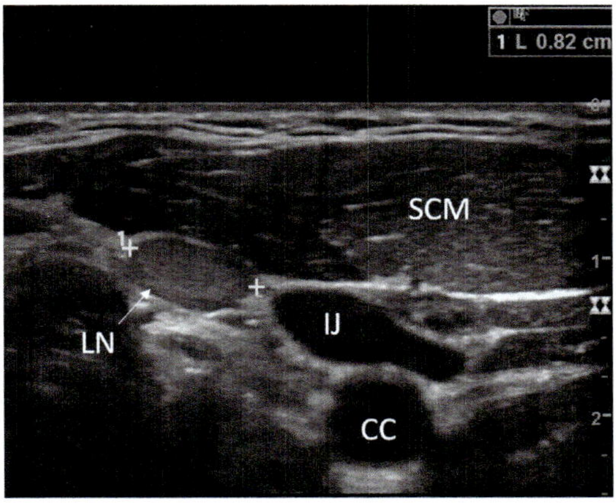


**Fig. 2.** Small lymph node on ultrasound detected when thyroglobulin increased from less than 0.1 ng/mL to 2.8 ng/mL. On transverse view, the lymph node demonstrated loss of a fatty hilum, increased echogenicity, and a rounded shape. FNA revealed recurrent papillary thyroid cancer. CC, common carotid artery; IJ, internal jugular vein; LN, lymph node; SCM, sternocleidomastoid muscle.

neck and are the most common location of thyroid cancer nodal metastases. The boundaries of level 6 are the hyoid bone superiorly, the common carotid artery laterally, and the sternal notch inferiorly. Level 7 includes the superior mediastinal nodes behind the sternum, inferior to the sternal notch and

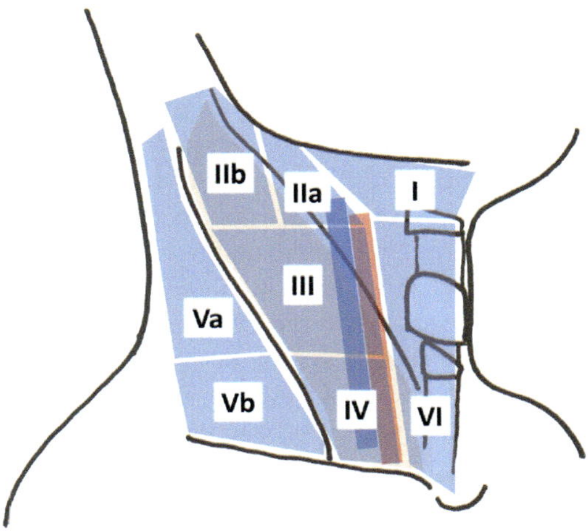


**Fig. 3.** Lymph node levels in the neck.

superior to the aortic arch. The lateral neck includes levels 2 to 5. Levels 2 through 4 run along the jugular vein, lateral to the carotid artery and deep to the sternocleidomastoid from the skull base superiorly to the clavicle inferiorly and are where thyroid cancer tends to metastasize laterally. Level 2 is separated from level 3 by an imaginary horizontal line at the level of the hyoid bone, and level 3 is separated from level 4 by a similar line extending from the cricoid cartilage. Level 5 begins at the posterior border of the sternocleidomastoid and extends to the border of the trapezius muscle. Level 1 is bound by the hyoid bone inferiorly and the mandible. Levels 1 and 5 are rarely involved in thyroid cancer. The lymphatic drainage of the thyroid is variable, but most thyroid cancer involving the lymph nodes spreads to the central neck before moving to the lateral neck. Tumors in the superior poles of the thyroid, however, can "skip" the central neck and metastasize directly to the lateral compartments [23].

## Central neck dissection

### *Indications*

Any patient undergoing a thyroidectomy for thyroid cancer should have a thorough lymph node evaluation preoperatively and intraoperatively. Any clinically evident disease in level 6 lymph nodes should prompt a formal dissection of the central compartment. If grossly abnormal or suspicious central neck nodes are discovered at the time of the initial operation, it is appropriate to perform a central neck dissection without biopsy confirmation. Patients should be made aware of this possibility during the consent process. A frozen section can be useful to distinguish reactive nodes from nodes with metastatic disease in ambiguous situations, but cannot rule out micrometastases.

### *Technique*

Exposure to the central neck is generally the same as that for an open thyroidectomy. After a transverse incision between the sternal notch and the cricoid cartilage, subplatysmal flaps are raised. The median raphe is separated, and the sternohyoid and sternothyroid muscles are retracted laterally. These strap muscles can be divided if necessary for greater exposure. Thyroidectomy facilitates the exposure of the deeper nodal tissue and can also make accessing inferior nodal tissue easier. However, nodes can also be removed en bloc with the thyroid. The recurrent nerve is exposed from its insertion into the cricothyroid muscle as low as possible into the thoracic inlet. On the right, nodal tissue resides lateral, medial, and deep to the recurrent nerve. On the left, the esophagus tends to occupy the space deep to the nerve so most nodal tissue is either lateral or medial to the nerve. Caution is required to avoid devascularizing the parathyroid glands during this dissection. Any parathyroid glands unable to be preserved can be set aside in saline for reimplantation. It is also important to remove the pretracheal nodal tissue superior to the thyroid along its developmental path of descent from the base of the tongue, anterior to the larynx. In the case of bulky nodal disease, dissection can be carried down into level 7.

*Special considerations–prophylactic*
Prophylactic central neck dissection at the time of thyroidectomy for thyroid cancer is controversial. The American Joint Committee on Cancer 8th Edition Staging System for differentiated thyroid cancer added a category specifically for clinically unremarkable cervical lymph nodes on dedicated ultrasound or palpation [24], which will allow population-based registries to record outcomes for patients with a nodal assessment but not sampling. Some physicians recommend prophylactic central neck dissection given high rates of occult disease in the central nodes and the difficulty of identifying such nodes with ultrasound. One meta-analysis found the rate of central nodal metastases in differentiated thyroid cancer to be as high as 48%, and the sensitivity of ultrasound to detect central nodal metastases as low as 0.33 [17]. Yet, other physicians suggest that prophylactic dissections are unnecessary for low-risk disease [25,26]. Recurrence rates remain much lower in patients with low-risk disease than estimated rates of microscopic nodal disease, and a nodal evaluation is not associated with a decreased risk of recurrence in population-based data [27]. Lastly, a recent randomized trial showed similar oncologic outcomes including thyroglobulin levels up to 1 year after thyroidectomy with or without prophylactic neck dissection [28].

*Special considerations–medullary*
Patients with medullary cancer, sporadic or familial, without evidence of nodal disease should undergo a total thyroidectomy with a prophylactic bilateral central neck dissection at the initial operation [29]. This recommendation stems from the findings that more than 80% of patients with medullary thyroid cancer have ipsilateral level 6 nodal metastases at their initial operation and more than 40% have contralateral level 6 disease. The technique is similar to that for well-differentiated thyroid cancer. Although the proportion of patients with medullary thyroid cancer receiving the appropriate extent of nodal dissection at their initial operation is increasing, nearly a quarter of patients receive less than a total thyroidectomy with bilateral central neck dissection [5]. For patients who receive less than the optimal extent of surgery at the onset, calcitonin levels are helpful guides as to whether or not the residual disease is present [12]. Detectable calcitonin levels after total thyroidectomy and bilateral central neck dissection might also be an early indicator of disease outside of the central compartment.

## Lateral neck dissection

*Indications*
Regardless of the type of thyroid cancer, when thyroid tissue is confirmed in a lateral neck lymph node during the initial evaluation of a thyroid nodule or during follow-up for thyroid cancer, a compartment-based dissection is indicated. The disease should be confirmed on each side before a dissection for the respective side. The ATA recommends an initial comprehensive modified radical neck dissection of nodal levels IIa, III, IV, and Vb at minimum, but

more extensive dissections may be required based on the extent of the disease [21].

*Technique*

A long transverse incision with extensive subplatysmal flaps or an incision along the anterior border of the sternocleidomastoid muscle provides ample access to levels II through V. The sternocleidomastoid is mobilized and the omohyoid is either divided or retracted off the nodal tissue below. Although a radical neck dissection involves resection of the sternocleidomastoid, internal jugular vein, and the spinal accessory nerve, these structures are almost always able to be preserved in thyroid cancer. Dissection begins inferiorly at the level of the clavicle. The internal jugular vein is skeletonized as are the muscles deep to the nodal tissue. On the left, care should be taken to identify and ligate the thoracic duct both where it enters the nodal tissue from behind the clavicle and where it enters the jugular vein. The phrenic nerve runs along the anterior scalene muscle and should be identified and protected (Fig. 4). Dissection is carried superiorly and laterally until the spinal accessory nerve is identified or further if the gross nodal disease is still present. In general, a substantial margin of grossly unremarkable nodes is favorable to optimize the ratio of positive to negative lymph nodes. Care should be taken to remove the nodal tissue between the jugular vein and the common carotid as well as nodes behind the vein and those overlying the bifurcation of the carotid. The hypoglossal nerve

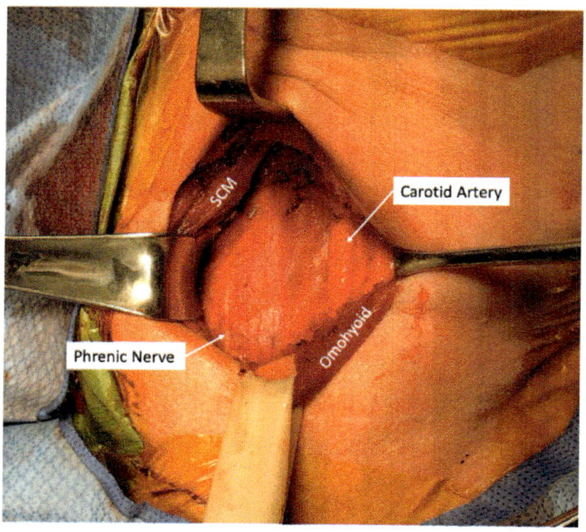


**Fig. 4.** Image showing a completed right level IIa to Vb neck dissection for recurrent papillary thyroid cancer. The superior retractor is at the angle of the mandible, the left retractor is reflecting the sternocleidomastoid (SCM), the right retractor is reflecting the mobilized internal jugular vein, and the Penrose drain is encircling the omohyoid muscle. All the nodal tissue beneath the SCM and around the internal jugular vein to the carotid has been removed. The phrenic nerve is visible running along the anterior scalene muscle.

crosses the carotid artery at the level of the bifurcation and should be preserved.

### Reoperative neck dissection

*Indications*

Although targeting recurrent thyroid cancer in scarred fields presents challenges, reoperative neck dissections are safe and effective in both the central and lateral compartments [30–32]. The disease should be confirmed with an FNA biopsy or thyroglobulin or calcitonin washout before re-exploring a reoperative field. In contrast to the initial dissection, a compartment-based comprehensive dissection is often problematic because of the loss of normal tissue planes. Therefore, a reoperative dissection often involves a more targeted approach.

*Technique*

When recurrence is identified, care should be taken to ensure that the targeted lesion can be identified during exploration. Finding small lesions can be challenging even if the lesion is readily identifiable on ultrasound or CT. It is helpful to make a map of the known lesion or lesions with a skin marker and an ultrasound in the operating room just before incision. Ultrasound-guided injection of a scant amount of isosulfan blue into the involved lymph node or local recurrence can also aid in intraoperative identification. If nodal disease is easily identified with ultrasound, an intraoperative ultrasound can be performed after the resection to confirm all positive disease has been removed.

## EVALUATION OF OUTCOMES

### Complications

Complications from neck dissections tend to correlate with the extent of the dissection. For central neck dissections, hypoparathyroidism can occur from injuring, devascularizing or inadvertently removing parathyroid glands. One large retrospective review identified a higher risk of transient and permanent hypoparathyroidism with central neck dissections over that associated with a total thyroidectomy alone [33]. On the contrary, a randomized trial identified no difference in rates of hypoparathyroidism between total thyroidectomy alone or with central neck dissection indicating that central neck dissection is safe with high volume surgeons [28]. Injury to the recurrent laryngeal nerve is also a concern, although many nerves are at risk during central and lateral neck dissection. A list of these nerves, their location in the neck, and the symptoms from an injury are in Table 2. Although functional deficits result from injury to motor nerves, some sensory nerves or branches can be injured and cause decreased sensation to parts of the neck and shoulder. Injury to the greater auricular nerve is rare during a neck dissection for thyroid cancer, but causes numbness to an area behind the ear and may even include part of the earlobe.

Injury to the thoracic duct can result in a lymphatic leak or potentially a chylothorax. Attempts to manage lymphatic leaks conservatively may include

**Table 2**
Structures at risk for injury during neck dissection

| Structure | Location | Possible symptoms and consequences |
|---|---|---|
| Recurrent laryngeal nerve | Level VI, VII | Weak or hoarse voice, aspiration |
| External branch of the superior laryngeal nerve | Level VI | Decreased pitch and voice projection |
| Spinal accessory nerve | Level II, V | Difficulty shrugging or turning neck |
| Hypoglossal nerve | Level II | Deviation of tongue |
| Phrenic nerve | Level III, IV | Diaphragmatic dysfunction |
| Vagus nerve | Level II, III, IV | Weak or hoarse voice, aspiration |
| Brachial plexus | Level IV, V | Varies |
| Thoracic duct | Left Level IV | Lymphatic leak |
| Parathyroid glands | Level VI, VII | Hypocalcemia |

elimination of long-chain fatty acids from the diet and drainage, but often an injury to the thoracic duct requires re-exploration and ligation. Administering cream into the patient's stomach with a nasogastric tube during exploration can aid in identification of the thoracic duct.

Hematomas, although rare, are more common when a thyroidectomy is combined with a neck dissection than for a thyroidectomy alone [34]. When compressive symptoms occur, hematomas should be evacuated immediately to prevent airway compromise. Infection is rare after neck dissections for thyroid cancer.

## Completeness of resection

Lymph node dissections for thyroid cancer should, at a minimum, aim to remove all macroscopic disease, but ideally be compartment-based and remove a "margin" of benign nodes. One helpful marker in determining the likelihood of a complete resection is the lymph node ratio, or the number of positive nodes divided by the total number of nodes removed. In general, higher ratios are associated with increased recurrence rates after central and lateral neck dissections [35–37].

Tumor markers can also gauge the completeness of resection, direct further management and estimate the risk of recurrence. For well-differentiated thyroid cancer, unstimulated thyroglobulin levels checked 6 weeks after resection accurately identify the presence of persistent disease and help direct patients to no additional treatment, adjuvant treatment with radioactive iodine or additional resection [11]. Postoperative thyroglobulin also helps predict the likelihood of additional structural recurrence after reoperative cases [38,39]. Unfortunately, many patients have persistently detectable thyroglobulin levels after reoperative neck dissections underscoring the importance of a complete and thorough initial operation [30,39]. For medullary thyroid cancer, calcitonin and CEA levels can serve as early indicators of persistent or recurrent disease after resection [12,40,41].

### Recurrence

Although the presence of nodal metastases in thyroid cancer can be associated with a higher risk of disease recurrence [27,42,43], biochemical remission is achieved in most patients who present with regional nodal metastases after a total thyroidectomy and compartment-based nodal dissection [44]. Furthermore, at a median follow-up of nearly 3 years, two-thirds of these patients will remain disease-free [45]. Patients with well-differentiated thyroid cancer with 5 or fewer positive lymph nodes are considered to have a low risk of recurrence as long as nodal involvement is with micrometastatic disease (metastases measuring <2 mm). Patients with more than 5 positive lymph nodes or metastases measuring between 2 mm and 3 cm have an intermediate risk for recurrence, whereas those with positive lymph nodes greater than 3 cm have a high risk of recurrence. Unlike initial nodal dissections, reoperative neck dissections are less likely to achieve biochemical remission, but the median decrease in preoperative thyroglobulin levels can be as high as 98%, indicating that reoperative neck dissections are effective at reducing disease burden [30].

### Survival

Most patients with well-differentiated thyroid cancer will not die from their disease. Although nodal metastases are associated with worse cancer-specific mortality, most patients with nodal metastases experience long-term survival [42]. In one study of more than 100 patients presenting with regional metastases in the lateral neck, no cancer-specific mortality was observed within 3 years of follow-up [45].

## LONG-TERM RECOMMENDATIONS

### Surveillance

In general, patients with thyroid cancer metastatic to the regional lymph nodes experience higher rates of recurrence than those without nodal involvement. As such, these patients should be followed up closely for recurrence with tumor markers and imaging at regular intervals. As neither thyroglobulin nor calcitonin is 100% sensitive, imaging should occur at regular intervals even when tumor markers are undetectable.

### Adjuvant RAI

For patients with well-differentiated thyroid cancer and nodal involvement, adjuvant radioactive iodine should be considered. However, patients without structural or biochemical evidence of disease and micrometastatic disease in less than 5 lymph nodes might not require adjuvant therapy [24]. Nevertheless, these patients are best treated with a multidisciplinary approach.

## SUMMARY

Regional nodal metastases are common in patients presenting with thyroid cancer. Therefore, lymph node examination and imaging during the evaluation of a thyroid nodule is imperative. Furthermore, attention to the nodal compartments is a vital component of follow-up for patients with a history of thyroid cancer. Compartment-based nodal dissections in both the central and lateral neck are safe and effective at reducing disease burden. Although lymph node metastases are associated with an increased risk of recurrence and cancer-specific mortality, a thorough lymph node dissection is associated with decreased recurrence and long-term survival.

## FUTURE DIRECTIONS

Arguably, the biggest debate in thyroid cancer in recent years has been over the optimal extent of the initial operation including the role of prophylactic central neck dissection. Additional population-level data are needed to determine both short- and long-term outcomes for patients with thyroid cancer as well as outcomes for lobectomy with ipsilateral central neck dissection. These studies would be facilitated by revising ICD-10 diagnosis codes to include subtypes of well-differentiated thyroid cancer. The role of radiofrequency ablation in the management of thyroid cancer is also an area that deserves additional investigation.

## CLINICS CARE POINTS

- Regional lymph node metastases are common in patients with thyroid cancer.
- Thorough assessment of regional lymph nodes should be included in the evaluation of any thyroid nodule, and ultrasound is both sensitive and specific in identifying lymph node metastases.
- Complications are uncommon for high-volume surgeons.
- Lymph node dissections for thyroid cancer should be compartment-based to help lower the ratio of positive to total lymph nodes removed.
- Lymph node metastases are associated with a higher risk of thyroid cancer recurrence, but, lymph node dissections are able to provide biochemical remission in most patients.
- When evaluating thyroid nodules or thyroid cancer, look for evidence of lymph node metastases with a preoperative ultrasound.
- Obtain a thyroglobulin washout during fine needle aspiration of suspicious lymph nodes to help detect metastases in well-differentiated thyroid cancer.
- During a node dissection for thyroid cancer, use a compartment-based approach rather than "berry-picking" abnormal nodes.
- Include levels IIa through Vb when performing the initial lateral neck lymph node dissection for thyroid cancer.
- When monitoring patients with thyroid cancer for recurrent disease, look for increases in tumor markers and abnormal nodes on imaging.

## DISCLOSURE

Dr. Pitt is funded by K08CA230204 from the National Institutes of Health/National Cancer Institute.

## References


[1] Lim H, Devesa SS, Sosa JA, et al. Trends in thyroid cancer incidence and mortality in the United States, 1974-2013. JAMA 2017;317(13):1338–48.
[2] Siegel RL, Miller KD, Jemal A. Cancer statistics, 2020. CA Cancer J Clin 2020;70(1):7–30.
[3] Randle RW, Rosen JE. Thyroid cancer mortality in an aging population. Bull Am Coll Surg 2019;104(2):37–40.
[4] Stulak JM, Grant CS, Farley DR, et al. Value of preoperative ultrasonography in the surgical management of initial and reoperative papillary thyroid cancer. Arch Surg 2006;141(5): 489–94 [discussion 494-6].
[5] Randle RW, Balentine CJ, Leverson GE, et al. Trends in the presentation, treatment, and survival of patients with medullary thyroid cancer over the past 30 years. Surgery 2017;161(1):137–46.
[6] American Thyroid Association Guidelines Task Force, Kloos RT, Eng C, et al. Medullary thyroid cancer: management guidelines of the American Thyroid Association. Thyroid 2009;19(6):565–612.
[7] Ghanem M, Olson MT, Zeiger MA. Approach to thyroid nodules. In: Textbook of Endocrine Surgery: 3rd edition. In: Clark OH, Duh QY, Kebebew E, Gosnell JE, Shen WT, editors. Jaypee Brothers Medical Publishers; 2016. p. 121–30.
[8] Schmid D, Ricci C, Behrens G, et al. Adiposity and risk of thyroid cancer: a systematic review and meta-analysis. Obes Rev 2015;16(12):1042–54.
[9] Bates MF, Lamas MR, Randle RW, et al. Back so soon? Is early recurrence of papillary thyroid cancer really just persistent disease? Surgery 2018;163(1):118–23.
[10] Kim HK, Ha EJ, Han M, et al. Reoperations for structurally persistent or recurrent disease after thyroidectomy. Sci Rep 2020;10(1):12376.
[11] McDow AD, Shumway CM, Pitt SC, et al. Utility of early postoperative unstimulated thyroglobulin in influencing decision making in patients with papillary thyroid carcinoma. Ann Surg Oncol 2019;26(12):4002–7.
[12] Randle RW, Bates MF, Schneider DF, et al. Survival in patients with medullary thyroid cancer after less than the recommended initial operation. J Surg Oncol 2018;117(6):1211–6.
[13] Haugen BR, Alexander EK, Bible KC, et al. 2015 American Thyroid Association Management Guidelines for adult patients with thyroid nodules and differentiated thyroid cancer: the american thyroid association guidelines task force on thyroid nodules and differentiated thyroid cancer. Thyroid 2016;26(1):1–133.
[14] Kuna SK, Bracic I, Tesic V, et al. Ultrasonographic differentiation of benign from malignant neck lymphadenopathy in thyroid cancer. J Ultrasound Med 2006;25(12):1531–7, quiz 1538-40.
[15] Rosário PWS, de Faria S, Bicalho L, et al. Ultrasonographic differentiation between metastatic and benign lymph nodes in patients with papillary thyroid carcinoma. J Ultrasound Med 2005;24(10):1385–9.
[16] Jiang L, Lee CY, Sloan DA, et al. Variation in the quality of thyroid nodule evaluations before surgical referral. J Surg Res 2019;244:9–14.
[17] Zhao H, Li H. Meta-analysis of ultrasound for cervical lymph nodes in papillary thyroid cancer: diagnosis of central and lateral compartment nodal metastases. Eur J Radiol 2019;112: 14–21.
[18] Lee CY, Snyder SK, Lairmore TC, et al. Utility of surgeon-performed ultrasound assessment of the lateral neck for metastatic papillary thyroid cancer. J Oncol 2012;2012:973124.
[19] Choi JS, Kim J, Kwak JY, et al. Preoperative staging of papillary thyroid carcinoma: comparison of ultrasound imaging and CT. AJR Am J Roentgenol 2009;193(3):871–8.
[20] Lesnik D, Cunnane ME, Zurakowski D, et al. Papillary thyroid carcinoma nodal surgery directed by a preoperative radiographic map utilizing CT scan and ultrasound in all primary and reoperative patients. Head Neck 2014;36(2):191–202.

[21] Stack BC, Ferris RL, Goldenberg D, et al. American Thyroid Association consensus review and statement regarding the anatomy, terminology, and rationale for lateral neck dissection in differentiated thyroid cancer. Thyroid 2012;22(5):501–8.
[22] Kahramangil B, Kose E, Donmez M, et al. Thyroglobulin washout from cervical lymph node fine needle aspiration biopsies in patients with differentiated thyroid cancer: an analysis of different expressions to use in post-total thyroidectomy follow-up. Surgery 2020;167(1): 34–9.
[23] Park JH, Lee YS, Kim BW, et al. Skip lateral neck node metastases in papillary thyroid carcinoma. World J Surg 2012;36(4):743–7.
[24] Tuttle M, Morris LF, Haugen B, et al. Thyroid-differentiated and anaplastic carcinoma (Chapter 73). In: Amin MB, Edge SB, Greene F, et al. *AJCC Cancer Staging Manual*, 8th edition. New York: Springer International Publishing; 2017.
[25] Gambardella C, Tartaglia E, Nunziata A, et al. Clinical significance of prophylactic central compartment neck dissection in the treatment of clinically node-negative papillary thyroid cancer patients. World J Surg Oncol 2016;14(1):247.
[26] Calò PG, Pisano G, Medas F, et al. Total thyroidectomy without prophylactic central neck dissection in clinically node-negative papillary thyroid cancer: is it an adequate treatment? World J Surg Oncol 2014;12:152.
[27] Gan T, Huang B, Chen Q, et al. Risk of recurrence in differentiated thyroid cancer: a population-based comparison of the 7th and 8th editions of the American joint committee on cancer staging systems. Ann Surg Oncol 2019;26(9):2703–10.
[28] Sippel RS, Robbins SE, Poehls JL, et al. A randomized controlled clinical trial no clear benefit to prophylactic central neck dissection in patients with clinically node negative papillary thyroid cancer. Ann Surg 2020;272(3):496–503.
[29] Wells SA, Asa SL, Dralle H, et al. Revised American Thyroid Association guidelines for the management of medullary thyroid carcinoma. Thyroid 2015;25(6):567–610.
[30] Hughes DT, Laird AM, Miller BS, et al. Reoperative lymph node dissection for recurrent papillary thyroid cancer and effect on serum thyroglobulin. Ann Surg Oncol 2012;19(9): 2951–7.
[31] Clayman GL, Agarwal G, Edeiken BS, et al. Long-term outcome of comprehensive central compartment dissection in patients with recurrent/persistent papillary thyroid carcinoma. Thyroid 2011;21(12):1309–16.
[32] Tufano RP, Bishop J, Wu G. Reoperative central compartment dissection for patients with recurrent/persistent papillary thyroid cancer: efficacy, safety, and the association of the BRAF mutation. Laryngoscope 2012;122(7):1634–40.
[33] Giordano D, Valcavi R, Thompson GB, et al. Complications of central neck dissection in patients with papillary thyroid carcinoma: results of a study on 1087 patients and review of the literature. Thyroid 2012;22(9):911–7.
[34] Fan C, Zhou X, Su G, et al. Risk factors for neck hematoma requiring surgical re-intervention after thyroidectomy: a systematic review and meta-analysis. BMC Surg 2019;19(1):98.
[35] Chéreau N, Buffet C, Trésallet C, et al. Recurrence of papillary thyroid carcinoma with lateral cervical node metastases: predictive factors and operative management. Surgery 2016;159(3):755–62.
[36] Barczyński M, Konturek A, Stopa M, et al. Nodal recurrence in the lateral neck after total thyroidectomy with prophylactic central neck dissection for papillary thyroid cancer. Langenbecks Arch Surg 2014;399(2):237–44.
[37] Ryu IS, Song CI, Choi S-H, et al. Lymph node ratio of the central compartment is a significant predictor for locoregional recurrence after prophylactic central neck dissection in patients with thyroid papillary carcinoma. Ann Surg Oncol 2014;21(1):277–83.
[38] Lee HS, Roh J-L, Gong G, et al. Risk factors for re-recurrence after first reoperative surgery for locoregional recurrent/persistent papillary thyroid carcinoma. World J Surg 2015;39(8): 1943–50.

[39] Yim JH, Kim WB, Kim EY, et al. The outcomes of first reoperation for locoregionally recurrent/persistent papillary thyroid carcinoma in patients who initially underwent total thyroidectomy and remnant ablation. J Clin Endocrinol Metab 2011;96(7):2049–56.
[40] Machens A, Dralle H. Surgical cure rates of sporadic medullary thyroid cancer in the era of calcitonin screening. Eur J Endocrinol 2016;175(3):219–28.
[41] Miyauchi A, Matsuzuka F, Hirai K, et al. Prospective trial of unilateral surgery for nonhereditary medullary thyroid carcinoma in patients without germline RET mutations. World J Surg 2002;26(8):1023–8.
[42] Liu F-H, Kuo S-F, Hsueh C, et al. Postoperative recurrence of papillary thyroid carcinoma with lymph node metastasis. J Surg Oncol 2015;112(2):149–54.
[43] Medas F, Canu GL, Boi F, et al. Predictive factors of recurrence in patients with differentiated thyroid carcinoma: a retrospective analysis on 579 patients. Cancers (Basel) 2019;11(9): 1230.
[44] Hughes DT, Miller BS, Cohen MS, et al. Outcomes of total thyroidectomy with therapeutic central and lateral neck dissection with a single dose of radioiodine in the treatment of regionally advanced papillary thyroid cancer and effects on serum thyroglobulin. Ann Surg Oncol 2014;21(5):1647–52.
[45] O'Neill CJ, Coorough N, Lee JC, et al. Disease outcomes and nodal recurrence in patients with papillary thyroid cancer and lateral neck nodal metastases. ANZ J Surg 2014;84(4): 240–4.

Advances in Surgery 55 (2021) 147–157
ADVANCES IN SURGERY

# Multimodal Pain Control in Surgery 2020

Hannah Decker, MD[a], Christopher L. Wu, MD[b,c], Elizabeth Wick, MD[a,*]

[a]Department of Surgery, University of California at San Francisco, 513 Parnassus Avenue HSW 1601, San Francisco, CA 94143, USA; [b]Department of Anesthesiology, Hospital for Special Surgery, 535 East 71st, Street, New York, NY 10021, USA; [c]Department of Anesthesiology, Weill Cornell Medicine, New York, NY, USA

**Keywords**

• Surgery • Acetaminophen • Opioid-sparing • Regional analgesia
• Non-steroidal anti-inflammatory agents

**Key points**

- The opioid crisis persists in the United States in 2020.
- Multimodal analgesia—pain management regimens consisting of a combination of mechanistically synergistic analgesic agents—should be adopted for all surgical patients.
- For many patients, it is appropriate to use opioids as part of a multimodal regimen.
- Appropriate, patient-centered pain management is an essential component of surgical care.

## INTRODUCTION

The opioid epidemic is a major public health crisis in the United States, costing the health care system more than $1 trillion since 2001 and projected to exceed another $500 billion over the next 3 years. Addressing new persistent opioid use after surgical care is of such importance it is now considered a postoperative complication, much like venous thromboembolism or surgical site infection. An estimated 5% to 19% of opioid naïve patients continue to use opioids after the immediate postoperative period, after both major and minor procedures. Furthermore, one in four opioid prescriptions filled in the United

*Corresponding author. *E-mail address:* Elizabeth.wick@ucsf.edu

https://doi.org/10.1016/j.yasu.2021.05.011
0065-3411/21/

States is provided for acute pain after procedural care, and surgeons are considered gatekeepers to opioid prescriptions. Substantial efforts have been made on both the local and national levels to better understand and address overprescribing after both acute and elective surgical cases. The epidemic is thought to have started in the 1980s, when pain, including expected postoperative surgical pain, came to be known as the "fifth vital sign." Undertreatment of pain garnered national attention as an indicator of poor surgical quality and many reports cited physician insensitivity to pain and disparities in pain management related to gender, age, and race. During this era, opioid prescription formed the backbone of programs to optimize pain management for hospitalized patients. Now, as we work to stem the flow of opioids, it is important we do not forget the center of this epidemic and the reason behind the prescription of opiates—the patient's pain.

In light of the opioid epidemic, use of multimodal analgesia, the concurrent utilization of multimodal nonopioid analgesics and techniques to provide perioperative analgesia while decreasing opioid use and opioid-related side-effects, has become increasingly important. Importantly, it is recognized that nonopioid analgesia, especially nonsteroidal anti-inflammatory drugs (NSAIDs), is as effective as some opioid analgesia and that multimodal analgesia is better than opioid analgesia alone. A database analysis of more than 1.5 million total hip/knee arthroplasties noted that, over a period from 2006 to 2016, the use of multimodal analgesia increased while opioid-only analgesia concurrently decreased [1]. Using more types of analgesia was associated with stepwise positive effects, including significantly fewer respiratory and gastrointestinal complications. NSAIDs appeared to be the most effective multimodal analgesic modality used [1]. Furthermore, the use of multimodal analgesia is associated with a stepwise reduction in opioid use and opioid-related complications, including critical respiratory failure in high-risk populations such as patients with obstructive sleep apnea (OSA) [2].

Multimodal analgesia is a cornerstone of enhanced recovery programs (ERPs) and likely one of the main processes that drives reduced length of stay and improved patient experience for patients on colorectal ERPs. Multimodal analgesia is based on the premise that the concurrent use of primarily nonopioid analgesics can have additive, if not synergistic, effects that produce superior analgesia while decreasing opioid use and opioid-related side-effects. A multimodal analgesic regimen can be designed such that the physiologic and pharmacologic benefits are maximized and the adverse effects are minimized to facilitate the patient's recovery and return to baseline function. There is an imperative to spread the best practices in multimodal modal analgesia to all surgical procedures, as appropriate. Ultimately, sustainable and spreadable success in reducing opioid analgesia for diverse surgical procedures will require a holistic approach, which includes increased adoption of multimodal analgesia based on clear and published guidelines. The goal of this review is to highlight the fundamentals of multimodal analgesia for surgical patients with a particular focus on new innovations in the past couple of years.

## DISCUSSION

### Nonsteroidal anti-inflammatory agents

NSAIDs are one of the most important nonopioid analgesic agents for multimodal analgesic regimens. Despite the presence of an analgesic ceiling effect, NSAIDs provide extremely effective analgesia equivalent to that seen with opioids. In Fig. 1, the number needed to treat to reach 50% pain relief compared with placebo is less for ibuprofen than that for morphine, based on systematic reviews of randomized, double-blind, single-dose studies.

NSAIDs may be associated with several adverse effects including platelet dysfunction, gastrointestinal tract irritation, and renal dysfunction. When properly administered, NSAIDs are not associated with an increase in postoperative bleeding. A systematic review (15 studies, 3064 patients) investigating the incidence of bleeding and hematoma formation with the use of NSAIDs in plastic surgery found no statistically significant difference in the incidence of hematoma or increased bleeding with NSAID use [3]. Another meta-analysis (27 studies, 2314 patients) in surgical patients found no difference in postoperative bleeding in patients receiving ketorolac [4]. A post-marketing study of more than 10,000 doses of ketorolac found no increase in operative site or gastrointestinal tract bleeding [5].

NSAIDs are typically administered either orally or intravenously as part of a perioperative multimodal regimen; however, investigational administration of extended-release NSAIDs topically (in conjunction with a local anesthetic) has been reported with the hope of reducing postsurgical pain for approximately 72 hours using novel extended-release polymer technology [6]. Although topical/transdermal NSAIDs have not been studied extensively for pain control in the perioperative period, topical NSAIDs in more chronic pain settings may be comparable alternatives to oral NSAIDs and may be associated with fewer serious adverse events [7,8].

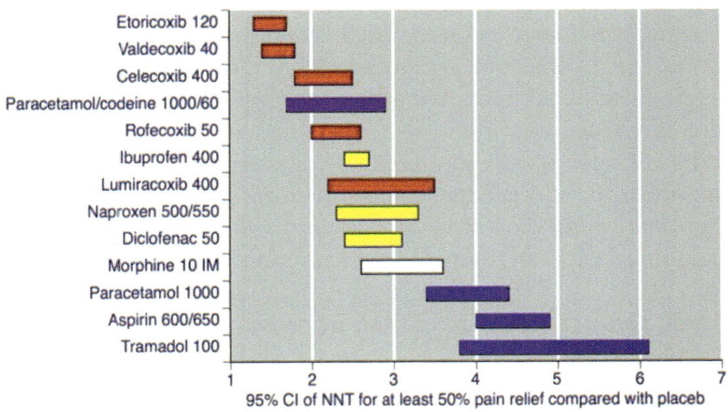


**Fig. 1.** Oxford league table representing the number of patients needed to treat to reach 50% pain relief for usual doses of analgesics in patients with acute pain. *Adapted from* http://www.bandolier.org.uk/booth/painpag/Acutrev/Analgesics/lftab.html.

### Acetaminophen

In terms of analgesia for postoperative pain control, acetaminophen is less potent than NSAIDs (see Fig. 1). However, acetaminophen is an important part of most multimodal analgesic regimens. High-quality evidence suggests that a single dose of acetaminophen provides around 4 hours of effective analgesia for about 36% of patients with acute postoperative pain [9–11]. When administered before incision, acetaminophen may provide preventive analgesia, a reduction in 24-h opioid consumption, and a lower incidence of postoperative vomiting [12].

Although the precise mechanism of action of acetaminophen is unknown, it presumably acts in part through inhibition of cyclo-oxygenase, like that for NSAIDs. Acetaminophen should be administered concurrently with NSAIDs in multimodal analgesic pathways as pooled estimates suggest that a combination of acetaminophen and an NSAID may offer superior analgesia compared with either drug alone [13]. A recent network meta-analysis suggests that morphine consumption reduction was greatest with the combination of acetaminophen and an NSAID and superior to either agent used alone [14]. There is insufficient data demonstrating a significant benefit in reducing pain and opioid consumption for intravenous versus oral formulations of acetaminophen [15].

### Gabapentinoids

Gabapentinoids (gabapentin and pregabalin) were originally introduced as anticonvulsants and subsequently used for the treatment of neuropathic pain such as diabetic neuropathy. Due in part to the success seen in the treatment of neuropathic pain, gabapentin was used as a nonopioid analgesic for the treatment of postoperative pain. Numerous meta-analyses of single-dose preoperative gabapentin (typically in dosages of 600–1200 mg) across a variety of surgical procedures suggest that the preoperative administration of gabapentin results in lower pooled visual analog scores for pain and opioid consumptions up to 24 hours postoperatively [16]. Similar results are seen with a single dose of preoperative administration of pregabalin [17]. Perioperative use of gabapentinoids is also associated with a significant reduction in postoperative nausea and vomiting [18]. It should be noted that the preoperative administration of gabapentinoids may not provide analgesia across all surgical types as recent data indicate that gabapentin did not decrease postoperative pain or cumulative morphine consumption after total knee or hip arthroplasty [19].

As a result, gabapentinoids have been incorporated into several multimodal analgesic regimens and ERPs [20]. Despite the enthusiasm for the utilization of gabapentinoids in multimodal analgesic regimens, earlier meta-analyses did note that the preoperative administration of gabapentinoids was associated with a significantly higher risk of dizziness, visual disturbances, and postoperative sedation compared with control [16,18]. Part of the difficulty in interpreting the data on gabapentinoids in the perioperative period is that much of the available evidence is of low quality and as such, the clinically relevant beneficial effect of gabapentin is unknown [21].

More recent studies suggest that the perioperative use of gabapentinoids, including use as part of a multimodal analgesic regimen, may be associated with increased respiratory adverse events including respiratory depression [22]. An investigation of a bedtime dose of gabapentin 300 mg in 8 nonobese older men noted that the apnea–hypopnea index was higher in those who received gabapentin versus placebo arm (and the authors concluded that gabapentin worsened sleep breathing acutely compared with placebo) [23]. In the most recent meta-analysis (281 trials, 24,682 participants), gabapentinoids were associated with a nonclinically significant lower postoperative pain intensity at 6, 12, and 24 h postoperatively and no effect was observed on chronic pain [2]. Although the use of gabapentinoids was associated with a lower risk of postoperative nausea and vomiting, these agents were associated with more dizziness and visual disturbance and the authors stated that their results do not support the routine use of pregabalin or gabapentin for the management of postoperative pain in adult patients [2]. Finally, in December 2019, the Food and Drug Administration (FDA) required updates to the labeling of gabapentinoids to include new warnings of potential respiratory depressant effects.

### N-methyl-D-aspartate antagonists

The N-methyl-D-aspartate (NMDA) receptor antagonists are drugs that inhibit the action of NMDA receptors, which play a central role in the development of chronic pain. Clinically available nonopioid NMDA antagonists include ketamine, magnesium, and dextromethorphan [24]. Ketamine, which traditionally has been used as an intraoperative anesthetic, is probably the most common NMDA antagonist used in multimodal regimens, where it is typically administered perioperatively as an infusion in subanesthetic doses. Used in this fashion, perioperative intravenous ketamine most likely reduces postoperative pain, opioid consumption, and, to a smaller extent, postoperative nausea and vomitting (PONV) [25]. There was no difference in central nervous system adverse events between with ketamine or control (25) and a recent large randomized controlled trial noted that a single subanesthetic dose of ketamine did not decrease delirium in older adults after major surgery [26]. Whether perioperative ketamine may decrease chronic postsurgical pain is not clear at this time; however, a meta-analysis of available trials did note that low-dose ketamine (<1 mg/kg) was associated with a decrease in the hyperalgesic area around the incision [27].

When given, magnesium is typically administered as an infusion in the perioperative period and is associated with a decrease in postoperative pain and opioid consumption. Magnesium can be a useful part of a multimodal analgesic regimen as a recent meta-analysis indicated that the use of intravenous magnesium as part of multimodal analgesia may reduce opioid consumption in the first 24 hours postoperatively and delay the time to the first request for analgesia in patients undergoing noncardiac surgery [26].

Dextromethorphan is not commonly used in multimodal analgesia but pooled estimates from clinical trials indicate that perioperative dextromethorphan reduces the opioid consumption at 24 to 48 hours and pain scores up to 24 hours postoperatively [28]. A recent experimental study in humans suggested that low-dose dextromethorphan (30 mg) is antihyperalgesic on the areas of primary and secondary hyperalgesia and reverses peripheral and central neuronal sensitization [29].

Although the NMDA antagonists may be a valuable component of a multimodal analgesic regimen, the available data are of relatively low quality and additional studies will be needed to determine the role for each NMDA antagonist in multimodal analgesia. Specifically, the precise dosing, timing of administration, and elucidation of their effect on outcomes and adverse events need to be investigated further.

### Local anesthetics

Local anesthetics are typically administered as the primary anesthetic agent in regional anesthesia–analgesic techniques. However, these nonopioid drugs can also be administered intravenously (IV) or transdermally as part of a multimodal analgesic regimen. Perioperative IV lidocaine may decrease pain and improve recovery of gastrointestinal function after abdominal surgery. A recent meta-analysis (9 RCTs, 405 patients) suggests that the use of IV lidocaine may reduce time to first bowel movement, ileus, pain scores, and length of stay compared with placebo [30]. IV lidocaine may also be effective in decreasing acute pain, reducing postoperative analgesic requirements, and accelerating recovery of gastrointestinal function in patients undergoing laparoscopic colorectal surgery [31]. A more recent meta-analysis found a significant reduction in time to defecation, hospital length of stay, and early postoperative pain, although these differences may not have been clinically relevant [32]. An international consensus recently suggested an initial dose of no more than 1.5 mg/kg of IV lidocaine (calculated using ideal body weight) be given as an infusion over 10 min followed by an infusion of no more than 1.5 mg/kg/h for no longer than 24 hours [33]. Further evidence is necessary to fully elucidate the role of IV lidocaine in multimodal analgesia in light of the substantial study heterogeneity and variable quality of methodology present in available studies [32].

Lidocaine may also be delivered transdermally via a patch. Although a meta-analysis of 5 RCTs found no significant difference in postoperative opioid consumption, postoperative pain intensity, or length of hospital stay between transdermal lidocaine or placebo, there are limitations (small sample size, unblinded studies, clinical heterogeneity between studies, and incomplete reported data for adjunct analgesics) in available studies [34]. Although transdermal lidocaine does not consistently reduce opioid consumption after surgery and has not been shown to improve patient function, several recent RCTs concluded transdermal lidocaine can reduce acute pain associated with a laparoscopic trocar or cannula insertion. As such, transdermal lidocaine may be considered after surgery in selected surgery types and carries a low risk of toxicity.

### Regional anesthesia/analgesia

The use of regional anesthesia–analgesia with local anesthetic-based solutions is an integral part of many multimodal analgesic regimens. Regional anesthesia, which typically includes neuraxial (epidural) and peripheral (upper/lower extremity, abdominal) nerve blocks, lowers opioid consumption and provides superior analgesia along with physiologic benefits, which may translate into improved patient outcomes including cardiovascular, pulmonary, and gastrointestinal morbidity. For instance, epidural analgesia, regardless of analgesic agent, location of catheter placement, and type and time of pain assessment, provided better postoperative analgesia compared with systemic opioids postoperatively. A meta-analysis of epidural analgesia (125 trials, 9044 patients) noted that the risk of death was decreased with epidural analgesia and that epidural analgesia significantly decreased the risk of atrial fibrillation, supraventricular tachycardia, deep vein thrombosis, respiratory depression, atelectasis, pneumonia, ileus, and PONV.

Similarly, the use of peripheral nerve blocks and catheters provide superior analgesia compared with systemic opioids and may provide some benefits in rehabilitation in orthopedic patients. Although the analgesic duration of single-shot peripheral nerve blocks is limited by the duration of the local anesthetic used, the use of additives such as dexamethasone may prolong the duration of postoperative analgesia.

The benefits of regional anesthesia–analgesia may be particularly important as part of a multimodal analgesic regimen in ERP pathways as the improved analgesia, decreased opioid consumption, earlier return of bowel function, and decreased morbidity may facilitate patient recovery and convalescence. The use of regional anesthesia–analgesia has been recommended as part of several national ERP pathways [35–37]. The decrease in perioperative opioids with regional anesthesia–analgesia part of an ERP pathway does not come at the expense of adequate analgesia as many patients with regional anesthesia–analgesia have lower pain scores [38]. Although there are many benefits of regional anesthesia–analgesia, not all surgical cases are amenable to these techniques and there are adverse events associated with regional anesthesia including hypotension, pruritus, urinary retention, and motor blockade, particularly with epidural analgesia. Patients who are anticoagulated may not be candidates for epidural analgesia [39–50].

With the increasing use of ultrasound technology, many newer regional blocks have been implemented. The erector spinae plane block is an interfascial block that may provide analgesia for thoracic and abdominal surgical procedures. The quadratus lumborum block is another interfascial block that may provide analgesia for abdominal procedures. The mechanisms of action for these newer blocks are still not thoroughly understood and their eventual role in multimodal analgesia is yet to be determined as high-quality randomized controlled trials will be needed.

## SUMMARY

In summary, although multimodal analgesia has been available for years, the opioid pandemic and the enhanced recovery after surgery movement has moved it to the forefront. Every single surgical patient–to both optimize analgesia and modulate opioid exposure–should be treated with a multimodal approach. No longer is it appropriate to exclusively use opioids for analgesia. Surgeons should be integral parts of the team that executes a multimodal analgesia approach from the operating room until the time of discharge. As pain management has been more complex and nuanced, it is essential that providers stay up to date and modify approach as more evidence is available. This is best exemplified by the recent warnings about the potential adverse side-effects of gabapentinoids as adjuncts, particularly in older adults.

## CLINICS CARE POINTS

- It is no longer appropriate to use opioids alone for perioperative analgesia. The data support a multimodal approach using multiple nonopioid agents to reduce patient exposure to opioids and opioid-related risks.
- Combining agents with different mechanisms of action appears to have the greatest effect on reducing patient pain. The combination of NSAIDs and acetaminophen has been shown to be equivalent or better than morphine to treat postoperative pain.
- NSAIDs are one of the most effective analgesic agents, although have been associated with platelet dysfunction, gastrointestinal tract irritation, and renal dysfunction. Despite the theoretical risk, systematic reviews have not found an association between NSAIDs and postoperative bleeding.
- Although there was initial enthusiasm for incorporating gabapentin into multimodal regimen, surgeons must use care as perioperative use may be associated with respiratory depression as well as dizziness and visual disturbances. These effects are most notable in older patients.
- Regional anesthesia lowers opioid consumption and provides superior physiologic analgesia than opioids. Epidural analgesia has been associated with a decreased risk of postoperative death and lower rates of cardiac, pulmonary, and gastrointestinal complications. Although not appropriate for all surgeries in all patient populations, such as those requiring anticoagulation, strong consideration should be given to this kind of analgesia.
- Although NMDA agonists are a promising potential adjunct in treating perioperative pain, their optimal timing and dosing is still being studied.

### Disclosure

The authors have nothing to disclose.

### References

[1] Memtsoudis SG, Poeran J, Zubizarreta N, et al. Association of multimodal pain management strategies with perioperative outcomes and resource utilization: a population-based study. Anesthesiology 2018;128(5):891–902.

[2] Cozowicz C, Poeran J, Zubizarreta N, et al. Non-opioid analgesic modes of pain management are associated with reduced postoperative complications and resource utilisation: a retrospective study of obstructive sleep apnoea patients undergoing elective joint arthroplasty. Br J Anaesth 2019;122(1):131–40.
[3] Walker NJ, Jones VM, Kratky L, et al. Hematoma risks of nonsteroidal anti-inflammatory drugs used in plastic surgery procedures: a systematic review and meta-analysis. Ann Plast Surg 2019;82(6S Suppl 5):S437–45.
[4] Gobble RM, Hoang HL, Kachniarz B, et al. Ketorolac does not increase perioperative bleeding: a meta-analysis of randomized controlled trials. Plast Reconstr Surg 2014;133(3):741–55.
[5] Strom BL, Berlin JA, Kinman JL, et al. Parenteral ketorolac and risk of gastrointestinal and operative site bleeding: a postmarketing surveillance study. J Am Med Assoc 1996;275(5):376–82.
[6] Ottoboni T, Quart B, Pawasauskas J, et al. Mechanism of action of HTX-011: a novel, extended-release, dual-acting local anesthetic formulation for postoperative pain. Reg Anesth Pain Med 2019; https://doi.org/10.1136/rapm-2019-100714.
[7] Zacher J, Altman R, Bellamy N, et al. Topical diclofenac and its role in pain and inflammation: an evidence-based review. Curr Med Res Opin 2008;24(4):925–50.
[8] Klinge SA, Sawyer GA. Effectiveness and safety of topical versus oral nonsteroidal anti-inflammatory drugs: a comprehensive review. Phys Sportsmed 2013;41(2):64–74.
[9] McNicol ED, Ferguson MC, Haroutounian S, et al. Single dose intravenous paracetamol or intravenous propacetamol for postoperative pain. Cochrane Database Syst Rev 2016;2016(5):CD007126.
[10] Yang L, Du S, Sun Y. Intravenous acetaminophen as an adjunct to multimodal analgesia after total knee and hip arthroplasty: a systematic review and meta-analysis. Int J Surg 2017;47: 135–46.
[11] Apfel CC, Turan A, Souza K, et al. Intravenous acetaminophen reduces postoperative nausea and vomiting: a systematic review and meta-analysis. Pain 2013;154(5):677–89.
[12] Doleman B, Read D, Lund JN, et al. Preventive acetaminophen reduces postoperative opioid consumption, vomiting, and pain scores after surgery: systematic review and meta-analysis. Reg Anesth Pain Med 2015;40(6):706–12.
[13] Ong CK, Seymour RA, Lirk P, et al. Combining paracetamol (acetaminophen) with nonsteroidal antiinflammatory drugs: a qualitative systematic review of analgesic efficacy for acute postoperative pain. Anesth Analg 2010;110(4):1170–9.
[14] Martinez V, Beloeil H, Marret E, et al. Non-opioid analgesics in adults after major surgery: systematic review with network meta-analysis of randomized trials. Br J Anaesth 2017;118(1):22–31.
[15] Sun L, Zhu X, Zou J, et al. Comparison of intravenous and oral acetaminophen for pain control after total knee and hip arthroplasty: A systematic review and meta-analysis. Medicine (Baltimore) 2018;97(6):e9751.
[16] Hurley RW, Cohen SP, Williams KA, et al. The analgesic effects of perioperative gabapentin on postoperative pain: a meta-analysis. Reg Anesth Pain Med 2006;31(3):237–47.
[17] Zhang J, Ho KY, Wang Y. Efficacy of pregabalin in acute postoperative pain: a meta-analysis. Br J Anaesth 2011;106(4):454–62.
[18] Grant MC, Lee H, Page AJ, et al. The effect of preoperative gabapentin on postoperative nausea and vomiting: a meta-analysis. Anesth Analg 2016;122(4):976–85.
[19] Kang J, Zhao Z, Lv J, et al. The efficacy of perioperative gabapentin for the treatment of postoperative pain following total knee and hip arthroplasty: a meta-analysis. J Orthop Surg Res 2020;15(1):332.
[20] Chiu C, Aleshi P, Esserman LJ, et al. Improved analgesia and reduced post-operative nausea and vomiting after implementation of an enhanced recovery after surgery (ERAS) pathway for total mastectomy. BMC Anesthesiol 2018;18(1):41.

[21] Cavalcante AN, Sprung J, Schroeder DR, et al. Multimodal analgesic therapy with gabapentin and Its association with postoperative respiratory depression. Anesth Analg 2017;125(1):141–6.
[22] Fabritius ML, Geisler A, Petersen PL, et al. Gabapentin for post-operative pain management - a systematic review with meta-analyses and trial sequential analyses. Acta Anaesthesiol Scand 2016;60(9):1188–208.
[23] Piovezan RD, Kase C, Moizinho R, et al. Gabapentin acutely increases the apnea-hypopnea index in older men: data from a randomized, double-blind, placebo-controlled study. J Sleep Res 2017;26(2):166–70.
[24] Verret M, Lauzier F, Zarychanski R, et al. Canadian Perioperative Anesthesia Clinical Trials (PACT) Group. Perioperative use of gabapentinoids for the management of postoperative acute pain: a systematic review and meta-analysis. Anesthesiology 2020;133(2):265–79.
[25] Food and Drug Administration. FDA In Brief: FDA requires new warnings for gabapentinoids about risk of respiratory depression. Available at: https://www.fda.gov/news-events/fda-brief/fda-brief-fda-requires-new-warnings-gabapentinoids-about-risk-respiratory-depression. Accessed November 14, 2020.
[26] Wick EC, Grant MC, Wu CL. Postoperative multimodal analgesia pain management with nonopioid analgesics and techniques: a review. JAMA Surg 2017;152(7):691–7.
[27] Brinck EC, Tiippana E, Heesen M, et al. Perioperative intravenous ketamine for acute postoperative pain in adults. Cochrane Database Syst Rev 2018;12(12):CD012033.
[28] Avidan MS, Maybrier HR, Abdallah AB, et al, PODCAST Research Group. Intraoperative ketamine for prevention of postoperative delirium or pain after major surgery in older adults: an international, multicentre, double-blind, randomised clinical trial. Lancet 2017;390(10091):267–75.
[29] Thompson T, Whiter F, Gallop K, et al. NMDA receptor antagonists and pain relief: a meta-analysis of experimental trials. Neurology 2019;92(14):e1652–62.
[30] Ng KT, Yap JLL, Izham IN, et al. The effect of intravenous magnesium on postoperative morphine consumption in noncardiac surgery: a systematic review and meta-analysis with trial sequential analysis. Eur J Anaesthesiol 2020;37(3):212–23.
[31] King MR, Ladha KS, Gelineau AM, et al. Perioperative dextromethorphan as an adjunct for postoperative pain: a meta-analysis of randomized controlled trials. Anesthesiology 2016;124(3):696–705.
[32] Martin E, Narjoz C, Decleves X, et al. Dextromethorphan analgesia in a human experimental model of hyperalgesia. Anesthesiology 2019;131(2):356–68.
[33] Cooke C, Kennedy ED, Foo I, et al. Meta-analysis of the effect of perioperative intravenous lidocaine on return of gastrointestinal function after colorectal surgery. Tech Coloproctol 2019;23(1):15–24.
[34] Wei S, Yu-Han Z, Wei-Wei J, et al. The effects of intravenous lidocaine on wound pain and gastrointestinal function recovery after laparoscopic colorectal surgery. Int Wound J 2020;17(2):351–62.
[35] Rollins KE, Javanmard-Emamghissi H, Scott MJ, et al. The impact of peri-operative intravenous lidocaine on postoperative outcome after elective colorectal surgery: a meta-analysis of randomised controlled trials. Eur J Anaesthesiol 2020;37(8):659–70.
[36] Foo I, Macfarlane AJR, Srivastava D, et al. The use of intravenous lidocaine for postoperative pain and recovery: international consensus statement on efficacy and safety. Anaesthesia 2020; https://doi.org/10.1111/anae.15270.
[37] Bai Y, Miller T, Tan M, et al. Lidocaine patch for acute pain management: a meta-analysis of prospective controlled trials. Curr Med Res Opin 2015;31(3):575–81.
[38] Smoker J, Cohen A, Rasouli MR, et al. Transdermal lidocaine for perioperative pain: a systematic review of the literature. Curr Pain Headache Rep 2019;23(12):89.
[39] Block BM, Liu SS, Rowlingson AJ, et al. Efficacy of postoperative epidural analgesia: a meta-analysis. JAMA 2003;290(18):2455–63.

[40] Pöpping DM, Elia N, Van Aken HK, et al. Impact of epidural analgesia on mortality and morbidity after surgery: systematic review and meta-analysis of randomized controlled trials. Ann Surg 2014;259(6):1056–67.
[41] Richman JM, Liu SS, Courpas G, et al. Does continuous peripheral nerve block provide superior pain control to opioids? A meta-analysis. Anesth Analg 2006;102(1):248–57.
[42] Ilfeld BM. Continuous peripheral nerve blocks: an update of the published evidence and comparison with novel, alternative analgesic modalities. Anesth Analg 2017;124(1): 308–35.
[43] Kirksey MA, Haskins SC, Cheng J, et al. Local anesthetic peripheral nerve block adjuvants for prolongation of analgesia: a systematic qualitative review. PLoS One 2015;10(9): e0137312.
[44] Soffin EM, Gibbons MM, Ko CY, et al. Evidence Review Conducted for the Agency for Healthcare Research and Quality Safety Program for Improving Surgical Care and Recovery: focus on anesthesiology for total knee arthroplasty. Anesth Analg 2019;128(3): 441–53.
[45] Grant MC, Gibbons MM, Ko CY, et al. Evidence review conducted for the AHRQ Safety Program for Improving Surgical Care and Recovery: focus on anesthesiology for gynecologic surgery. Reg Anesth Pain Med 2019; https://doi.org/10.1136/rapm-2018-100071.
[46] Ban KA, Gibbons MM, Ko CY, et al. Evidence Review Conducted for the Agency for Healthcare Research and Quality Safety Program for Improving Surgical Care and Recovery: focus on anesthesiology for colorectal surgery. Anesth Analg 2019;128(5):879–89.
[47] Grant MC, Sommer PM, He C, et al. Preserved analgesia with reduction in opioids through the use of an acute pain protocol in enhanced recovery after surgery for open hepatectomy. Reg Anesth Pain Med 2017;42(4):451–7.
[48] Horlocker TT, Wedel DJ, Rowlingson JC, et al. Regional anesthesia in the patient receiving antithrombotic or thrombolytic therapy: American Society of Regional Anesthesia and Pain Medicine Evidence-Based Guidelines (Third Edition). Reg Anesth Pain Med 2010;35(1): 64–101.
[49] De Cassai A, Bonvicini D, Correale C, et al. Erector spinae plane block: a systematic qualitative review. Minerva Anestesiol 2019;85(3):308–19.
[50] Xu M, Tang Y, Wang J, et al. Quadratus lumborum block for postoperative analgesia after cesarean delivery: a systematic review and meta-analysis. Int J Obstet Anesth 2020;42: 87–98.

Advances in Surgery 55 (2021) 159–174

ADVANCES IN SURGERY

ELSEVIER
MOSBY

# What is the Current Role of Hyperthermic Intraperitoneal Chemotherapy in Colorectal Cancer?

Catherine H. Davis, MD, MPH, H. Richard Alexander Jr, MD*

Rutgers Cancer Institute of New Jersey, 195 Little Albany Street, New Brunswick, NJ 08901, USA

**Keywords**

- Colorectal cancer • Peritoneal carcinomatosis • Peritoneal metastasis
- Cytoreductive surgery • HIPEC

**Key points**

- In well-selected patients in experienced centers, cytoreductive surgery (CRS) and hyperthermic intraperitoneal chemotherapy (HIPEC) can be performed for colorectal peritoneal metastasis with acceptable morbidity and are associated with prolonged survival.
- HIPEC using oxaliplatin after CRS has not been shown to result in improved outcome compared with CRS alone.
- The outcomes after CRS and HIPEC using oxaliplatin versus mitomycin C are conflicting.
- The optimal sequencing and duration of systemic chemotherapy around CRS and HIPEC have not yet been established.

## CLINICAL BACKGROUND

Among patients with colorectal cancer (CRC), 30% to 40% develop peritoneal metastases (PMs) in the course of their disease process [1–3], and approximately 10% of patients with colon cancer and 3% of patients with rectal cancer present with synchronous PMs [4]. The peritoneum is the third most common location for metastases, following the liver and lungs, but portends the worst prognosis [2]. Historically, treatment of colorectal PMs was palliative in nature and median survival with systemic chemotherapy is between 5 months and 13 months [5].

*Corresponding author. *E-mail address:* Ha364@cinj.rutgers.edu
Twitter: @CDavisMD (C.H.D.)

https://doi.org/10.1016/j.yasu.2021.05.012
0065-3411/21/

PMs are believed to develop through a sequence of events called the tumor cell entrapment hypothesis. First, down-regulation of E-cadherin causes shedding of tumor cells into the peritoneal fluid, which then bind to mesothelial cells, followed by FAS-mediated apoptosis of mesothelial cells. Finally, tumor cells enter into the submesothelial space, where they may proliferate into individual peritoneal deposits [6,7].

PMs may present with abdominal pain, distension, or weight loss; however, the disease process often is asymptomatic at diagnosis and the full extent of disease is difficult to determine on cross-sectional imaging [7]. Risk factors associated with the development of PMs from colorectal adenocarcinoma include advanced T stage, lymph node metastases, synchronous ovarian metastases, poor tumor differentiation, colonic origin, incomplete resection of index tumor, mucinous adenocarcinoma, signet ring histology, emergency surgery at time of diagnosis, and younger age [8]. In the most recent edition of the *TNM Classification of Malignant Tumours* (8th edition, 2017), PM is classified as M1c (as opposed to M1a, metastasis to 1 organ, and M1b, metastasis to more than 1 organ) and makes the overall cancer stage 4C [9].

Sadeghi and colleagues [10] showed in the EVOCAPE 1 study that patients with larger burden of PMs have the shortest survival. Patients with less than 5-mm peritoneal implants localized to 1 part of the abdomen had a mean survival of 14.3 months; those with diffusely distributed less than 5-mm implants had a mean survival of 8.4 months; patients with implants between 5 mm and 2 cm in size had a mean survival of 6 months; and patients with large malignant cakes (>2 cm in size) had a mean survival of 4.4 months. Outcome also is influenced by tumor histology, with PMs from mucinous carcinoma having a more favorable prognosis than either adenocarcinoma or signet ring cell cancers [11].

Sugarbaker was 1 of the first to advocate the concept of cytoreductive surgery (CRS) and heated intraperitoneal chemotherapy (HIPEC) [12,13]. As of 2018, an estimated 430 centers treated 3800 patients with colorectal PMs with CRS and HIPEC in a single year [14]. Despite seemingly widespread treatment with CRS and HIPEC, the procedure has not been universally accepted, is not performed uniformly using the same technique between all centers, and is by some still considered "experimental" due to lack of robust randomized data. In addition, there is potential for significant morbidity and mortality of the procedure [15].

## CYTOREDUCTIVE SURGERY AND HYPERTHERMIC INTRAPERITONEAL CHEMOTHERAPY TECHNIQUE

Disease burden is codified using the peritoneal cancer index (PCI) (Fig. 1) [16]. The PCI describes lesion size and location by defined region in the abdomen. Increasing PCI has been shown in multiple retrospective reviews to be an independent predictor of poor outcome after CRS and HIPEC [16–20]. Based on data showing significantly different overall survival (OS) and disease-free survival (DFS) between patients with PCI less than 20 versus those with PCI greater than or equal to 20 (OS 19 months vs 62 months, respectively; and

DFS 19 months vs 42 months, respectively), many surgeons recommend against CRS and HIPEC for patients with PCI greater than 20 [17]. Later, the Peritoneal Surface Disease Severity Score (PSDSS) was developed to stratify patients with PMs and help guide appropriate therapy [21]. The PSDSS is based on PCI and clinical symptomatology, including weight loss, abdominal pain, and ascites, as well as tumor histopathology (Table 1). PSDSS also has been shown in retrospective studies to correspond to survival outcomes [22].

Cytoreduction consists of removal of all peritoneal tumor deposits. Thus, the operation must be tailored to the disease burden and involved organs in each individual patient. In a survey of 19 expert surgeons from 19 different countries in the Peritoneal Surface Oncology Group International, only 1 surgeon responded that they routinely performed a total parietal peritonectomy, even of unaffected peritoneum; the other surgeons responded that they only resect diseased peritoneum [14]. Routine omentectomy was performed, however, by all 19 experts. Furthermore, 9/19 surgeons perform routine bilateral oophorectomy in all patients and an additional 6 surgeons reported they routinely do so only in postmenopausal women. Most surgeons commonly resected intra-abdominal organs as part of CRS include small bowel (58%), omentum (55%), colon (31%), ovaries (18%), spleen (9%), gallbladder (9%), uterus (7%), rectum (7%), appendix (5%), kidney (5%), and liver (5%) [23]. Additionally, many surgeons believe that simultaneous colorectal resection combined with CRS and HIPEC is a reasonable approach in carefully selected patients [24]. Complete cytoreduction (CCR) (an R0 resection) is an important prognostic factor in patients undergoing surgical treated for PMs [16]. This was confirmed in the French study by Elias and colleagues [19], which demonstrated distinct survival advantages for patients based on CCR (Fig. 2).

After CRS, HIPEC is performed in an attempt to address the remaining microscopic disease. HIPEC may be performed in open or closed technique using mitomycin C or oxaliplatin, the cytotoxic effect of which is potentiated by heat (Fig. 3) [25]. In a 2014 survey of all cancer centers performing HIPEC in the United States, a majority of surgical oncologists favored closed technique for treatment of patients with colorectal PMs [26].

## HISTORICAL PERSPECTIVE: SURVIVAL AFTER CYTOREDUCTIVE SURGERY AND HYPERTHERMIC INTRAPERITONEAL CHEMOTHERAPY FOR PATIENTS WITH COLORECTAL CANCER PERITONEAL METASTASIS

Survival in patients with colorectal PMs has been reported multiple times over the past 15 years often in the context of comparing systemic chemotherapy to CRS and HIPEC. A comprehensive list of study outcomes following CRS and HIPEC for CRC PM can be found in Table 2. Most of these studies have consisted of retrospective reviews, perhaps 3 of the most significant of which were performed by Glehen and colleagues in 2004, [16] Elias and colleagues in 2010 [19], and Chua in 2013 [27]. Glehen and colleagues [16] studied 506 patients undergoing CRS with perioperative intraperitoneal chemotherapy with an

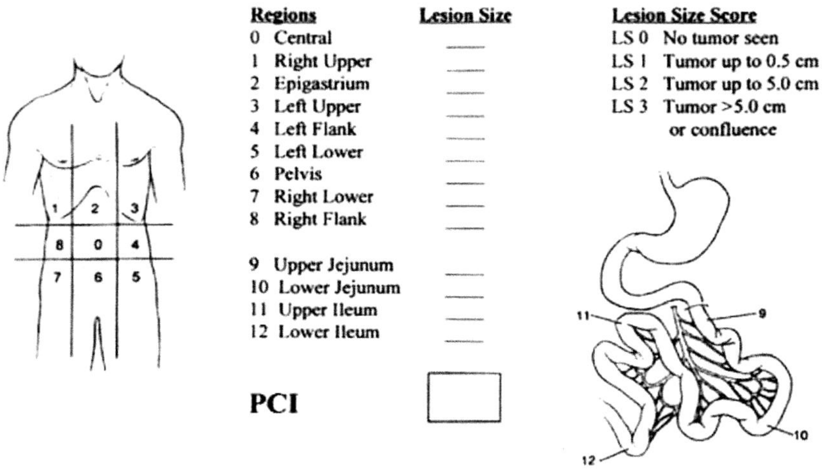


**Fig. 1.** PCI [16].

overall median survival of 32 months and 5-year survival rate of 40%. Perioperative mortality was 4.0%. In a multivariate analysis, CCR, treatment with a second procedure, extent of PMs, lymph node involvement, age, tumor differentiation, synchronous resection of liver metastasis, treatment with preoperative systemic chemotherapy, and treatment with adjuvant systemic chemotherapy were identified as independent prognostic factors. Specifically, patients with CCR-0 versus CCR-1 and CCR-2 patients had median survival of 32.4 months versus 24 months and 8.4 months, respectively; 73% of patients experienced recurrences, 42% of which were peritoneal. In the French retrospective multicenter analysis by Elias and colleagues [19], median OS of 523

**Table 1**
Peritoneal Surface Disease Severity Score

| Peritoneal carcinomatosis index | Tumor grade/ histopathology/ nodal status | Clinical symptoms |
|---|---|---|
| PCI <10 = 1 point | Well–moderately differentiated, N0 = 1 point | Asymptomatic = 0 points |
| PCI 10–20 = 3 points | Moderately differentiated, N1–N2 = 3 points | Mild symptoms = 1 point |
| PCI >20 = 7 points | Poorly differentiated or signet ring = 9 points | Severe symptoms = 6 points |

patients with CRC PM undergoing CRS and HIPEC was 30 months, 5-year OS was 27%, and 5-year DFS was 10%. Perioperative mortality was 3.3%. Factors associated with better prognosis in multivariate analysis included complete CRS, lower PCI, no invaded lymph nodes, and the use of adjuvant chemotherapy. Neither the grade of disease nor the presence of liver metastases had a significant prognostic impact in this study. Finally, in 2013 systematic review by Chua and colleagues [27], 1084 patients receiving CRS and HIPEC for CRC PM were found to have a median OS of 33 months and 5-year OS of 40%. Patients with CRC PM receiving palliative surgery and/or systemic chemotherapy had a median OS of 12.5 months and 5-year OS of 13%.

Two randomized studies have also been completed to compare CRS and HIPEC with systemic chemotherapy [28,29]. The first study, from Verwaal and colleagues [29] in the Netherlands, compared 54 patients undergoing CRS and HIPEC with mitomycin C to 51 patients treated with systemic chemotherapy alone and found a 22.2-month median survival in the surgery group compared with a 12.6-month survival in the chemotherapy group ($P = .028$) and progression-free survival of 12.6 versus 7.7 months, respectively ($P = .020$) (Fig. 4). Criticisms of this study included its high perioperative mortality rate (8%), outdated systemic chemotherapy regimen, and that 20% of patients included had appendiceal cancer. The Swedish Peritoneal Study compared 24 patients with colorectal and appendiceal cancers undergoing CRS and HIPEC to 24 patients undergoing systemic chemotherapy in a randomized controlled trial [28]. In this study, 2-year OS was 54% in the surgery arm and 38% in the chemotherapy arm ($P = .04$). OS rates after 5 years were 33% ($n = 8$) and 4% ($n = 1$), respectively ($P = .02$). Median OS was 25 months versus 18 months, respectively, and hazard ratio was 0.51 (95% CI, 0.27–0.96; $P = .04$).

In a study of American College of Surgeons National Quality Improvement Program (ACS-NSQIP) data for patients of any primary (8% colorectal) undergoing CRS and HIPEC, 30-day mortality was 2.3%, and the main cause of death was sepsis followed by respiratory complications [30]. A large review of CRS and HIPEC in CRC demonstrated that mortality was higher for patients 70 years of age or older (1-month mortality 13.6% vs 3.9% in patients <70; 3-month mortality 27.4% vs 10.2%, respectively) [31]. Additionally, nutrition status as defined by the preoperative Subjective Global Assessment was predictive of survival outcome [32].

## TOXICITY AND MORBIDITY ASSOCIATED WITH CYTOREDUCTIVE SURGERY AND HYPERTHERMIC INTRAPERITONEAL CHEMOTHERAPY

Toxicity, or morbidity, of CRS and HIPEC long has been a major concern for both surgeons performing the procedure as well as the procedure's critics. Furthermore, there have been conflicting reports in the medical literature about the rate and severity of postoperative morbidity from CRS and HIPEC. A retrospective review of 25 patients in 2006 demonstrated a 24% major

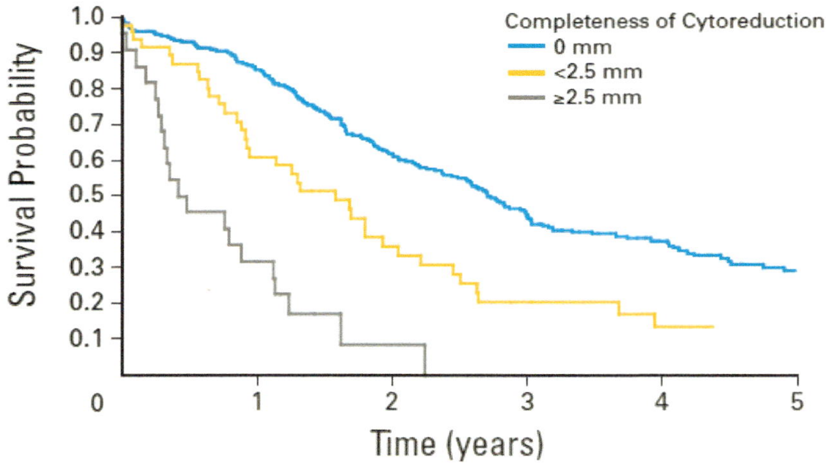


**Fig. 2.** Relationship between survival and CCR [19].

postoperative morbidity rate [33], a review of 121 patients performed in 2008 by Shen and colleagues [23] reported a 30-day postoperative morbidity rate of 42%, and a 2010 review of 523 patients by Elias and colleagues [19] reported grade 3 to 4 complications in 31% of patients. Of these, 11% required reoperation, 9% had an enteric fistula, 4% had "profound" abscess, 6% had

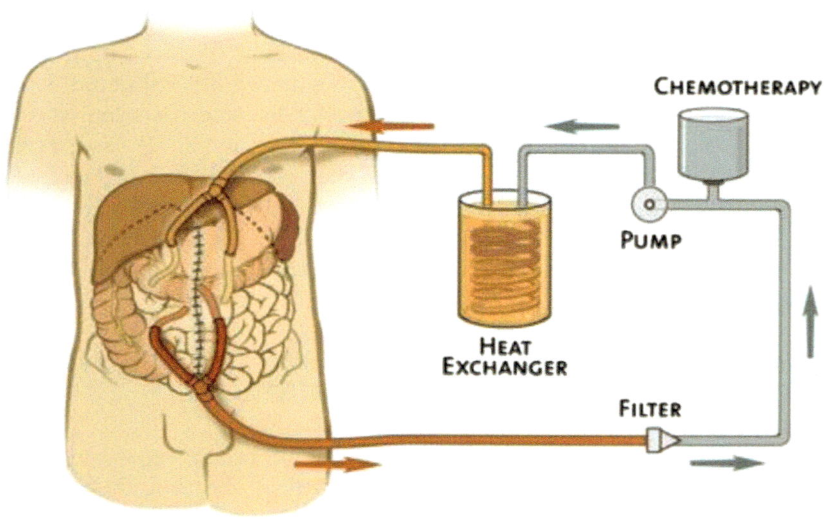


**Fig. 3.** HIPEC circuit schematic [23].

hemorrhage, and 12% had grade 3 to grade 4 hematologic toxicity. The median hospitalization in this study was 18 days [19]. In this multicenter analysis, PCI and treatment center were the only 2 factors found associated with morbidity and mortality. The Swedish Peritoneal Study was a randomized trial of 48 patients comparing CRS and HIPEC to systemic chemotherapy [28]. The study found equal morbidity in the 2 arms; 50% of the patients in the systemic chemotherapy arm experienced grade 3 to grade 4 complications, including neutropenia, allergic reaction, venous thromboembolism, neuropathy, pancytopenia, thrombocytopenia, nausea requiring hospitalization, and ileus. Patients in the surgery arm experienced ileus, intraabdominal infection, wound dehiscence, hemorrhage, enterocutaneous fistula, wound infection, bowel perforation by the intraperitoneal catheter, anastomotic leak, vena cava tear, and renal failure. Seven of the 24 patients in the surgery arm required reoperation [28]. Finally, the largest study of postoperative outcomes following CRS and HIPEC used the ACS-NSQIP database and demonstrated equivalent 30-day postoperative outcomes to patients undergoing other major oncologic operations, including pancreaticoduodenectomy, esophagectomy, and major hepatectomy [34]. Overall morbidity was 32.9%, with a reoperation rate of 9.8% and readmission rate of 11.4%. Respiratory complications were found particularly common (ventilator use >48 hours, 5.2%; pneumonia 4.8%; and unplanned reintubation, 4.6%). These complications were attributed to the massive resuscitation required during the procedure, leading to postoperative fluid shifts, which affected postoperative pulmonary function [34].

The cost implications of postoperative complications following CRS and HIPEC were studied by Simkens and colleagues in 2018 [35]. In a study of 161 patients, 27% experienced minor complications, and 31% experienced severe complications. The 31% patients who experienced severe complications accounted for 56% of all hospital costs for the 161-patient cohort, which translated to a 320% higher cost than patients with no postoperative complications. Analysis found that 43% of all admission costs of the cohort were attributed to treatment of complications.

Given the significant potential for morbidity and mortality during CRS and HIPEC, postoperative quality of life is an important outcome. Two studies focused on quality of life following CRS and HIPEC. A prospective cohort of 115 patients answered the 36-item Short Form survey at defined intervals postoperatively [36]. There was a consistent decline in quality of life during the first 3 postoperative months, but patients returned to their preoperative baseline by 6 months postoperatively. Lower PCI and CCR-0 corresponded to higher quality of life. A second prospective study of 90 patients similarly demonstrated decreased quality of life in the early postoperative period with improvement by postoperative month 6 [37] (Fig. 5). Although pain, appetite loss, and constipation improved to baseline by postoperative month 1, fatigue, diarrhea, dyspnea, and sleep disturbance persisted and did not return to baseline until 6 months. Nausea and vomiting improved by 6 months but unfortunately worsened over time thereafter.

**Table 2**
Survival outcomes in cytoreductive surgery and hyperthermic intraperitoneal chemotherapy, selected series

| Author, Year | N | Overall Survival (Months) | Five-year (%) | Notes |
|---|---|---|---|---|
| Cashin et al, 2016 [28] | 24 | 25 | 33 | |
| Chua et al, 2013 [27] | 1084 | 33 | 40 | |
| da Silva and Sugarbaker, 2006 [18] | 70 | 33 | 32 | |
| Elias et al, 2009 [5] | 46 | 62.7 | 51 | Versus 13% 5-y OS and 23.9-mo median survival in systemic chemotherapy arm |
| Elias et al, 2010 [19] | 523 | 30.1 | 27 | 5-y DFS 10% |
| Elias et al, 2011 [55] | 146 | 41 | 42 | |
| Franko et al, 2010 [56] | 67 | 34.7 | | |
| Glehen et al, 2004 [16] | 506 | 32 | 40 | |
| Shen et al, 2008 [23] | 121 | 34 | 26 | |
| Ung et al, 2013 [57] | 211 | 47 | 42 | |
| Verwaal et al, 2008 [29] | 54 | 22.3 | 45 | Progression-free survival 12.6 mo |
| Zanon et al, 2006 [33] | 25 | 30.3 | | Progression-free survival 17.3 mo |

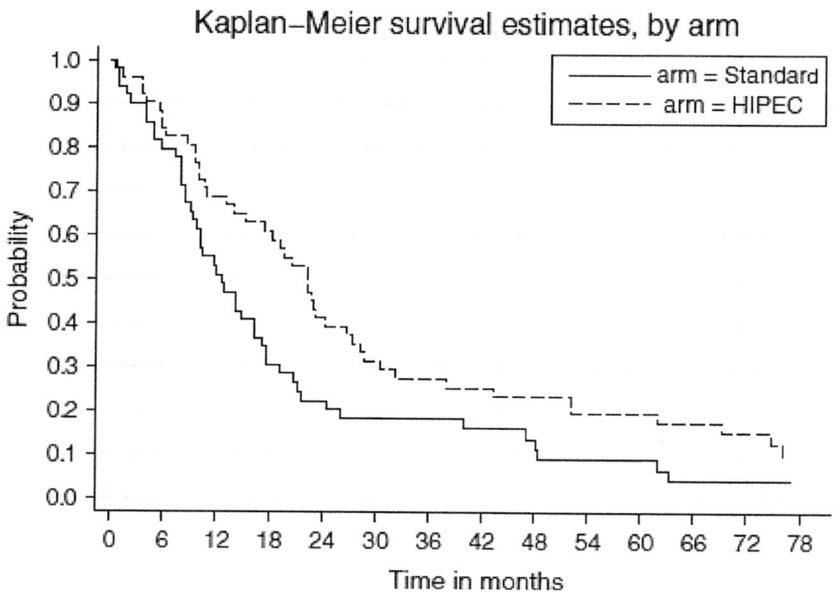


**Fig. 4.** Survival estimates in patients treated with CRS and HIPEC versus systemic chemotherapy [29].

In cost-effectiveness analyses, the cost-effectiveness ratio for treatment with CRS and HIPEC compared with systemic chemotherapy was $91,034 per quality-adjusted life-year gained, which, given $100,000 as a conservative threshold, deems CRS and HIPEC a cost-effective treatment [38].

## CURRENT STATUS OF CYTOREDUCTIVE SURGERY AND HYPERTHERMIC INTRAPERITONEAL CHEMOTHERAPY IN COLORECTAL CANCER PERITONEAL METASTASIS

Currently, there are several areas of debate within the field of CRS and HIPEC in patients with CRC PM. These include the use of mitomycin C versus oxaliplatin as first-choice chemotherapeutic agent in HIPEC, the optimal timing and duration of systemic chemotherapy around CRS and HIPEC, the therapeutic contribution (if any) of HIPEC after CRS, and the role of prophylactic HIPEC in high-risk patients.

### Mitomycin C versus oxaliplatin

One majorly debated aspect of HIPEC is the use of mitomycin C versus oxaliplatin as the superior chemotherapeutic agent. Both agents interfere with DNA synthesis as cell-cycle alkylating agents and have limited systemic absorption due to their large molecular weight. Tissue penetration (maximum of 2 mm with hyperthermia) is comparable between the 2 agents. Oxaliplatin typically has a shorter perfusion time (30 minutes vs 90 minutes, respectively) and does not induce neutropenia, like mitomycin C (Table 3) [25,39]. Multiple retrospective reviews comparing patients receiving mitomycin C versus oxaliplatin have been performed with varying conclusions (Table 4). Bakkers and colleagues reported a median OS of 30.7 months in the mitomycin C group versus 46.6 months in patients receiving oxaliplatin; however, when adjusting for confounders, there was no difference between groups [40]. Similarly, Hompes and colleagues [41], van Eden and colleagues [42], and Woeste and colleagues [43] did not find any survival difference between patients receiving mitomycin C versus oxaliplatin [41–43]. The largest of these studies, performed by Prada-Villaverde and colleagues, included 539 patients and reported no difference in OS between groups (32.7 months for mitomycin C and 31.4 months for oxaliplatin). In a subgroup of PSDSS I/II patients with low disease burden who received CCR, however, mitomycin C did appear to increase survival: 54.3 months versus 28.2 months, respectively ($P = .012$). Finally, an Australian study performed by Leung and colleagues [44] did report a survival advantage in patients receiving oxaliplatin at 56 months versus 29 months OS (hazard ratio 0.59; 95% CI, 0.37–0.91). In subgroup analysis, this advantage was most strong for women, tumors with moderate to well grade differentiation, non–signet ring pathology, and patients with PCI between 10 and 15. Although 1 study found no difference in postoperative complications between the 2 groups [42], 1 study found that postoperative complications were significantly higher in patients treated with oxaliplatin [43], and another found complications to be higher in the mitomycin C group [41].

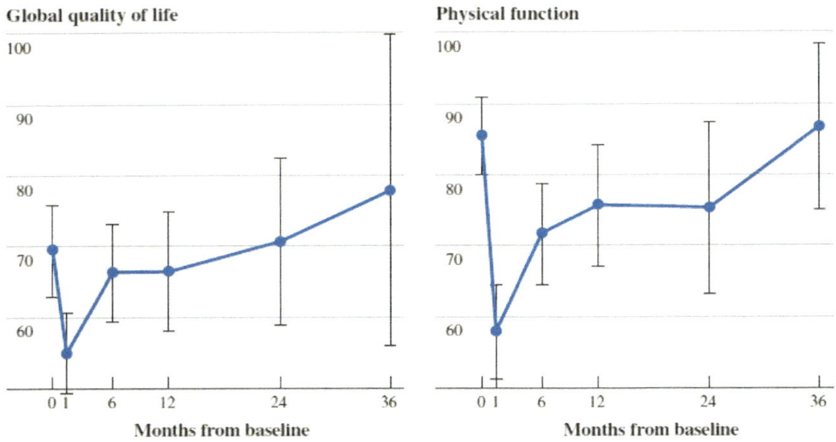


**Fig. 5.** Quality of life following CRS and HIPEC [37].

## Use of systemic chemotherapy with cytoreductive surgery and hyperthermic intraperitoneal chemotherapy

Although CRS versus systemic chemotherapy has been compared, the authors believe the question should not be whether 1 is superior to the other, but how the 2 modalities can be optimally integrated. To that end, the role of neoadjuvant chemotherapy (NAC) has been examined. First, a systematic review and meta-analysis by Waite and Youssef in 2017 [45] reported that there was insufficient evidence at the time to determine the role of NAC in patients with CRC PM undergoing CRS and HIPEC. In the Swedish Peritoneal Study, prolonged systemic chemotherapy prior to CRS and HIPEC was found to be of limited benefit, with a smaller proportion of patients with resectable disease after 6 months of chemotherapy compared with those undergoing up-front surgery

**Table 3**
Technical differences of mitomycin C versus oxaliplatin in hyperthermic intraperitoneal chemotherapy

| | Mitomycin C | Oxaliplatin |
|---|---|---|
| HIPEC method | Closed | Open |
| Medication dosage | 40 mg | 460 mg/m$^2$ oxaliplatin, 20 mg/m$^2$ leucovorin IV, 400 mg/m$^2$ 5-FU IV |
| Medication timing | 30 mg at time 0, 10 mg at 60 min, or 40 mg at time 0 | IV 5-FU/leucovorin 1 h prior to start of HIPEC, oxaliplatin at time 0 |
| Perfusate volume | 3–4 L | 2 L/m$^2$ |
| Inflow temperature | 42°C | 42°C |
| Perfusion duration | 90 min | 30 min |

(15% vs 79%, respectively; $P<.001$) [28]. Similarly, Gilly and colleagues [46] reported a decreased OS in patients receiving NAC compared with those receiving upfront CRS and HIPEC. However, 2 subsequent studies did report benefit to NAC in CRC PM: Devilee and colleagues [47] found NAC to be an independent predictor of improved OS, and Ceelen and colleagues [48] found benefit to NAC in patients receiving bevacizumab as part of their treatment regimen. Most recently, a multi-institutional retrospective review was performed in 2020 that showed after controlling for confounders, NAC was not associated with improved OS or DFS [49]. There also was no increased grade III/IV complications, readmissions, or mortality, however, with NAC, either. A Dutch randomized controlled trial currently is being performed to determine the role for NAC prior to CRS and HIPEC for CRC PM [50].

## Cytoreductive surgery and hyperthermic intraperitoneal chemotherapy versus cytoreductive surgery alone

There is much debate over the use of HIPEC following CRS and whether this actually translates to improved oncologic outcomes. Two major studies recently have been published, both demonstrating no improved outcome with the addition of HIPEC [51,52]. The PRODIGE-7 trial is the first phase III study questioning the specific role of HIPEC in CRS; it included 265 patients with CRC PM from 17 French centers [52]. After CCR, this study randomized patients to HIPEC versus no HIPEC. After a median follow-up of 64 months, the median OS was 41.7 months for patients in the HIPEC arm, and 41.2 months in the non-HIPEC arm. The unexpectedly high survival rate in the non-HIPEC arm strongly supports the role of CRS in the patients' outcome. HIPEC with oxaliplatin had no effect on OS or recurrence-free survival, although a subgroup analysis shows significantly better OS and recurrence-free survival rates for patients presenting with a medium PCI, between 11 and 15 (41.6 months vs 32.7 months, respectively in the CRS alone arm). The number of patients in this subgroup, however, was very small and the OS of the CRS alone group was worse than expected suggesting that this small subgroup analysis may not be representative of the general population. Furthermore, the 60-day complication rate was significantly higher for patients in the HIPEC arm (24.1% vs 13.6%, respectively). Next, Baratti and colleagues reported a nonrandomized study of 96 patients with CRC PM, 48 of whom underwent CRS and systemic chemotherapy, and the other 48 of whom underwent CRS and HIPEC with mitomycin C [51]. Median OS was 39.3 months in the non-HIPEC group and 34.8 months in the HIPEC group ($P = .702$). In the 2 groups, severe morbidity was not different between the groups, 29% and 27%, respectively. Although these 2 studies demonstrate no survival benefit with the addition of HIPEC, patients in both of these studies were treated with systemic NAC, which may have impacted any effect of intraperitoneal chemotherapy [40].

**Table 4**
Studies on outcomes of mitomycin C versus oxaliplatin in hyperthermic intraperitoneal chemotherapy for colorectal cancer

| | | Disease-free Survival (Months) | | Overall Survival (Months) | | |
|---|---|---|---|---|---|---|
| Study | N | Mitomycin C | Oxaliplatin | Mitomycin C | Oxaliplatin | Conclusion |
| Bakkers and colleagues, 2020 [40] | 297 | | | 30.7 | 46.6 | No statistically significant difference |
| Hompes and colleagues, 2014 [41] | 95 | 13.8 | 12.2 | 26.5 | 37.1 | No statistically significant difference |
| Leung and colleagues, 2017 [44] | 212 | | | 29 | 56 | Favors oxaliplatin |
| Prada-Villaverde and colleagues, 2014 [39] | 539 | | | 32.7 | 31.4 | No OS difference; however, patients with low disease burden favor MMC |
| van Eden and colleagues, 2018 [42] | 177 | 12.5 | 13.1 | 37.2 | 29.4 | No statistically significant difference |
| Woeste and colleagues, 2020 [43] | 48 | | | 56.9 | 68.2 | No statistically significant difference |

### Hyperthermic intraperitoneal chemotherapy as prophylactic therapy

PMs for T4 CRCs are reported to be 15.6% at 12 months and 36.7% at 36 months following surgical resection. Thus, HIPEC has been proposed as a prophylactic treatment of patient with T4 colorectal tumors [25]. A 2015 randomized controlled trial studying oxaliplatin-based HIPEC for the prevention of CRC PM in patients with T4 or perforated CRCs, the COLOPEC study, failed to find a survival benefit to HIPEC [53]. A second study (PROPHYLCHIP) similarly failed to find survival benefit using second-look surgery with HIPEC for high-risk CRC patients [54]. A third randomized controlled trial, the HIPEC-T4 study, currently is ongoing to evaluate the role of mitomycin C–based HIPEC for the prevention of CRC PM in patients with T4 CRCs [25].

## SUMMARY

CRC PM is a complex disease process, which presents significant clinical challenges. In well-selected patients in experienced centers, CRS and HIPEC can be performed with acceptable morbidity and are associated with prolonged survival. HIPEC using oxaliplatin after CRS, however, does not result in improved outcome compared with CRS alone. In retrospective studies, the outcomes after CRS and HIPEC using oxaliplatin or mitomycin C are conflicting, indicating that additional clinical trials testing HIPEC with mitomycin C are needed. In patients with CRC PM who have exhausted all systemic chemotherapy options, the use of CRS and HIPEC as a salvage therapy has not been tested and should be offered only in the context of a clinical trial. The use of CRS and HIPEC as prophylactic therapy in high-risk patients does not appear to be effective. The optimal sequencing and duration of systemic chemotherapy around CRS and HIPEC have not been established, and additional studies to define and standardize the optimal parameters around patient selection and management are a high clinical priority.

## CLINICS CARE POINTS

- Patients with colorectal PM are treated best with CRS and HIPEC in high-volume centers experienced in treatment of peritoneal carcinomatosis.
- Patients with colorectal PM have survival benefit from CRS and HIPEC.
- There is no current good evidence to support CRS and HIPEC versus CRS alone or the use of oxaliplatin versus mitomycin C as the chemotherapeutic agent of choice.
- HIPEC should not be used as prophylactic therapy in high-risk patients, such as those with perforated or T4 colorectal tumors.

## DISCLOSURE

The authors have nothing to disclose.

## References


[1] Jayne DG, Fook S, Loi C, et al. Peritoneal carcinomatosis from colorectal cancer. Br J Surg 2002;89(12):1545–50.

[2] Segelman J, Granath F, Holm T, et al. Incidence, prevalence and risk factors for peritoneal carcinomatosis from colorectal cancer. Br J Surg 2012;99(5):699–705.

[3] Koppe MJ, Boerman OC, Oyen WJ, et al. Peritoneal carcinomatosis of colorectal origin: incidence and current treatment strategies. Ann Surg 2006;243(2):212–22.

[4] Cotte E, Peyrat P, Piaton E, et al. Lack of prognostic significance of conventional peritoneal cytology in colorectal and gastric cancers: results of EVOCAPE 2 multicentre prospective study. Eur J Surg Oncol 2013;39(7):707–14.

[5] Elias D, Lefevre JH, Chevalier J, et al. Complete cytoreductive surgery plus intraperitoneal chemohyperthermia with oxaliplatin for peritoneal carcinomatosis of colorectal origin. J Clin Oncol 2009;27(5):681–5.

[6] Sugarbaker PH. Cytoreductive surgery and hyperthermic intraperitoneal chemotherapy in the management of gastrointestinal cancers with peritoneal metastases: progress toward a new standard of care. Cancer Treat Rev 2016;48:42–9.

[7] Narasimhan V, Ooi G, Michael M, et al. Colorectal peritoneal metastases: pathogenesis, diagnosis and treatment options - an evidence-based update. ANZ J Surg 2020;90(9): 1592–7; https://doi.org/10.1111/ans.15796, Epub 2020 Mar 4. PMID: 32129577.

[8] Sánchez-Hidalgo JM, Rodríguez-Ortiz L, Arjona-Sánchez Á, et al. Colorectal peritoneal metastases: Optimal management review. World J Gastroenterol 2019;25(27):3484–502.
[9] UICC. TNM classification of malignant tumours. 8th Edition ed. Springer-Verlag Berlin Heidelberg: Wiley; 2017.
[10] Sadeghi B, Arvieux C, Glehen O, et al. Peritoneal carcinomatosis from non-gynecologic malignancies: results of the EVOCAPE 1 multicentric prospective study. Cancer 2000;88(2):358–63.
[11] Razenberg LG, van Gestel YR, Lemmens VE, et al. The prognostic relevance of histological subtype in patients with peritoneal metastases from colorectal cancer: a nationwide population-based study. Clin Colorectal Cancer 2015;14(4):e13–9.
[12] Sugarbaker PH, Jablonski KA. Prognostic features of 51 colorectal and 130 appendiceal cancer patients with peritoneal carcinomatosis treated by cytoreductive surgery and intraperitoneal chemotherapy. Ann Surg 1995;221(2):124–32.
[13] Fernández-Trigo V, Stuart OA, Stephens AD, et al. Surgically directed chemotherapy: heated intraperitoneal lavage with mitomycin C. Cancer Treat Res 1996;81:51–61.
[14] Bushati M, Rovers KP, Sommariva A, et al. The current practice of cytoreductive surgery and HIPEC for colorectal peritoneal metastases: Results of a worldwide web-based survey of the Peritoneal Surface Oncology Group International (PSOGI). Eur J Surg Oncol 2018;44(12): 1942–8.
[15] Esquivel J, Piso P, Verwaal V, et al. American Society of Peritoneal Surface Malignancies opinion statement on defining expectations from cytoreductive surgery and hyperthermic intraperitoneal chemotherapy in patients with colorectal cancer. J Surg Oncol 2014;110(7):777–8.
[16] Glehen O, Kwiatkowski F, Sugarbaker PH, et al. Cytoreductive surgery combined with perioperative intraperitoneal chemotherapy for the management of peritoneal carcinomatosis from colorectal cancer: a multi-institutional study. J Clin Oncol 2004;22(16):3284–92.
[17] Burnett A, Lecompte MA, Trabulsi N, et al. Peritoneal carcinomatosis index predicts survival in colorectal patients undergoing HIPEC using oxaliplatin: a retrospective single-arm cohort study. World J Surg Oncol 2019;17(1):83.
[18] da Silva RG, Sugarbaker PH. Analysis of prognostic factors in seventy patients having a complete cytoreduction plus perioperative intraperitoneal chemotherapy for carcinomatosis from colorectal cancer. J Am Coll Surg 2006;203(6):878–86.
[19] Elias D, Gilly F, Boutitie F, et al. Peritoneal colorectal carcinomatosis treated with surgery and perioperative intraperitoneal chemotherapy: retrospective analysis of 523 patients from a multicentric French study. J Clin Oncol 2010;28(1):63–8.
[20] Faron M, Macovei R, Goéré D, et al. Linear relationship of peritoneal cancer index and survival in patients with peritoneal metastases from colorectal cancer. Ann Surg Oncol 2016;23(1):114–9.
[21] Pelz JO, Stojadinovic A, Nissan A, et al. Evaluation of a peritoneal surface disease severity score in patients with colon cancer with peritoneal carcinomatosis. J Surg Oncol 2009;99(1):9–15.
[22] Chua TC, Morris DL, Esquivel J. Impact of the peritoneal surface disease severity score on survival in patients with colorectal cancer peritoneal carcinomatosis undergoing complete cytoreduction and hyperthermic intraperitoneal chemotherapy. Ann Surg Oncol 2010;17(5):1330–6.
[23] Shen P, Thai K, Stewart JH, et al. Peritoneal surface disease from colorectal cancer: comparison with the hepatic metastases surgical paradigm in optimally resected patients. Ann Surg Oncol 2008;15(12):3422–32.
[24] Baratti D, Sammartino P, Kusamura S, et al. Past, present and future of adjuvant HIPEC in patients at high risk for colorectal peritoneal metastases. Eur J Surg Oncol 2020;46(5): 737–9.
[25] Arjona-Sánchez A, Barrios P, Boldo-Roda E, et al. HIPECT4: multicentre, randomized clinical trial to evaluate safety and efficacy of Hyperthermic intra-peritoneal chemotherapy

(HIPEC) with Mitomycin C used during surgery for treatment of locally advanced colorectal carcinoma. BMC Cancer 2018;18(1):183.
[26] Turaga K, Levine E, Barone R, et al. Consensus guidelines from The American Society of Peritoneal Surface Malignancies on standardizing the delivery of hyperthermic intraperitoneal chemotherapy (HIPEC) in colorectal cancer patients in the United States. Ann Surg Oncol 2014;21(5):1501–5.
[27] Chua TC, Esquivel J, Pelz JO, et al. Summary of current therapeutic options for peritoneal metastases from colorectal cancer. J Surg Oncol 2013;107(6):566–73.
[28] Cashin PH, Mahteme H, Spång N, et al. Cytoreductive surgery and intraperitoneal chemotherapy versus systemic chemotherapy for colorectal peritoneal metastases: A randomised trial. Eur J Cancer 2016;53:155–62.
[29] Verwaal VJ, Bruin S, Boot H, et al. 8-year follow-up of randomized trial: cytoreduction and hyperthermic intraperitoneal chemotherapy versus systemic chemotherapy in patients with peritoneal carcinomatosis of colorectal cancer. Ann Surg Oncol 2008;15(9):2426–32.
[30] Jafari MD, Halabi WJ, Stamos MJ, et al. Surgical outcomes of hyperthermic intraperitoneal chemotherapy: analysis of the american college of surgeons national surgical quality improvement program. JAMA Surg 2014;149(2):170–5.
[31] Tabrizian P, Jibara G, Shrager B, et al. Outcomes for cytoreductive surgery and hyperthermic intraperitoneal chemotherapy in the elderly. Surg Oncol 2013;22(3):184–9.
[32] Vashi PG, Gupta D, Lammersfeld CA, et al. The relationship between baseline nutritional status with subsequent parenteral nutrition and clinical outcomes in cancer patients undergoing hyperthermic intraperitoneal chemotherapy. Nutr J 2013;12:118.
[33] Zanon C, Bortolini M, Chiappino I, et al. Cytoreductive surgery combined with intraperitoneal chemohyperthermia for the treatment of advanced colon cancer. World J Surg 2006;30(11):2025–32.
[34] Foster JM, Sleightholm R, Patel A, et al. Morbidity and mortality rates following cytoreductive surgery combined with hyperthermic intraperitoneal chemotherapy compared with other high-risk surgical oncology procedures. JAMA Netw Open 2019;2(1):e186847.
[35] Simkens GA, Rovers KP, van Oudheusden TR, et al. Major influence of postoperative complications on costs of cytoreductive surgery and HIPEC in patients with colorectal peritoneal metastases. Medicine (Baltimore) 2018;97(10):e0042.
[36] Steffens D, Koh C, Ansari N, et al. Quality of Life After Cytoreductive Surgery and Hyperthermic Intraperitoneal Chemotherapy: Early Results from a Prospective Cohort Study of 115 Patients. Ann Surg Oncol 2020;27(10):3986–94; https://doi.org/10.1245/s10434-020-08443-4, Epub 2020 Apr 13. PMID: 32285283.
[37] Tsilimparis N, Bockelmann C, Raue W, et al. Quality of life in patients after cytoreductive surgery and hyperthermic intraperitoneal chemotherapy: is it worth the risk? Ann Surg Oncol 2013;20(1):226–32.
[38] Hamilton TD, MacNeill AJ, Lim H, et al. Cost-effectiveness analysis of cytoreductive surgery and HIPEC compared with systemic chemotherapy in isolated peritoneal carcinomatosis from metastatic colorectal cancer. Ann Surg Oncol 2019;26(4):1110–7.
[39] Prada-Villaverde A, Esquivel J, Lowy AM, et al. The American Society of Peritoneal Surface Malignancies evaluation of HIPEC with Mitomycin C versus Oxaliplatin in 539 patients with colon cancer undergoing a complete cytoreductive surgery. J Surg Oncol 2014;110(7):779–85.
[40] Bakkers C, van Erning FN, Rovers KP, et al. Long-term survival after hyperthermic intraperitoneal chemotherapy using mitomycin C or oxaliplatin in colorectal cancer patients with synchronous peritoneal metastases: A nationwide comparative study. Eur J Surg Oncol 2020;46(10 Pt A):1902–7; https://doi.org/10.1016/j.ejso.2020.04.018, Epub 2020 Apr 18. PMID: 32340819.
[41] Hompes D, D'Hoore A, Wolthuis A, et al. The use of Oxaliplatin or Mitomycin C in HIPEC treatment for peritoneal carcinomatosis from colorectal cancer: a comparative study. J Surg Oncol 2014;109(6):527–32.

[42] van Eden WJ, Kok NFM, Woensdregt K, et al. Safety of intraperitoneal Mitomycin C versus intraperitoneal oxaliplatin in patients with peritoneal carcinomatosis of colorectal cancer undergoing cytoreductive surgery and HIPEC. Eur J Surg Oncol 2018;44(2):220–7.
[43] Woeste MR, Philips P, Egger ME, et al. Optimal perfusion chemotherapy: A prospective comparison of mitomycin C and oxaliplatin for hyperthermic intraperitoneal chemotherapy in metastatic colon cancer. J Surg Oncol 2020 Jun;121(8):1298–305; https://doi.org/10.1002/jso.25920, Epub 2020 Apr 1. PMID: 32239529.
[44] Leung V, Huo YR, Liauw W, et al. Oxaliplatin versus Mitomycin C for HIPEC in colorectal cancer peritoneal carcinomatosis. Eur J Surg Oncol 2017;43(1):144–9.
[45] Waite K, Youssef H. The role of neoadjuvant and adjuvant systemic chemotherapy with cytoreductive surgery and heated intraperitoneal chemotherapy for colorectal peritoneal metastases: a systematic review. Ann Surg Oncol 2017;24(3):705–20.
[46] Gilly FN, Cotte E, Brigand C, et al. Quantitative prognostic indices in peritoneal carcinomatosis. Eur J Surg Oncol 2006;32(6):597–601.
[47] Devilee RA, Simkens GA, van Oudheusden TR, et al. Increased survival of patients with synchronous colorectal peritoneal metastases receiving preoperative chemotherapy before cytoreductive surgery and hyperthermic intraperitoneal chemotherapy. Ann Surg Oncol 2016;23(9):2841–8.
[48] Ceelen W, Van Nieuwenhove Y, Putte DV, et al. Neoadjuvant chemotherapy with bevacizumab may improve outcome after cytoreduction and hyperthermic intraperitoneal chemoperfusion (HIPEC) for colorectal carcinomatosis. Ann Surg Oncol 2014;21(9):3023–8.
[49] Beal EW, Suarez-Kelly LP, Kimbrough CW, et al. Impact of neoadjuvant chemotherapy on the outcomes of cytoreductive surgery and hyperthermic intraperitoneal chemotherapy for colorectal peritoneal metastases: a multi-institutional retrospective review. J Clin Med 2020;9(3).
[50] Rovers KP, Bakkers C, Simkens GAAM, et al. Perioperative systemic therapy and cytoreductive surgery with HIPEC versus upfront cytoreductive surgery with HIPEC alone for isolated resectable colorectal peritoneal metastases: protocol of a multicentre, open-label, parallel-group, phase II-III, randomised, superiority study (CAIRO6). BMC Cancer 2019;19(1):390.
[51] Baratti D, Kusamura S, Azmi N, et al. Colorectal peritoneal metastases treated by perioperative systemic chemotherapy and cytoreductive surgery with or without Mitomycin C-based HIPEC: a comparative study using the Peritoneal Surface Disease Severity Score (PSDSS). Ann Surg Oncol 2020;27(1):98–106.
[52] Quenet FED, Roca L, et al. A UNICANCER phase III trial of hyperthermic intra-peritoneal chemotherapy (HIPEC) for colorectal peritoneal carcinomatosis (PC): PRODIGE 7. J Clin Oncol 2018;36(18).
[53] Klaver CE, Musters GD, Bemelman WA, et al. Adjuvant hyperthermic intraperitoneal chemotherapy (HIPEC) in patients with colon cancer at high risk of peritoneal carcinomatosis; the COLOPEC randomized multicentre trial. BMC Cancer 2015;15:428.
[54] Goéré D, Glehen O, Quenet F, et al. Second-look surgery plus hyperthermic intraperitoneal chemotherapy versus surveillance in patients at high risk of developing colorectal peritoneal metastases (PROPHYLOCHIP-PRODIGE 15): a randomised, phase 3 study. Lancet Oncol 2020;21(9):1147–54.
[55] Elias D, Honoré C, Dumont F, et al. Results of systematic second-look surgery plus HIPEC in asymptomatic patients presenting a high risk of developing colorectal peritoneal carcinomatosis. Ann Surg 2011;254(2):289–93.
[56] Franko J, Ibrahim Z, Gusani NJ, et al. Cytoreductive surgery and hyperthermic intraperitoneal chemoperfusion versus systemic chemotherapy alone for colorectal peritoneal carcinomatosis. Cancer 2010;116(16):3756–62.
[57] Ung L, Chua TC, David LM. Peritoneal metastases of lower gastrointestinal tract origin:a comparative study of patient outcomes following cytoreduction and intraperitoneal chemotherapy. J Cancer Res Clin Oncol 2013;139(11):1899–908.

Advances in Surgery 55 (2021) 175–195
ADVANCES IN SURGERY
ELSEVIER
MOSBY

# Machine Perfusion in Liver Transplantation

Malcolm MacConmara, MB BCh, Parsia A. Vagefi, MD*
Division of Surgical Transplantation, Department of Surgery, University of Texas Southwestern Medical Center, 5959 Harry Hines Boulevard, Dallas, TX 75390-8567, USA

**Keywords**

• Liver transplantation • Machine perfusion • Donor liver

**Key points**

- Enhanced donor preservation techniques hold the potential to expand the donor pool and thus reduce the disparity between organ supply and demand.
- Advances in machine perfusion for donor liver preservation during the previous decade have allowed this technology to be integrated into clinical practice.
- Normothermic machine perfusion (NMP) offers a superior platform for donor liver assessment and preservation.
  - Randomized controlled trial data indicate that NMP results in fewer liver discards and less early allograft dysfunction.
  - Ischemia-reperfusion injury is mitigated.
  - Biliary complications are reduced.
- Donation after cardiac death donors, advanced age donors (>70 years old), and steatotic donor grafts all show significant benefit from NMP.
- The NMP platform has potential to allow for ex vivo treatments to enhance donor livers prior to transplant.

**Video content accompanies this article at http://www.advancessurgery.com.**

## INTRODUCTION

Many advances have been made in immunosuppression, surgical technique, anesthesia, and perioperative care since the first liver transplant performed by Thomas Starzl in 1963 [1]. In concert, these improvements have allowed

*Corresponding author. *E-mail address:* Parsia.Vagefi@UTSouthwestern.edu

https://doi.org/10.1016/j.yasu.2021.05.013

liver transplantation to become the optimal treatment of patients with end-stage liver disease, hepatic malignancies not amenable to resection, and metabolic liver diseases [2].

Donor liver scarcity has become increasingly problematic [3]; however, it was not until this past decade that advances were made in donor organ preservation with the development of machine perfusion devices suitable for clinical use [4,5]. Machine perfusion provides enhanced options for organ preservation and offers great promise to expand the number of donor livers suitable for transplant. The field of liver transplant rapidly is embracing the use of machine perfusion, bringing with it paradigm shifts in donor organ selection and utilization, while providing a novel platform to assess and optimize the donor liver prior to implantation [6,7].

This review summarizes current clinical practice and describes the novel opportunities that are emerging to enhance donor livers using ex vivo therapeutics.

## HISTORY OF ORGAN PRESERVATION

Since the successful adoption of liver transplantation, the preservation method for donor livers was limited to static cold storage (SCS) [8]. Using this approach, donor organs were cooled rapidly and flushed in situ to remove blood from the allograft prior to being placed in a cold solution and transported on ice within coolers. The approach was simple and portable [8]. SCS, however, did not arrest cellular metabolism or prevent ischemic injury, and recipients were subjected to the deleterious effects of ischemia-reperfusion (IR) injury upon reestablishment of perfusion during the transplant procedure [9]. These limitations increasingly were encountered as the donor pool expanded to include donors of advanced age, donation after cardiac death (DCD) donors, and liver allografts with increasing fat content–all of which portended a greater degree of IR injury following reperfusion in the recipient [10,11].

### Early experimental work with machine perfusion

Ex vivo perfusion that permitted extended tissue preservation and provided an environment to repair damaged organs is not a new concept [12]; Alexis Carrel and Charles Lindenberg in 1935 produced a prefusion device they believed would allow rejuvenation of human tissue ex vivo [13]. Despite much excitement, the rudimentary technology was not sufficient to support their goals.

The early liver transplants done by Thomas Starzl at the University of Colorado in the 1960s all were done using locally procured deceased donors. A device similar to cardiopulmonary bypass machine was designed to allow preservation of donor livers following procurement [14]. Starzl described the use of this blood-based prefusion circuit during his initial series of liver transplants; however, his system was unsuitable for transport outside the transplant center [14]. Instead, SCS was the only practical option for travel to donor procurement sites, and donor organ research became focused on optimizing the constituents of preservation solutions [15,16]. Throughout the next 40 years, enthusiasm for machine perfusion persisted, although in the absence of technological advancements, all devices remained cumbersome and impractical (Fig. 1). With few exceptions, machine perfusion remained a stationary, experimental tool in the research laboratory unfit for clinical use [17].

### Contemporary advances in machine perfusion

In the past decade, the rapid development of machine prefusion technology has allowed this long sought-after preservation strategy to become a reality [4,5]. Solutions were found to allow portability, simplify control of perfusion parameters, and provide a physiologically normal environment for the donor liver [18]. Multiple, high-quality perfusion devices now are available from commercial manufacturers that offer the potential to improve preservation of donor livers, especially livers with marginal characteristics [5,19,20]. In Europe and the Unites States, machine perfusion is being integrated into donor organ management to address the disparity between demand for liver transplants and the limited availability of donor livers [21,22].

## TYPES OF MACHINE PERFUSION OF THE LIVER

Broadly, there are 2 categories–hypothermic machine perfusion (HMP), which circulates cold, oxygenated preservation solution, and normothermic machine perfusion (NMP), which preserves livers at near-physiologic temperatures using oxygenated blood, supporting active metabolism in the allograft (Fig. 2).

### Hypothermic perfusion

HMP is used extensively in kidney allograft preservation, and its use in liver preservation has been championed by several researchers in the United States and Europe. The liver is attached to the device and acellular perfusate then is circulated at temperatures between 2°C and 10°C. Hypothermic conditions slow metabolic processes, while the addition of oxygen to the perfusate may further attenuate reperfusion injury. Single-perfusion (portal only) and dual-perfusion (portal and hepatic artery) systems are under investigation. Dual perfusion offers potential advantage by delivering oxygenated perfusate to

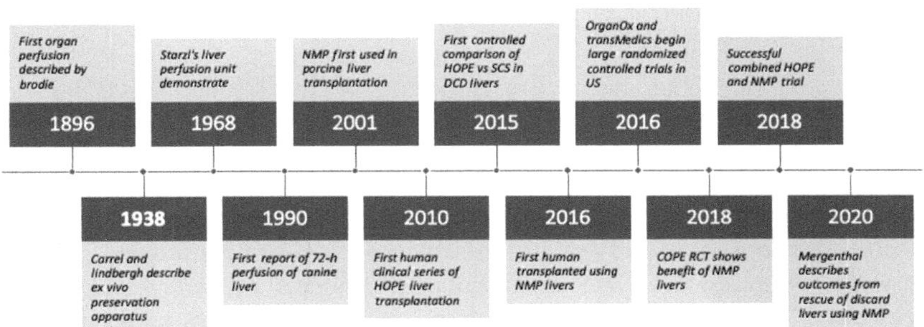


**Fig. 1.** History and milestones in liver machine perfusion.

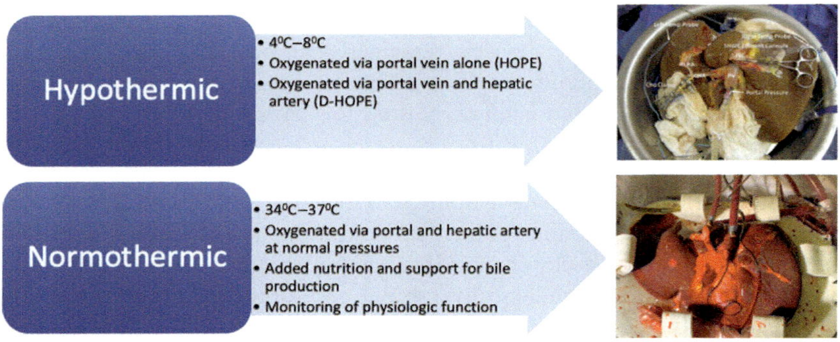


**Fig. 2.** Comparison of HMP and NMP.

the biliary tree, thus attempting to mitigate ischemic injury to the biliary tree [23].

### Normothermic machine perfusion

In NMP, the liver is placed on a circuit that perfuses the organ typically via the portal vein and hepatic artery with oxygenated blood at a temperature of 34°C to 37°C [24]. The liver is monitored as it performs normal metabolic functions and can be assessed using serial sampling of the circulating fluid. Bile production also is monitored easily.

### Advantages of machine perfusion

The advantages of machine profusion consist of (1) prolongation of traditional preservation limits, (2) optimized preservation of the liver, (3) improved monitoring and assessment, and (4) possibility for ex vivo manipulation of the organ.

## TECHNIQUE OF MACHINE PERFUSION

Most NMP devices are brought to donor site and the donor liver is placed on the circuit directly after procurement. Recently, investigators have sought to determine if transport with SCS, followed by machine perfusion once the graft has returned to the transplant center, can be used as an alternative method [25].

### Preparation for perfusion

Back-table preparation is performed to remove surrounding tissue and to prepare the donor vessels. Appropriately sized cannulae then are secured in the (1) portal vein, (2) hepatic artery, (3) inferior vena cava (IVC), and (4) bile duct in preparation for perfusion. In the event of aberrant arterial anatomy, arterial inflow is reconstructed at the procurement site. Current devices use either closed (both suprahepatic IVC and infrahepatic IVC are cannulated) or open (only the suprahepatic IVC is cannulated) systems to collect and return perfusate to the circuit. The liver is placed inside a sterile container and connected to the circuit. Upon initiation of perfusion warm oxygenated blood containing nutrition, anticoagulation, anti-inflammatory agents, and antibiotics are pumped through the donor liver (Video 1). Flows and pressures within the hepatic artery and portal vein are adjusted to achieve physiologic levels (Fig. 3). Adjustments are made according to real-time hemodynamic data and sampling of the perfusate. Typically, arterial flow increases as the liver warms and initial high resistance dissipates [26].

### Assessment of donor organs

The donor liver may be assessed by sampling the perfusate directly and determining changes in liver biochemistry, pH, lactate levels, and glucose. In addition, the graft remains immediately accessible for biopsy and histologic examination while on the circuit [26]. Lactate levels within stored packed red blood cell concentrate, and thus the perfusate, typically are elevated. Serial measurements of lactate levels during perfusion are employed, with a decreasing trend used as confirmation of suitability of the liver graft for transplantation [26,27]. Bile is another potential source of prognostic data for determining graft suitability, and the cannulated common bile duct allows for continuous assessment of bile production. Bile biochemistry also is under evaluation to determine its prognostic value, especially when assessing livers procured from DCD donors [26,28].

## CLINICAL TRIALS

Multiple clinical trials using HMP and NMP in Europe in the past 10 years have helped to develop practices of machine perfusion (Table 1).

### Hypothermic machine perfusion

*Early clinical research*

Guarrera and colleagues [4] reported the first prospective clinical trial using HMP in 2009. The study compared 20 HMP-preserved liver allografts with a matched group of SCS livers. It reported lower transaminase levels, shorter hospital lengths of stay, and fewer biliary complications in the HMP group, although early allograft dysfunction (EAD) was not different. In a follow-up

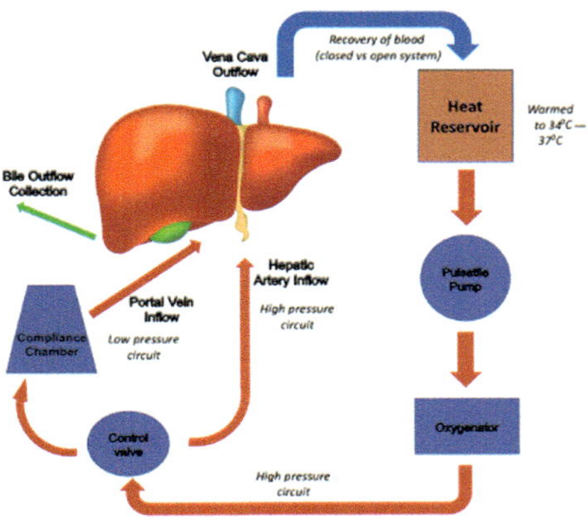


| NMP variable | Normal Range |
|---|---|
| Temperature | 34°C–37°C |
| Portal Vein Flow | 700–1700 mL/min |
| Portal Vein Pressure (mean) | 2–8 mm Hg |
| Hepatic Artery Flow | 300–700 mL/min |
| Hepatic Artery Pressure (mean) | 60–80 mm Hg |
| Bile Production | Variable (2–20 mL/hr) |

**Fig. 3.** Machine perfusion circuit and perfusion parameters.

**Table 1**
Summary of completed clinical trials using hypothermic machine perfusion and normothermic machine perfusion

| Perfusion type | Trial Name, Year | Study design | Primary Endpoints | Major Findings |
|---|---|---|---|---|
| HMP | Guarrera et al [4], 2010 | Prospective with retrospectively matched control | Patient and graft survival at 30 d, 90 d, and 1 year post-transplant | Lower rates of EAD in HMP compared with SCS, Similar patient survival, lower biliary complications in HMP, shorter hospital stay in HMP |
| HMP | Schlegel et al [33], 2019 | Prospective nonrandomized trial with matched control cohort | Lactate clearance at the end of transplant, ICU and hospital length of stay, complications, patient and graft survival | Similar graft survival despite extended donor warm ischemia in HOPE compared with DBD, decreased graft loss in HOPE DCD compared with control DCD, higher graft survival in HOPE DCD vs control DCD |
| HMP | van Rijn et al [23], 2017 | Prospective case-control study | Graft survival at 6 mo | Higher graft survival in DHOPE group vs control |
| HMP | Dutkowski et al [31], 2015 | Prospective, multicenter trial with matched control | Incidence and severity of biliary complications with 1 y of transplantation | Decreased intrahepatic cholangiopathy, biliary complications, and higher 1-y graft survival in HOPE DCD livers vs control |
| NMP | Ravikumar et al [5], 2016 | Prospective single-arm trial | 30-d graft survival | Similar 30-d graft survival NMP vs SCS, median AST lower in first 7 d in NMP group |
| NMP | Selzner et al [18], 2016 | Prospective single arm with matched control group | 90-d patient and graft survival | NMP vs SCS—lower transaminase on days 1–3 postoperative, no difference in international normalized ratio, bilirubin, no difference in ICU stay or hospital stay, no difference in patient or graft survival |
| NMP | Bral et al [41], 2017 | Prospective nonrandomized study with matched controls | Graft survival at 30 d post-transplant | No difference in graft survival, graft function similar to control |

| | | | | |
|---|---|---|---|---|
| NMP | Ghinolfi et al [44], 2019 | Pilot, open, single-center, randomized trial | Graft and patient survival at 6 mo | No difference in graft and patient. Use of NMP with older liver grafts is associated with histologic evidence of reduced IR injury. |
| NMP | Nasralla et al [21], 2018 | Multicenter RCT | Peak AST levels | 50% lower level of graft injury, 50% lower rate of organ discard, and 54% longer mean preservation time |
| NMP | Mergental et al [48], 2020 | Prospective single-arm study | Objective assessment of viability, graft utilization, transplant outcomes | 71% of discard livers achieved viability, 100% graft survival at 90 d, 18% retransplant rate for biliary complications |

study, the same team utilized HMP in a series of 31 marginal livers initially declined for all recipients and reported similar rates of EAD and patient survival at 1-year compared with a matched control cohort using SCS [29].

*Donation after cardiac death donors and dual hypothermic oxygenated machine perfusion*

Dutkowski and colleagues [30] described favorable outcomes a small series of 8 high-risk DCD livers with extended warm ischemia time that underwent HMP with oxygenated perfusion. They found no evidence of intrahepatic biliary complications. In a follow-up multicenter trial, they evaluated 25 DCD livers treated with HMP and compared their outcomes with 50 SCS DCD donors and 50 SCS brain death donor livers [31]. The HMP preserved group had superior outcomes to SCS preserved DCD livers with fewer biliary complications and improved 1-year graft survival. They found that outcomes were as good as DBD donors preserved with SCS. Patrono and colleagues [32] reported a reduction in EAD and acute kidney injury in an observational study of 25 DBD liver grafts that underwent dual hypothermic oxygenated machine perfusion (D-HOPE). Significantly, donor eligibility required greater than 80 years of age, body mass index greater than 30Kg/m2, macrosteatosis, or an expectation of prolonged preservation time. Schlegel and colleagues [33] examined long-term outcomes in 50 DCD livers treated with hypothermic oxygenated machine perfusion (HOPE) and demonstrated significantly improved 5-year graft survival with HOPE over DCDs treated with SCS.

*Ongoing clinical trials*

Two large randomized trials currently are active in European transplant centers [34,35]. The NCT01317342 trial uses single portal perfusion (HOPE) with a primary outcome of alanine aminotransferase (ALT) levels post-transplant. The NCT02584283 trial is using dual perfusion (D-HOPE) and its primary endpoint is the incidence of nonanastomotic biliary strictures. In the United States, the PILOT study (NCT03484455) is actively recruiting subjects in this randomized controlled trial to study the effect of the HMP LifePort liver device (Organ Recovery Systems) on EAD [36] (Table 2).

## Normothermic machine perfusion

*Early clinical research*

Peter Friend has pioneered the contemporary use of NMP [5,6,17,21,37–40]. Following encouraging preclinical results by his team at Oxford University, Ravikumar and colleagues [5] reported the first phase 1 clinical series using NMP in 2016. In addition to their primary goal of demonstrating the safety and feasibility of NMP technology, significant reduction in aspartate aminotransferase (AST) was noted in the 20 NMP recipients compared with matched controls. Additional single-center series supported the safety of NMP [41].

*Randomized clinical trials*

The first phase 3 randomized controlled trial was completed by the Consortium for Organ Preservation in Europe [21]. This multicenter trial

**Table 2**
Summary of currently active trials using hypothermic machine perfusion and normothermic machine perfusion

| Perfusion Type | Trial Name | Year | Study Design | Primary Outcome |
|---|---|---|---|---|
| HMP | HOPE for Human Extended Criteria and Donation after Brain Death Donor Liver Allografts [74] NCT03124641 | 2017 | Open, prospective, multicenter, randomized controlled trial | Peak and change in peak ALT within 7 d |
| HMP | Sequential Hypo- and Normo-thermic Perfusion to Preserve Extended Criteria Donor Livers for Transplantation [75] NCT04023773 | 2020 | Prospective single-arm trial | Patient and graft survival at 1 mo post-transplant |
| HMP | Study to Evaluate Performance of the Organ Recovery Systems LifePort Liver Transporter System, a Machine Perfusion System, for Liver Transplant (PILOT) [36] NCT03484455 | 2019 | Multicenter randomized controlled trial | Rate of EAD |
| NMP | Preserving and Assessing Donor Livers for Transplantation (PROTECT) TransMedics [42] NCT02522871 | 2015 | Multicenter randomized controlled trial | Incidence of early liver allograft dysfunction, incidence of liver graft related serious adverse events up to 30 d |
| NMP | WP01—Normothermic Liver Preservation [43] NCT02775162 | 2016 | Multicenter rancomized controlled trial | EAD |
| NMP | Safety and Feasibility of Normothermic Machine Perfusion to Preserve and Evaluate Orphan Livers [76] NCT03456284 | 2020 | Prospective single-arm pilot study | Patient survival at 30 d, primary nonfunction at 30 d |

(*continued on next page*)

**Table 2 (*continued*)**

| Perfusion Type | Trial Name | Year | Study Design | Primary Outcome |
|---|---|---|---|---|
| NMP | Efficacy of Ex-situ Normothermic Perfusion Versus Cold Storage in the Transplant With Steatotic Liver Graft (ORGANOXLAFE) [77] NCT03930459 | 2019 | Single-center randomized controlled trial | Peak transaminases at days 1, 3, 5, and 7 post-transplant |

randomized 335 livers to preservation with NMP or SCS. Their findings, reported by Nasralla and colleagues in 2018 [21] showed decreased postreperfusion syndrome (12.4% vs 33%, respectively; $P = .0002$) and EAD (10.1% vs 29.9%, respectively; $P = .0002$) after transplant in the NMP group compared with the SCS group. Furthermore, lower discard rates were noted in livers randomized to the NMP group (11.7% vs 24.1%, $P = .008$). There was no difference in biliary complications, 1-year graft survival, or 1-year overall survival between the NMP and SCS groups.

*Ongoing clinical trials*

Two large, multicenter, US-based, randomized clinical trials began in 2016 [42,43]. PROTECT (NCT02522871) used the TransMedics Organ Care System (OCS) for liver NMP whereas WP01 (NCT02775162) used the OrganOx metra. PROTECT recruited 300 patients at 17 centers in the United States, randomizing to 2 study arms: liver graft preservation by SCS and graft preservation by the OCS NMP pump. Their primary endpoints were EAD and incidence of graft related severe adverse events within the first 30 days. The WP01 study enrolled 267 patients across 15 centers in the United States. The primary endpoint of this study was EAD. Both trials recently have completed enrollment and results are expected in early 2021. In addition to assessment of allograft dysfunction, it is expected that these studies will provide important outcome data related to the effect of NMP on IR injury, biliary complications, and organ utilization as well as patient and graft survival (see Table 2).

*Extended criteria trials*

Ghinolfi and colleagues [44] studied the potential benefit of NMP in older donors (>70 years old). In this small single-center trial, 20 patients were randomized to receive older livers preserved using NMP or SCS. No difference was noted in patient or graft survival (the primary endpoint); however, significant differences in histologic signs of reperfusion injury were observed.

Case reports of the successful transplantation of DCD donors with prolonged warm ischemia time or severe (greater than 50%) steatosis following

NMP have been described [45–47]. These reports have offered initial enthusiasm that NMP could expand the donor pool further to meet growing demand in wait-listed candidates. In the recently reported VITTAL trial, Mergental and colleagues [48] examined outcomes after using NMP to assess and resuscitate discarded donor livers. The trial enrolled 31 livers. Viability criteria, including homogeneous liver perfusion, lactate clearance, bile production, and glucose metabolism, were met in 22 (71%) of organs. These livers all had prolonged cold ischemia prior to NMP (>6 hours); 45% were from DCD donors and 41% had steatosis greater than 30%. Although 32% developed EAD, all grafts achieved 3-month survival. In subsequent follow-up, 4 (18%) developed biliary complications requiring retransplantation.

*Timing of machine perfusion*

Initiation of NMP at the donor site minimizes the deleterious effects of SCS. This process, however, produces logistic challenges and likely adds to the cost and duration of the procurement, especially in closed-circuit NMP devices [25]. The feasibility and safety of NMP following SCS have been studied in small uncontrolled series. Watson and colleagues [49] reported their experience using a protocol for NMP following greater than 6 hours of SCS in DCD donors. Graft loss from primary nonfunction or ischemic cholangiopathy complicated 3 of the 12 transplanted livers. In contrast, Shapiro and colleagues [25] found no adverse graft outcomes in 26 livers using a back-to-base protocol; however, their study enrolled lower-risk donor livers with shorter SCS time. Although further studies are needed, these results, taken together with the VITTAL trial, appear to demonstrate that, although some donor livers may tolerate SCS followed by NMP, a subset of liver allografts (primarily those considered of marginal status) can undergo unrecoverable injury despite NMP preservation. The VITTAL trial highlights the need not only for improved diagnostic capabilities to determine graft suitability once perfused but also for the ability to enhance marginal liver during NMP to allow the graft to achieve a status suitable for transplant.

## CURRENT STATUS OF CLINICAL PRACTICE IN THE UNITED STATES

There currently are 2 NMP devices in clinical use in the United States [5,19,20]. All devices currently are limited by the Food and Drug Administration (FDA) for use under the conditions of investigational device exemption (IDE). These study conditions limit donor types and recipient characteristics to prespecified criteria, thus restricting their widespread availability.

### Trends in normothermic machine perfusion application

The United Network for Organ Sharing began identifying all donor liver procurements in which machine perfusion devices were used at the beginning of 2016. Between 2016 and 2019, there were 220 NMP donor livers perfused, leading to 212 transplants. The number of livers perfused with NMP rose steadily of this period. The discard rate was 3.51%, representing a 73.5% decrease in discard compared with SCS donor livers procured during the same period.

### Normothermic machine perfusion of marginal organs

DCD donors (18.2% vs 6.9%, $P<.001$) and older donors (17.7% vs 12.2%,) were over-represented in the NMP group relative to SCS procurements [22]. Hepatitis C virus positive donors and liver with severe macrosteatosis (>30%) were not used frequently, presumably due to exclusion criteria of trials.

### Cost and organ allocation

Machine perfusion adds significantly to liver procurement costs after accounting for all disposables, blood products, and monitoring costs associated with the device [50]. Centers that adopt machine perfusion and the associated cost to their practice may benefit from an expanded donor pool for consideration. In addition, patients who receive an NMP preserved graft potentially may benefit from shorter wait times, less risk of complications or death on the wait list, lower rates of EAD, shorter intensive care unit (ICU) and hospital stays, and improved post-transplant outcomes [51].

Donor livers currently are offered to listed candidates based on sharing rules that account for blood group and severity of illness (Model for End-stage Liver Disease score). Recently, donor livers now are distributed across a larger geographic area, effectively increasing the need for air travel among procurement teams. NMP devices have the capacity to allow for increased travel distances and thus longer times from procurement to implantation, all the while mitigating the IR injury risk traditionally observed with SCS preservation. This technology has the potential to alter organ sharing patterns and the full impact will become increasingly apparent once devices receive FDA approval.

## BIOMARKERS

As NMP and HMP become increasingly prevalent, understanding which organs can be enhanced or rescued for clinical transplant will be necessary to allow efficient use of the devices. In addition, the duration of perfusion, perfusate constituents, and specific device requirements for each donor liver will be important. The development of biomarkers to guide perfusion practices accurately and confirm suitability for transplant reliably is an essential requirement. Biomarker research currently is impeded, however, by the considerable variability in donors, the quality of the perfused livers, and the multiple NMP types, perfusates, and protocols used.

### Current biomarkers

At present, surgeons can monitor multiple objective hemodynamic parameters during NMP that indicate graft functional status, in addition to subjective markers, such as graft appearance and feel [27].

#### *Lactate metabolism*

Lactate levels have been linked to liver function post-transplant, and most users have included perfusate lactate levels within their viability assessment, especially because it is easily measured with portable point-of-care instruments. The sensitivity of lactate clearance as a biomarker has been questioned;

however, it appears that failure to clear lactate is specific for poor graft function [26,27].

*Transaminase levels*
Trends in transaminase levels are used as a hepatocellular marker of injury post-transplant. During perfusion, the rate of increase of AST/ALT appears to be of greatest importance [21,26]. ALT is considered more accurate because AST release from blood can confound assays [52]. ATP production, metabolic profiling, and circulating RNA/DNA offer promise as indicators, but the extensive processing required limits their clinical applicability at this time [53].

*Biliary system viability*
The volume of bile produced during perfusion provides limited prognostic value. Recent reports from the VITTAL trial and other single-center series have attempted to define criteria, including alkalinization of the bile, glucose levels, and rate of bile production, to identify marginal livers at risk of bile duct pathology post-transplant [28,48]. Histologic examination of the bile duct after NMP suggest that peribiliary gland injury is an important marker for ischemic cholangiopathy [54].

## Novel biomarkers

*microRNAs*
miRNAs are a group of small noncoding RNAs known to regulate post-transcriptional activity and have been associated with liver injury. Several specific miRNAs (miR-122, miR-146b, and miR-223) have been found in animal models or IR models of liver injury to be highly specific to hepatocytes and offer potential as future biomarkers during NMP [54].

*Cytokines*
Interleukin (IL)-17 is a proinflammatory cytokine secreted by $CD4^+$ T cells and associated with IR and has been shown to be elevated in animal models during warm ischemia injury [54]. Decreased levels of IL-33, a cytokine that promotes type 2 helper T-cell responses, have been found in livers with severe steatosis and is associated with primary nonfunction.

*Endothelin-1*
Serum levels of endothelin-1, a vasoconstrictor, have been associated with biliary strictures in liver transplant recipients and measurement during NMP may offer value as a predictor or biliary complications [55].

## Composite viability scores

Viability criteria based on combined objective measures have begun to emerge from large-volume centers (Table 3) [26–28,48]. These include criteria for EAD, primary nonfunction, and bile duct complications. It will be important to determine if these scoring systems are center-specific or if they can be extrapolated to other centers, other devices, or differing perfusion protocols.

**Table 3**
Viability assessment criteria

| Variable | Value |
|---|---|
| Perfusate | |
| Lactate | <2.5 trough or significant downtrend within 3–4 h, ≥4.4 mmol/L/kg/h drop from peak |
| Peak transaminases (AST, ALT) | <3000–6000 after 2–6 h |
| pH | >7.2.–7.3 without need for bicarbonate |
| Glucose | Trending down beyond 2 h |
| Mitochondrial flavin | <10,000 A U |
| ATP | Steady rise during perfusion |
| Bile | |
| Bicarbonate | >18 mmol/L |
| pH | >7.4 in first 4 h |
| Glucose | <3 mmol/L or <10 mmol less than perfusate glucose |
| Presence of bile production | Production but not volume may indicate viability |

## FUTURE ADVANCES

The clinical application of liver machine perfusion technology is expanding rapidly. Current devices represent the first wave of commercially available devices and future enhancements will incorporate additional tools for assessment and support of the liver. In the short term, advances likely will focus on refining existing perfusion technology and developing biomarkers. In the long term, machine perfusion devices likely will provide supportive ex vivo environments to permit therapeutic interventions to the liver prior to transplant.

### Expanding marginal livers

*Donation after cardiac death donors*

DCD livers are underutilized and represent a large reserve of potential donors. Transplant surgeons are reluctant to use DCD livers for fear of graft loss related to the higher risk of developing ischemic cholangiopathy [56]. Strict criteria related to warm ischemia (typically <30 minutes), obesity, age, and presence of additional risk factors result in only 25% of DCD donors being considered for transplant [57]. Nasralla and colleagues [21] demonstrated significantly improved outcomes in DCD donor grafts with NMP. The VITTAL trial has shown, however, that NMP by itself cannot prevent all cholangiopathy, even when metabolic and synthetic function has been restored [48]. The identification of bile duct-specific biomarkers is needed to assess the biliary tree during machine perfusion and thus determine the presence of irreversible damage that would prohibit transplantation.

*Steatotic livers*

The prevalence of steatotic donor livers has increased with ongoing increases in obesity and nonalcoholic fatty liver disease [58]. Severe steatosis promotes exaggerated injury responses and lessens the ability of the liver to withstand IR injury [11]. It long has been regarded as significant risk for primary graft nonfunction post-transplant. Methods to modify this risk using machine perfusion are being pursued using discarded donor livers with severe steatosis. Liu and colleagues [59] studied NMP in 10 discarded livers with various levels of steatosis, noting significant increase in perfusate triglyceride levels as well as decreased perfusate low-density lipoprotein and high-density lipoprotein. Allard and colleagues [60] examined 11 discarded livers undergoing NMP with a median macrosteatosis level of 40%. After 6 hours of perfusion, no differences were noted in microsteatosis or macrosteatosis on histologic examination. Upon completion of perfusion experiments, 4 of 11 livers were considered recovered and transplantable based on lactate clearance and continuous bile production. Vogel and colleagues [37] found similar absence of decreased steatosis levels for 13 discarded livers that underwent 24 hours of NMP. Boteon and colleagues [61] tested the addition of defatting enzymes in 10 discarded livers preserved using NMP. Half of the livers received the defatting cocktail had a significantly steeper drop in triglycerides at 6 hours and 12 hours. Macrosteatosis decreased by 40% compared with no change in the control group. Overall, the control group required significantly more sodium bicarbonate, reached lower levels of final lactate, and had a lower bile pH and a decreased volume of bile production. All defatted livers met viability criteria for transplantation, whereas only 40% of the control group met criteria. Ketogenesis was promoted, ATP levels increased, and perfusate triglycerides were increased in livers, which achieved viability criteria. Yeh and colleagues' [53] demonstration of impaired lipid metabolism, especially in discarded steatotic livers, supports maladaptive metabolic responses as the underlying mechanism for failure of these hepatocytes to tolerate organ procurement, preservation, and subsequent reperfusion.

## Enhancing livers

*Extracellular vesicles*

Paracrine effects from extracellular vesicles (derived from mesenchymal stem cells) increasingly are recognized as potent mechanisms to attenuate immune responses. The therapeutic potential of extracellular vesicles has been recently studied in ex vivo lung models, where reduction in proinflammatory cytokines and amelioration of IR injury was noted [62].

*RNA interference*

RNA interference (RNAi) treatments utilize this naturally occurring mechanism for suppression of gene expression [63]. Preclinical studies provide evidence for beneficial effects by interrupting Fas signaling and reducing hepatocellular injury in a rat liver transplant model [64]; however, cost, delivery, and nonspecific off-target effects limit its translation to clinical practice.

RNAi interventions utilizing NMP and HMP are being investigated in preclinical proof of concept experiments [64].

*Immunomodulation and cell therapy*

NMP has been found to reduce immune-mediated processes and it has been postulated that $CD4^{+}CD25^{+}FOXP3+$ regulatory T cells increase during perfusion orchestrating suppression of inflammatory responses [65]. Stimulation of resident regulatory cells may offer therapeutic options to reduce inflammation and necrotic and apoptotic responses [66]. In addition, with the liver isolated on NMP, an ideal environment is established for not only delivery of cellular therapies (regulatory T cells, mesenchymal stem cells, and so forth) within the perfusate but also assessment of their effects [66].

## Integration with other novel technologies

*Cryopreservation*

Advances in tissue and organ cryopreservation techniques have the potential to expand storage options for transplanted organs. Prolonged preservation using cryopreservation techniques could permit enhanced sharing strategies and reduce discard. The first subzero preservation of human livers recently was reported by Uygun and colleagues [67], in which discarded human organs were stored in a supercooled state without ice formation. NMP was integral during the preparation of organs by facilitating perfusion with cryoprotective agents. NMP was then used to rewarm the livers and assess their function.

*Xenotransplantation*

Xenotransplantation has seen significant progress in the past decade with reports of long-term survival in preclinical animal models and better understanding of the existing immunologic and coagulation barriers [68,69]. The unique ex vivo approach offered by NMP has multiple applications in future research and clinical preparation of xenografts. Xenografts can be perfused with human blood product to investigate early events post-xenotransplant, eliminating the need for costly and complex nonhuman primate experiments [70]. Future clinical use of xenografts would be facilitated by NMP assessment and optimization before transplant. Endothelial injury, inflammatory cytokine production, and Kupffer cell activation are the result of IR after organ procurement and transplant [71]. NMP can mitigate the risk of these IR-related injury responses and thus avoid triggering innate immune recipient responses to the xenograft.

*Bioengineering*

Another long-term potential application of NMP is artificial organ engineering [72]. Techniques are being developed that construct tissues and organs by bioprinting cells directly onto a matrix or by recellularization of a decellularized scaffold. In order to sustain metabolism during the process, NMP potentially could perfuse the developing organ with oxygen and nutrition, and, subsequently, NMP could serve as a tool to assess the success of the organogenesis [73].

## SUMMARY

Machine perfusion delivers significant advancement in preservation needed in the field of liver transplantation. Both NMP and HMP offer solutions to safely increase donor liver numbers to address growing patient demand. Biomarkers and clinical protocols will evolve to help promote widespread utilization. In the long term, NMP has the added potential to facilitate future technology aimed at enhancing donor livers using ex vivo therapeutics.

## CLINICS CARE POINTS

- Programmatic use of machine perfusion should be considered, especially when considering marginal donor liver offers.
- NMP reduces reperfusion syndrome, which may benefit liver transplant recipients.
- When monitoring livers during preservation, an important indicator of viability is reduction of perfusate lactate to less than 2.5 mmol/L.

Conflicts of interest
None. M. MacConmara is the site PI for PROTECT and Continuous Access Protocol clinical trials using the TransMedics OCS Liver device.

## SUPPLEMENTARY DATA

Supplementary data to this article can be found online at https://doi.org/10.1016/j.yasu.2021.05.013.

### References

[1] McKenna G, Klintmalm KG. History of liver transplantation. In: Busuttil RW, editor. Transplantation of the liver. 3rd edition. Elsevier; 2015. p. 2–22.
[2] Dienstag JL, Cosimi AB. Liver transplantation–a vision realized. N Engl J Med 2012;367(16):1483–5.
[3] Kwong A, Kim WR, Lake JR, et al. OPTN/SRTR 2018 annual data report: liver. Am J Transplant 2020;20(Suppl s1):193–299.
[4] Guarrera JV, Henry SD, Samstein B, et al. Hypothermic machine preservation in human liver transplantation: the first clinical series. Am J Transplant 2010;10(2):372–81.
[5] Ravikumar R, Jassem W, Mergental H, et al. Liver transplantation after Ex Vivo normothermic machine preservation: a phase 1 (first-in-man) clinical trial. Am J Transplant 2016;16(6): 1779–87.
[6] Ceresa CDL, Nasralla D, Coussios CC, et al. The case for normothermic machine perfusion in liver transplantation. Liver Transpl 2018;24(2):269–75.
[7] Quillin RC 3rd, Guarrera JV. Hypothermic machine perfusion in liver transplantation. Liver Transpl 2018;24(2):276–81.
[8] Todo S, Nery J, Yanaga K, et al. Extended preservation of human liver grafts with UW solution. JAMA 1989;261(5):711–4.
[9] Clavien PA, Harvey PR, Strasberg SM. Preservation and reperfusion injuries in liver allografts. An overview and synthesis of current studies. Transplantation 1992;53(5):957–78.

[10] de Vries Y, von Meijenfeldt FA, Porte RJ. Post-transplant cholangiopathy: classification, pathogenesis, and preventive strategies. Biochim Biophys Acta Mol Basis Dis 2018;1864(4 Pt B):1507–15.
[11] Cayuela NC, Negreti GP, Rasslan R, et al. Oxidative stress on ischemia/reperfusion injury in mice with non-alcoholic hepatic steatosis or steatohepatitis. Acta Cir Bras 2018;33(9): 753–61.
[12] Brodie TG. The perfusion of surviving organs. J Physiol 1903;29(3):266–75.
[13] Men in Black. Time Magazine 1938;31(24):40–4.
[14] Marchioro TL, Huntley RT, Waddell WR, et al. Extracorporeal perfusion for obtaining postmortem homografts. Surgery 1963;54:900–11.
[15] Olthoff KM, Millis JM, Imagawa DK, et al. Comparison of UW solution and Euro-Collins solutions for cold preservation of human liver grafts. Transplantation 1990;49(2):284–90.
[16] Takaoka F, Brown MR, Ramsay MA, et al. Intraoperative evaluation of EuroCollins and University of Wisconsin preservation solutions in patients undergoing hepatic transplantation. Transplantation 1990;49(3):544–7.
[17] Reddy S, Greenwood J, Maniakin N, et al. Non-heart-beating donor porcine livers: the adverse effect of cooling. Liver Transpl 2005;11(1):35–8.
[18] Selzner M, Goldaracena N, Echeverri J, et al. Normothermic ex vivo liver perfusion using steen solution as perfusate for human liver transplantation: First North American results. Liver Transpl 2016;22(11):1501–8.
[19] TransMedics. Liver preservation. Available at: https://www.transmedics.com/ocs-hcp-liver/ accessed on 06/17/2021.
[20] Minor T, Efferz P, Fox M, et al. Controlled oxygenated rewarming of cold stored liver grafts by thermally graduated machine perfusion prior to reperfusion. Am J Transplant 2013;13(6):1450–60.
[21] Nasralla D, Coussios CC, Mergental H, et al. A randomized trial of normothermic preservation in liver transplantation. Nature 2018;557(7703):50–6.
[22] MacConmara M, Hanish SI, Hwang CS, et al. Making every liver count: increased transplant yield of donor livers through normothermic machine perfusion. Ann Surg 2020;272(3):397–401.
[23] van Rijn R, Karimian N, Matton APM, et al. Dual hypothermic oxygenated machine perfusion in liver transplants donated after circulatory death. Br J Surg 2017;104(7):907–17.
[24] Jayant K, Reccia I, Virdis F, et al. The role of normothermic perfusion in liver transplantation (TRaNsIT Study): a systematic review of preliminary studies. HPB Surg 2018;2018: 6360423.
[25] Bral M, Dajani K, Leon Izquierdo D, et al. A back-to-base experience of human normothermic Ex Situ liver perfusion: does the chill kill? Liver Transpl 2019;25(6):848–58.
[26] Watson CJE, Kosmoliaptsis V, Pley C, et al. Observations on the ex situ perfusion of livers for transplantation. Am J Transplant 2018;18(8):2005–20.
[27] Mergental H, Stephenson BTF, Laing RW, et al. Development of clinical criteria for functional assessment to predict primary nonfunction of high-risk livers using normothermic machine perfusion. Liver Transpl 2018;24(10):1453–69.
[28] Matton APM, de Vries Y, Burlage LC, et al. Biliary bicarbonate, pH, and glucose are suitable biomarkers of biliary viability during Ex Situ normothermic machine perfusion of human donor livers. Transplantation 2019;103(7):1405–13.
[29] Guarrera JV, Henry SD, Samstein B, et al. Hypothermic machine preservation facilitates successful transplantation of "orphan" extended criteria donor livers. Am J Transplant 2015;15(1):161–9.
[30] Dutkowski P, Schlegel A, de Oliveira M, et al. HOPE for human liver grafts obtained from donors after cardiac death. J Hepatol 2014;60(4):765–72.
[31] Dutkowski P, Polak WG, Muiesan P, et al. First comparison of hypothermic oxygenated PErfusion versus static cold storage of human donation after cardiac death liver transplants:

an international-matched case analysis. Ann Surg 2015;262(5):764–70 [discussion: 70–1].
[32] Patrono D, Lavezzo B, Molinaro L, et al. Hypothermic oxygenated machine perfusion for liver transplantation: an initial experience. Exp Clin Transplant 2018;16(2):172–6.
[33] Schlegel A, Muller X, Kalisvaart M, et al. Outcomes of DCD liver transplantation using organs treated by hypothermic oxygenated perfusion before implantation. J Hepatol 2019;70(1):50–7.
[34] Hypothermic Oxygenated Perfusion (HOPE) of Human Liver Grafts. Available at: https://clinicaltrials.gov/ct2/show/NCT01317342. Accessed June 17, 2021.
[35] Dual Hypothermic Oxygenated Perfusion of DCD Liver Grafts in Preventing Biliary Complications After Transplantation (DHOPE-DCD). Available at: https://clinicaltrials.gov/ct2/show/NCT02584283. Accessed June 17, 2021.
[36] Study to Evaluate Performance of LifePort® Liver Transporter System, a Machine Perfusion System, for Liver Transplant (PILOT™). Available at: https://clinicaltrials.gov/ct2/show/NCT03484455.
[37] Vogel T, Brockmann JG, Quaglia A, et al. The 24-hour normothermic machine perfusion of discarded human liver grafts. Liver Transpl 2017;23(2):207–20.
[38] Ravikumar R, Leuvenink H, Friend PJ. Normothermic liver preservation: a new paradigm? Transpl Int 2015;28(6):690–9.
[39] Jamieson RW, Zilvetti M, Roy D, et al. Hepatic steatosis and normothermic perfusion-preliminary experiments in a porcine model. Transplantation 2011;92(3):289–95.
[40] Friend PJ. Advances in normothermic perfusion of the liver. Liver Transpl 2017;23(S1): S50–1.
[41] Bral M, Gala-Lopez B, Bigam D, et al. Preliminary single-center canadian experience of human normothermic Ex Vivo liver perfusion: results of a clinical trial. Am J Transplant 2017;17(4):1071–80.
[42] Preserving and Assessing Donor Livers for Transplantation (Liver PROTECT). Available at: https://clinicaltrials.gov/ct2/show/NCT02522871. Accessed June 17, 2021.
[43] WP01 - Normothermic Liver Preservation. Available at: https://clinicaltrials.gov/ct2/show/NCT02775162. Accessed June 17, 2021.
[44] Ghinolfi D, Rreka E, De Tata V, et al. Pilot, open, randomized, prospective trial for normothermic machine perfusion evaluation in liver transplantation from older donors. Liver Transpl 2019;25(3):436–49.
[45] Pavel MC, Reyner E, Molina V, et al. Evolution under normothermic machine perfusion of type 2 donation after cardiac death livers discarded as nontransplantable. J Surg Res 2019;235:383–94. Accessed June 17, 2021.
[46] Mergental H, Perera MT, Laing RW, et al. Transplantation of declined liver allografts following normothermic Ex-Situ evaluation. Am J Transplant 2016;16(11):3235–45.
[47] Manzia TM, Toti L, Quaranta C, et al. Liver transplantation with a normothermic machine preserved fatty ronagenarian liver: a case report. Int J Surg Case Rep 2019;57:163–6.
[48] Mergental H, Laing RW, Kirkham AJ, et al. Transplantation of discarded livers following viability testing with normothermic machine perfusion. Nat Commun 2020;11(1):2939.
[49] Watson CJE, Kosmoliaptsis V, Randle LV, et al. Normothermic perfusion in the assessment and preservation of declined livers before transplantation: hyperoxia and vasoplegia-important lessons from the first 12 cases. Transplantation 2017;101(5):1084–98.
[50] Raigani S, De Vries RJ, Carroll C, et al. Viability testing of discarded livers with normothermic machine perfusion: alleviating the organ shortage outweighs the cost. Clin Transplant 2020;34:e14069.
[51] Javanbakht M, Mashayekhi A, Trevor M, et al. Cost-utility analysis of normothermic liver perfusion with the OrganOx metra compared to static cold storage in the United Kingdom. J Med Econ 2020;23(11):1284–92.
[52] Woreta TA, Alqahtani SA. Evaluation of abnormal liver tests. Med Clin North Am 2014;98(1):1–16.

[53] Raigani S, Karimian N, Huang V, et al. Metabolic and lipidomic profiling of steatotic human livers during ex situ normothermic machine perfusion guides resuscitation strategies. PLoS One 2020;15(1):e0228011.
[54] op den Dries S, Westerkamp AC, Karimian N, et al. Injury to peribiliary glands and vascular plexus before liver transplantation predicts formation of non-anastomotic biliary strictures. J Hepatol 2014;60(6):1172–9.
[55] Dorobantu B, Popescu I, Dima S, et al. Molecular biomarkers as predictors for biliary complications following liver transplantation. A prospective study. J Gastrointestin Liver Dis 2017;26(3):253–9.
[56] Jay CL, Lyuksemburg V, Ladner DP, et al. Ischemic cholangiopathy after controlled donation after cardiac death liver transplantation: a meta-analysis. Ann Surg 2011;253(2):259–64.
[57] Fayek SA, Quintini C, Chavin KD, et al. The current state of liver transplantation in the United States: perspective from American Society of Transplant Surgeons (ASTS) Scientific Studies Committee and Endorsed by ASTS Council. Am J Transplant 2016;16(11):3093–104.
[58] Allen AM, Therneau TM, Larson JJ, et al. Nonalcoholic fatty liver disease incidence and impact on metabolic burden and death: a 20 year-community study. Hepatology 2018;67(5):1726–36.
[59] Liu Q, Nassar A, Buccini L, et al. Lipid metabolism and functional assessment of discarded human livers with steatosis undergoing 24 hours of normothermic machine perfusion. Liver Transpl 2018;24(2):233–45.
[60] Allard MA, Castro-Benitez C, Imai K, et al. Suitability of livers for transplantation when treated by normothermic machine perfusion. Clin Transplant 2018;32(6):e13256.
[61] Boteon YL, Attard J, Boteon A, et al. Manipulation of lipid metabolism during normothermic machine perfusion: effect of defatting therapies on donor liver functional recovery. Liver Transpl 2019;25(7):1007–22.
[62] Stone ML, Zhao Y, Robert Smith J, et al. Mesenchymal stromal cell-derived extracellular vesicles attenuate lung ischemia-reperfusion injury and enhance reconditioning of donor lungs after circulatory death. Respir Res 2017;18(1):212.
[63] Thijssen MF, Bruggenwirth IMA, Gillooly A, et al. Gene silencing with siRNA (RNA interference): a new therapeutic option during Ex Vivo machine liver perfusion preservation. Liver Transpl 2019;25(1):140–51.
[64] Bruggenwirth IMA, Martins PN. RNA interference therapeutics in organ transplantation: the dawn of a new era. Am J Transplant 2020;20(4):931–41.
[65] Jassem W, Xystrakis E, Ghnewa YG, et al. Normothermic Machine Perfusion (NMP) inhibits proinflammatory responses in the liver and promotes regeneration. Hepatology 2019;70(2):682–95.
[66] Karimian N, Yeh H. Opportunities for therapeutic intervention during machine perfusion. Curr Transplant Rep 2017;4(2):141–8.
[67] de Vries RJ, Tessier SN, Banik PD, et al. Supercooling extends preservation time of human livers. Nat Biotechnol 2019;37(10):1131–6.
[68] Patel MS, Louras N, Vagefi PA. Liver xenotransplantation. Curr Opin Organ Transplant 2017;22(6):535–40.
[69] Shah JA, Patel MS, Elias N, et al. Prolonged survival following pig-to-primate liver xenotransplantation utilizing exogenous coagulation factors and costimulation blockade. Am J Transplant 2017;17(8):2178–85.
[70] MacConmara M, Feizpour CA, Shubin A, et al. The role of machine perfusion in liver xenotransplantation. Curr Opin Organ Transplant 2020;25(5):477–82.
[71] Cimeno A, Barth RN, LaMattina JC. Advances in liver xenotransplantation. Curr Opin Organ Transplant 2018;23(6):615–20.
[72] Smith LJ, Li P, Holland MR, et al. FABRICA: a bioreactor platform for printing, perfusing, observing, & stimulating 3D tissues. Sci Rep 2018;8(1):7561.

[73] Chen AM, Lashmet M, Isidan A, et al. Oxygenation profiles of human blood, cell culture medium, and water for perfusion of 3D-bioprinted tissues using the FABRICA bioreactor platform. Sci Rep 2020;10(1):7237.

[74] HOPE for human extended criteria and donation after brain death donor (ECD-DBD) liver allografts (HOPE-ECD-DBD). Available at: https://clinicaltrials.gov/ct2/show/NCT03124641. Accessed June 17, 2021.

[75] Sequential hypo- and normo-thermic perfusion to preserve extended criteria donor livers for transplantation. Available at: https://clinicaltrials.gov/ct2/show/NCT04023773. Accessed June 17, 2021.

[76] Safety and feasibility of normothermic machine perfusion to preserve and evaluate orphan livers. Available at: https://clinicaltrials.gov/ct2/show/NCT03456284. Accessed June 17, 2021.

[77] Efficacy of Ex-situ Normothermic perfusion versus cold storage in the transplant with steatotic liver graft. (ORGANOXLAFE). Available at: https://clinicaltrials.gov/ct2/show/NCT03930459. Accessed June 17, 2021.

Advances in Surgery 55 (2021) 197–214

ADVANCES IN SURGERY

# What Is the Proper Technique for Primary Laparotomy Closure?

Charlotte Horne, MD*, Eric Pauli, MD

Penn State Hershey Medical Center, Milton S Hershey Medical Center, Mail Code H149, 500 University Drive, PO Box 850, Hershey, PA 17033, USA

**Keywords**

• Primary laparotomy closure • Small stitch technique • Hernia prevention

**Key points**

- Appropriate midline closure can decrease postoperative incisional hernia rates.
- Using a small stitch technique with a suture length to wound length ratio of 4:1 is most effective.
- Self-locking knots maximize suture strength.
- The benefit to the routine use of prophylactic mesh is still undetermined.

## INTRODUCTION

A midline laparotomy remains the most common open method of surgical access to the abdominal cavity. This incision allows adequate visualization of the entirety of the abdominal contents and avoids injury to vascular, muscular, or neurologic structures. Unfortunately, the Achilles heel of this incision remains the high rate of incisional hernias after its use. Despite an increased awareness of this issue, hernia rates have not significantly decreased in the modern surgical era, still occurring 10% to 40% of the time after midline laparotomy [1,2]. Incisional hernias not only result in decreased quality of life for the patient but they also represent a significant and enlarging economic burden to health care. Estimates from 2012 suggesting greater than $3 billion dollars is spent annually in the United States on management of hernia disease have subsequently risen to 7.3 billion dollars in 2018 [3,4].

While certain patient factors (obesity, smoking, diabetes, immunosuppression, and steroid use) increase the rate of incisional hernia after laparotomy

*Corresponding author. *E-mail address:* charlotte.m.horne@gmail.com

https://doi.org/10.1016/j.yasu.2021.05.014

[5–7], there are also numerous surgeon-controlled technical factors known to mitigate the risk of an incisional hernia formation. These factors include what abdominal wall layer(s) are closed, what suturing pattern is used, how large of a bite of tissue are taken, the distance of travel in between bites, and what suture gauge and needle size facilitate optimal closure. While each of these aspects of the closure may seem small and inconsequential, meticulous attention to these details has been shown to decrease incisional hernia rates [8–10]. Unfortunately, many surgeons still choose to close abdominal wall incisions based on their training and habits rather than with evidenced supported approaches.

Thoughtfully addressing these surgical knowledge gaps with an in-depth understanding of the healing process of a laparotomy incision as well as the relevant physics will hopefully allow more surgeons to select the appropriate suture material and needle size and use the appropriate closure technique to minimize the risk of hernia formation postoperatively. Many of the literature supported methods of fascial closure originated and are widely practiced in Europe but appear to be underutilized in the United States. To this end, the Americas Hernia Society launched its "Stop the Bulge" hernia prevention educational program in 2018 to address the knowledge and technical skills gap in North America.

In this article, we will present an evidence-based overview of the proper technique for laparotomy closure. Descriptions of the appropriate abdominal wall layers to reapproximate, the optimal suture type, suturing pattern, and needle types will be discussed. Additional consideration of the benefits of mesh implantation at the time of primary laparotomy closure will be given. Armed with this information, it is our hope that more surgeons use evidence-based laparotomy closure methodology to reduce the rate of incisional hernia formation.

## What layer(s) should be closed?

In order to determine what layer(s) to incorporate when closing a primary laparotomy, it is important to not only understand which layer(s) provide strength to the abdominal closure but also whether the addition of subsequent layers augments or detracts the strength of the closure. In addition, understanding the healing process of the laparotomy incision can further provide insight into advantages or disadvantages to incorporating layers into the closure.

When a midline incision is made, multiple layers are divided. From superficial to deep, a surgeon encounters the dermis and subcutaneous fat, the anterior and posterior sheath which fuse in the midline to form the lineal alba, preperitoneal fat, and finally the peritoneum. During closure, the surgeon must decide the most appropriate way to reapproximate these layers. The techniques most commonly performed include

a. Mass closure—incorporating multiple myofascial layers of abdominal wall in one layer
b. Layered closure—where multiple myofascial layers are closed in sequence

c. Single layer closure—where the anterior fascia/aponeurosis is closed with ideally no incorporation of fat or muscle

Historically, a mass closure technique was thought to be ideal because of the decreased incidence of early dehiscence. This was based on evidence from the study by Ellis and colleagues who analyzed midline closure after 1129 major laparotomies from 1975 to 1980 [9]. In their comparison of a layered closure to a mass closure, a mass closure was associated with a decreased incidence of burst abdomen. While they did note a higher incidence of incisional hernia with the mass closure technique, they hypothesized that this was likely due to an increased utilization of an absorbable suture in the mass closure group. However, evaluation of his technique demonstrated an increased rate of surgical site infection (SSI) and incisional hernia [8,11]. The increased rate of SSI is thought to be secondary to the compression of the large amount of tissue incorporated in the suture line [12]. The en mass method ultimately compresses a large amount of tissue which results in an increased amount of necrotic tissue in the closure. This necrotic tissue not only increases the risk of an SSI (which can increase the incidence of incisional hernias) but also is in and of itself an independent predictor of incisional hernia formation [11,12].

Another common technique for abdominal closure is a layered closure, where the peritoneum is closed initially as a separate layer, followed by approximation of the linea alba. Theoretically this technique has the benefit of minimizing the total amount of tissue compressed in one large bite while simultaneously permitting a multiple-layer closure. An evaluation into whether a separate peritoneal closure strengthens the laparotomy closure by Gurusamy and colleagues demonstrated no improvement in mortality, decrease in risk of burst abdomen, or decreased rates of incisional hernia [13,14]. In addition, using a layered method does not improve the tensile strength of the closure and is associated with a higher rate of wound dehiscence [9,13].

Based on the current evidence, the appropriate layer to close when closing a midline laparotomy is the aponeurosis only with minimal incorporation of muscle and subcutaneous tissue [15,16]. This layer has the capacity to withstand the tensile forces applied after laparotomy closure. Incorporation of additional muscle or subcutaneous tissue does not increase the strength of the closure but rather increases the risk of a SSI due to an increased amount of ischemic tissue in the closure [17].

## How should the linea alba be sutured?

The next question to address when closing a laparotomy is how exactly should the linea alba be approximated. To answer this, a surgeon must decide first whether to close in a continuous/running fashion or with interrupted sutures. Subsequently, one must then determine appropriate tissue bite size and the amount of travel in between bites.

A continuous suture technique is the most commonly used and the most effective method of midline laparotomy closure. Seiler and colleagues conducted a randomized controlled trial evaluating an interrupted technique with rapidly absorbable suture material and a continuous closure technique with slowly absorbable suture material [18]. Interestingly, they found no difference in hernia rates at 1 year between the groups [18]. However, a subsequent meta-analysis conducted by Diener and colleagues demonstrated decreased hernia incidence with a continuous closure method [1]. An interrupted technique is also more time-consuming to perform than a continuous closure [16]. Although suture material variation among studies represents a mitigation factor in data interpretation, a continuous/running method remains the recommend technique for fascial closure [15].

Traditionally, laparotomy incisions were closed with 1-cm bites of fascia with 1-cm travel between bites. This technique was first introduced by experimental studies that demonstrated increased strength with a wider bite, and as a result, this became the standard technique for midline laparotomy closure [19]. Initial evidence of the benefit of increasing the total amount of suture used to close a laparotomy dates back to the late 1970s. Jenkins evaluated how suture length to wound length (SL:WL) ratios changed when vertical stretching force was applied to a closure and how this changed the tension across the midline closure. Using principles of tensile strength, Jenkins demonstrated that when an incision is closed at a 4:1 SL:WL ratio (4 times as much suture material length used for the closure as the wound is long), there was a decreased tension across the stretched incision. The decrease in tension across the suture line notably resulted in decreased tissue ischemia [20].

This concept was further studied and subsequently popularized clinically by the Swedish surgeon Leif Israelsson. In a series of clinical trials, Israelsson and colleagues demonstrated that an SL:WL ratio of greater than 4:1, with tissue bites only 3 to 6 mm from the fascia edge, not only increased early postoperative wound strength but also resulted in a 3-fold reduction in the incisional hernia rate [8,21]. Israelsson went on to demonstrate in a prospective randomized controlled trial that when a 4:1 SL:WL ratio is achieved, there are significantly decreased infectious wound complications (5.2% vs 10.2%, $P = .02$) and significantly reduced hernia rates (5.6% vs 18.0%, $P < .01$) [8].

Despite the impressive results of Isralesson's well-designed studies, critics noted that the single center nature of the research, being conducted by surgeons with years of practice in this so-called "small bite" method, might not translate well to other surgeons. Fortunately, these concerns were not borne out. In 2015, Deerenberg and colleagues reported the results of the "STITCH Trial", a Dutch multicenter study of small bite methodology [15]. This double- blind randomized controlled trial showed that when a 4:1 SL:WL ratio is achieved with small tissue bites (0.5-mm bites from fascial edge with 0.5-mm travel between bites) there was a significant decrease in incidence of hernia formation at 1-year follow-up (13% vs 21%, $P = .05$) [15]. We recently investigated the technique for the prevention of incisional hernias in 86 patients who underwent heated intraperitoneal chemotherapy. Even in an extremely high-risk cohort, we found a significant reduction in the development of radiographically or clinically detectable incisional hernias

(13.0% vs 34.9%, $P = .048$) when compared with a standard laparotomy closure method [22,23].

*Suture material*

Multiple prospective randomized controlled trials and meta-analyses have demonstrated a decrease in incisional hernia rate with a small bite closure [8,15,21]. While the small bites themselves are part of this method, it is also important to understand the materials used in these trials. Generally, a size 2 to 0 slowly absorbable, monofilament suture on a small (20 mm) needle is used in a continuous running fashion. Alternately, a monofilament permanent suture of the same gauge can be used. Understanding why this material was selected in trials is integral to understanding the technique itself.

There are certainly numerous suture materials, suture gauges, and needle characteristics that can be used for fascial closure. Although seemingly inconsequential, these choices have been shown to alter the risk of SSI as well as incisional hernia rates after laparotomy [8]. Suture can either be nonabsorbable, slowly absorbable, or rapidly absorbable and can either be a braided or monofilament suture. Initial meta-analyses by Sajid and colleagues and Van't Riet and colleagues demonstrated that incisional hernia rates increase when rapidly absorbable suture is used [22,24]. More recently, a meta-analysis by Henriksen and colleagues failed to demonstrate differences in incisional hernia rates or SSI between rapidly absorbable, slowly absorbable, and permanent suture materials [25].

When choosing the appropriate suture material for closure, one must consider the evolving strength of the midline wound after closure. Initially, weaker type 3 collagen is produced [26]. It is not until 3 weeks later that this collagen begins to be remodeled to the stronger type 1 collagen [26,27]. As such, the absorption rate of many fast-absorbing sutures overlaps with a time when the midline wound remains week, creating a circumstance that may be herniogenic. The use of slowly absorbable or nonabsorbable suture for midline fascial closure is most appropriate as their strength characteristics are most compatible with the early phases of wound healing. Bloemen and colleagues compared a nonabsorbable (polypropylene) to slowly absorbable (polydioxanone) suture for closure in elective midline laparotomy closure finding no difference in incisional hernia rates, suture sinus formation, or SSI between the two groups [28,29]. However, other studies have demonstrated an increased risk of sinus or granuloma formation, increased risk of SSI, wound pain, and palpable knots when nonabsorbable sutures are used [25,30].

The main drawback with a multifilament suture is that the braided nature of the material harbors bacteria and limits macrophage penetration [30]. Combined, these two factors permit chronic suture infections to occur. In addition, some permanent sutures continue to lose their tensile strength over time [28]. The common misconception is that their strength is uniformly "permanent" over time, which is true for only a select few suture types (eg, polyester).

Ultimately these may serve as a nidus for potential infection without providing strength to the now healed wound. Owing to these factors, our preference is to use a slowly absorbable monofilament suture for laparotomy closure.

*Suture length*

When performing a 4:1 SL:WL closure with small bites, the length of the chosen suture material needs to be considered. The anticipated amount of suture needed to close can be calculated by measuring the length of the incision and multiplying by 4, while keeping in consideration the extra suture material that will be discarded as the tail ends of the knot when the suture is trimmed. For example, a 15-cm incision would require 60 cm of suture to be placed. This task can be reasonably accomplished with a 75-cm-long suture. An incision longer than this would require a longer suture to be used.

Commercially available suture lengths can vary based on location (both geographic- and hospital-specific). In Europe, for example, commercially available 150-cm-long sutures (2–0, monofilament, slow absorbing on a small taper tip needle) are widely available for the specific purpose of performing an 4:1 SL:WL closure of a full-length laparotomy incision. Such long sutures are not yet available in the United States (on small needles, in a 2–0 size, and so forth). To overcome this issue, we often times have to use two 75-cm-long sutures to close a full-length laparotomy incision while achieving a 4:1 SL:WL ratio. Note that when performing the closure in this fashion, we do not tie the sutures together in the mid portion of the wound but stop each suture independent of the other, a maneuver that reduces the chances of the sutures fracturing. Please see the *Knot Technique* section for additional details.

*Needle choice*

The type of needle used for fascial closure is less well studied than other elements of laparotomy closure, but we believe that needle choice is also a critical element of proper laparotomy closure. As demonstrated in Figs. 1 and 2, there are significant differences in needle size among common sutures used to close a laparotomy incision. In general, a taper tip needle is most commonly used instead of a cutting or reversing cutting needle. Even with the same gauge and suture material type, there can be a significant difference in needle width. The majority of the data analyzing laparotomy closure in the 4:1 SL:WL trials and "small bite" trials compared a 2 to 0 monofilament suture on a 20-mm taper tip needle to that of a 1 to 0 monofilament either single-stranded or double-stranded suture on a 38-mm taper tip needle [10–12]. A smaller needle was chosen for fascial closure as it facilitates a small bite with a small travel between bites. The 20-mm arc of the needle minimizes the excess tissue capable of being incorporated into the closure, making it harder to inadvertently include fat or muscle. Larger needles can be used (in particular, if a surgeon is electing to use a suture with a gauge greater than 2–0), but great care must be taken to not make the size of the bite match the size of the needle.

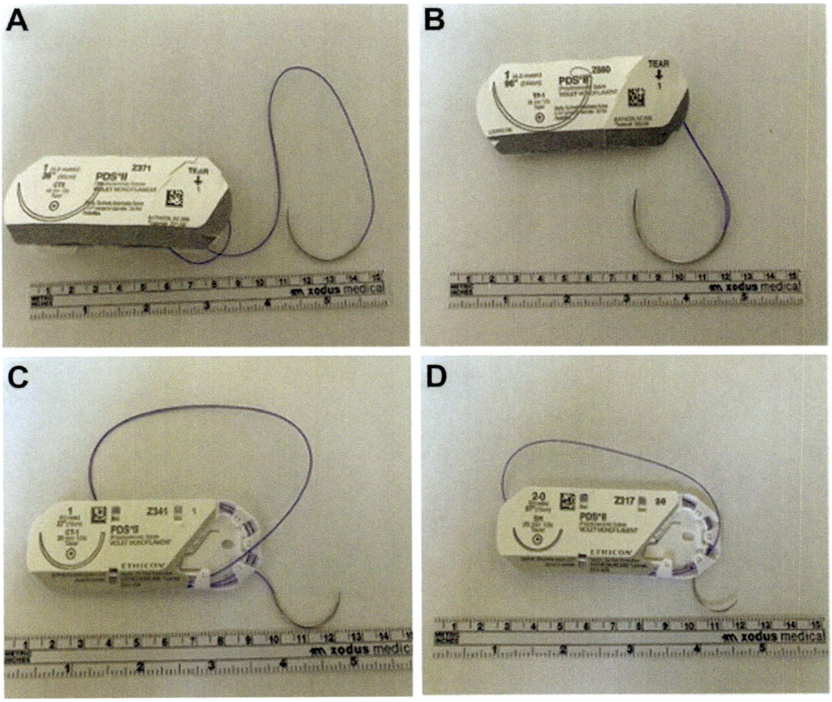


**Fig. 1.** Common sutures used to close laparotomy incisions. (*A*) 1.0 polydioxanone suture (PDS) on a 48-mm needle. (*B*) 1.0 PDS on a 65-mm needle. (*C*) 1.0 PDS on a 36-mm needle (*D*) 2.0 PDS on a 20-mm needle.

*Knot technique*

The types of knots used to secure the suture to the fascia also influence the strength of the closure for several reasons. In an ideal situation, knots should be secure, have a low profile, and prevent slippage. One of the drawbacks of a monofilament suture is that it is more difficult to tie secure knots [31]. To overcome this, multiple sequential knots must be placed to offset the tendency of these knots to come undone. This is notably different than multifilament sutures, where the interaction between the filaments in the two suture strands creates friction that prevents a tendency to come undone. The need for increased throws on the knots has the clear flaw of increasing the risk of SSI by creating a larger cluster of material that can harbor bacteria [32].

In addition, the type of knots being tied affects the actual strength of the suture material itself [32,33]. This has to do with the fact that the knot-suture interface is a potential location where sutures lines can fail. To this end, traditional sliding knots (eg, square knot, a surgeons' knot, and a granny knot) all result in dramatic reduction in the strength of the suture itself because the knots overlap with the running strand of suture. When tension is placed on the suture, these types of knots actually transmit pressure directly to a focal point

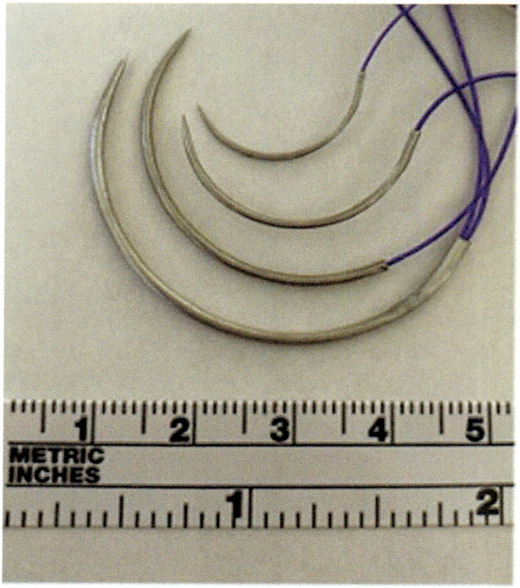


**Fig. 2.** Common needle sizes used to close a laparotomy incision. From largest to smallest: TP1, CTX, CT1, and SH.

on the suture itself, which can result in suture fracture at the interface with the knot and subsequent failure of the suture line. Self-locking anchor knots tighten to themselves, rather than to the running strand of suture they are helping to secure. This eliminates transmission of pressure to a focal point on the suture and thereby reducing the risk of suture failure. These types of knots are commonly used to secure fishing hooks to monofilament suture, to secure boats to docks, and to secure climbing equipment (including the climber).

Israelsson and colleagues studied the use of self-locking anchor knots for fascial closure and found them to be ideal; these knots did not slip, and they are smaller than conventional knots. More importantly, they identified significance differences in the effect of the knot on the suture itself. Traditional sliding knots decreased the strength of the suture by 40%, while the self-locking knots only decreased the strength of the suture by 5% to 10% [32]. These findings are further supported by Fong and colleagues who analyzed the tensile strength of a square knot, surgeons' knot, the Aberdeen (self-locking) knot, and a looped suture "knot" [33]. They found that the holding capacity of the looped suture was highest. Of the actual knots tied, however, the Aberdeen knot had the greatest holding capacity. There are multiple substantial drawbacks to the use of a looped suture outlined in the following paragraphs.

We use two knots during laparotomy closure. The closure is initiated by tying a half blood knot. As seen in Fig. 3, this knot is tied by first passing

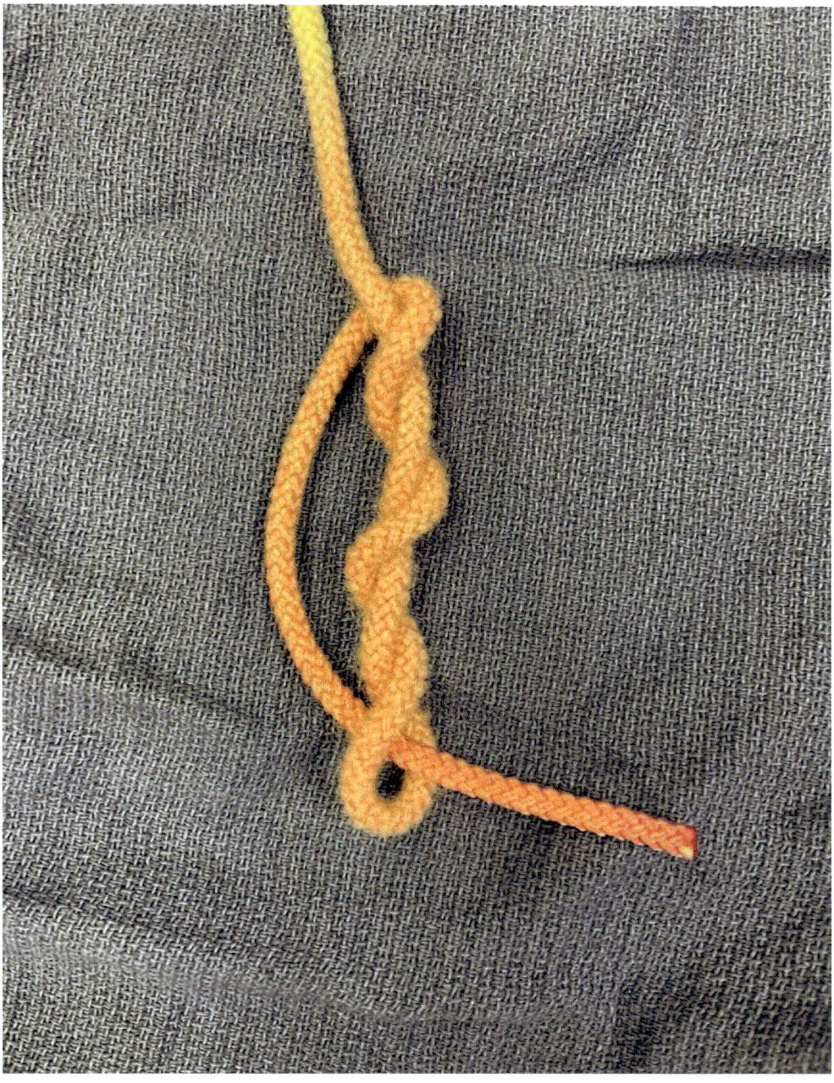

**Fig. 3.** A half-blood knot. The right strand of the suture is passed behind the left. It is wrapped around the left suture 3 times and then passed in front of the stitch and then back through the loop this created. The knot is then pulled tight and synched down.

the free tail end of the suture strand behind the longer end still attached to the needle. It is subsequently loosely wrapped around 3 times and then subsequently passed back through the initial loop created by the two ends of the suture imbedded in tissue. The long end of the suture (with needle attached) is pulled upward allowing the knot to tighten while minimizing the amount of suture tail to be discarded. Upon completion of the running closure, the suture is secured with an Aberdeen knot. This knot uses the loop and free end that are created at the completion of the laparotomy closure. This knot is formed by creating a loop, and the middle portion of the free end of the suture is pulled through (Fig. 4) creating a new loop. This process is repeated 3 total times. On the fourth throw, the suture is pulled all the way through which tightens the knot. Many surgeons are familiar with this type of knot as a method to complete a running subcutaneous skin closure.

The type of knots being used increases in importance when using the recommend 2- to 0-gauge suture (discussed in the following sections). While this suture gauge is sufficiently strong to withstand abdominal wall forces when a small bite method is used, it becomes insufficiently strong when traditional sliding knots are used. As such, we suggest that using self-locking knots is a *mandatory* component of appropriate fascial closure when using 2- to 0-gauge suture. When larger gauge suture is being used, the 40% reduction in burst strength with traditional sliding knots may not prohibit their use, but they still have all the other drawbacks listed previously. As such, we still recommend the use of self-locking knots even when larger gauge suture is being used.

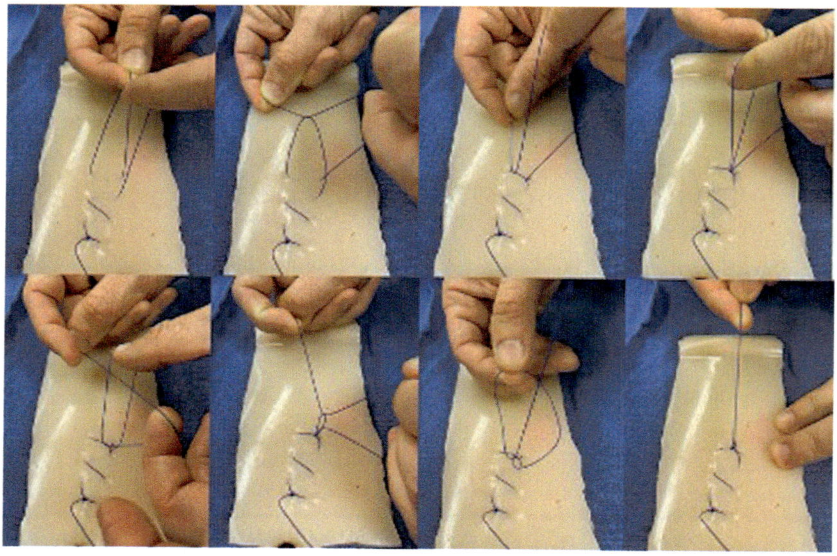

**Fig. 4.** Performing an Aberdeen knot. This knot is used at the end of the suture when the surgeon is left with a loop and a free end. To create his knot, a loop is made, and the free end is passed through, creating a new loop while the new loop is tightened. Traction is maintained on the working end. This process is repeated three times. The final throw involves the free end of the suture being pulled through to secure the knot.

*Suture gauge*

The gauge of suture chosen also has implications for the type of needle being used. Smaller suture gauges are available on smaller needles, and larger gauge sutures (or double-stranded sutures) are available on larger needles. Not only do these larger needles facilitate inappropriately large bites (as noted previously) but they also create large holes in the fascia. Fig. 5 demonstrates the change in caliber from the base to the swedge of the needle for commonly used facial closure sutures. Note that when comparing a 2-to-0 suture on an SH needle to a looped 1 suture on a TP1 needle, there is a full 1 mm difference in the size of the fascial holes created to pass the needle. Moreover, note that the TP-1 needle is ultimately capable of creating 1.76-mm holes in the fascia (at a minimum) for the sole purpose of passing not one but two strands of a suture with a burst strength much greater than what is required for fascial closure. We strongly discourage the use of this suture gauge/needle choice combination for any fascial closure. It has no demonstrable value in our opinion.

A 2-to-0 gauge is the appropriate size for a 4:1 SL:WL ratio laparotomy closure for multiple reasons. This suture gauge is fully capable of withstanding the abdominal wall forces when tension is distributed over many small bites and when appropriate knots are used. Most important, however, is that this suture is commonly mounted on a needle that facilitates a small stitch bite. Owing to the smaller size of the needle, it is technically challenging to take bites larger than 5-8 mm.

## PROPER FASCIAL CLOSURE TECHNIQUE

We recommend the following methodology be adopted for the closure of a primary laparotomy incision (Fig. 6). Before suturing, the edges of the fascia

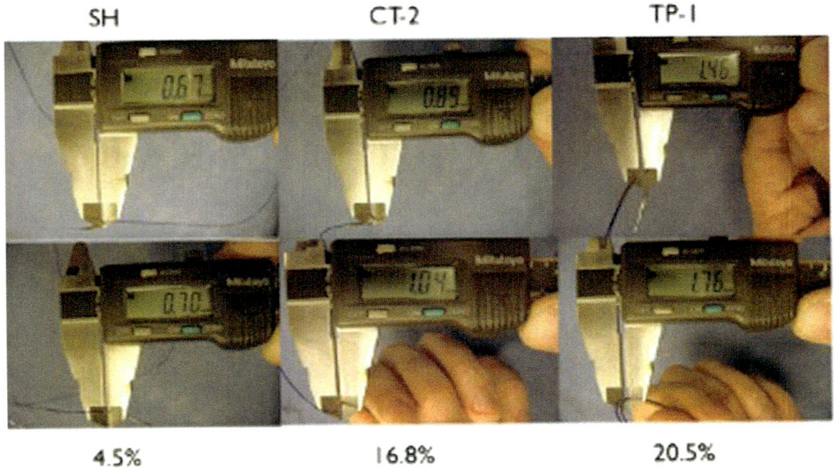


**Fig. 5.** Needle width at the proximal and distal point of the needle and associated maximal diameter of the hole made in the fascia in mm.

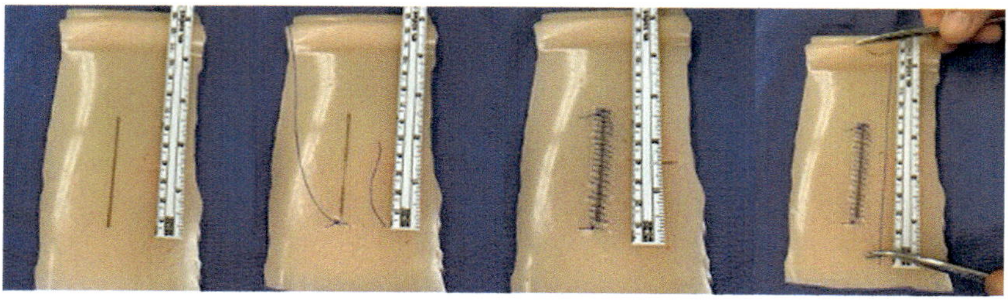

**Fig. 6.** Appropriate 4:1 closure technique. First the incision is measured to determine length of suture required. A self-locking knot is tied, and the remnant is cut and measured. The fascia is then reapproximated with a 5- to 8-mm bites with 5- to 8-mm travel between bites. Upon completion, the remnant suture is again measured to ensure a 4:1 SL:WL ratio.

should be identified circumferentially and, if necessary, should be cleared of subcutaneous fat to allow proper identification. The US population has a higher average body mass index (BMI) than the European populations in which the method was studied. While physics (and wound forces) are the same on both sides of the Atlantic, performing a 4:1 SL:WL ratio closure requires bites of fascia alone. The consequences of taking a bite (or bites) of only fat are high enough that we feel obligated to clearly delineate the fascia before attempting closure. We also use a Gelpi retractor placed just above the edges of the fascia to retract the fat locally facilitating closure.

With the fascia identified, we measure the length of the wound itself and multiple by 4 to determine the amount of suture needed to appropriately complete the closure method. We record this number and document it in the operative dictation. If there is no suture long enough to complete the closure, then two sutures can be used (one from superior and one from inferior). Beginning at the upper aspect of the fascia defect, we use a 2-0 slowly absorbing (polydioxanone) suture on an SH needle. The length of the suture is recorded. The suture is passed through tissue just above the apex of the fascial defect and is tied using a half blood knot while keeping the tail short to minimize suture loss. The suture to be discarded after the tail has been cut is measured, and its length is subtracted from the length of the original suture.

The laparotomy is then closed using a small-bite method that incorporates the fascia only. Bites 5-8 mm back from the fascia and 5-8 mm apart are taken using standard suturing methodology. At the end of the fascial defect, the closure is completed by tying an Aberdeen knot. The tail is trimmed, and the suture to be discarded is once again measured and its length subtracted from the length of the original suture length. Note that if a two-suture method is required, the sutures should each be secured with Aberdeen knots immediately adjacent to each other rather than tied to each other.

The amount of suture placed in the wound (original length − tail 1 length − tail 2 length) is compared with the amount calculated to achieve a 4:1 SL:WL ratio closure. If the ratio has been achieved, the operative dictation should reflect this. If the ratio has not been achieved, the suture is removed, and the laparotomy closure is repeated to achieve the 4:1 SL:WL ratio.

## Closure adjuncts

### *Prophylactic mesh placement*

Owing to the high incidence of incisional hernia formation after midline laparotomy, various adjuncts have been investigated for their ability to mitigate hernia formation. One of these adjuncts is the prophylactic placement of mesh at the time of primary laparotomy closure. The ability of mesh to prevent recurrent hernia formation is well established. While extrapolating a benefit for primary closures seems logical, there are many questions that need to be addressed to determine its true utility.

Mesh can be placed in an intraperitoneal, preperitoneal, retrorectus, or onlay position. Delineating where prophylactic mesh should be placed to provide the most benefit is imperative. Ideal placement would afford the lowest morbidity associated with mesh use while at the same time being technically easy to perform. In addition, a determination as to which type of mesh (biologic, biosynthetic, or synthetic) and which material construct provide the most benefit must be undertaken.

Studies involving prophylactic placement of a biologic mesh have not shown a benefit. Sarr and colleagues evaluated biologic mesh placement in obese patients undergoing closure of laparotomy incisions [34]. Sarr and colleagues placed Surgisis Gold (Cook Biotech, Inc, West Lafayette, IN) in a sublay position in patients undergoing bariatric surgery [34]. Not only did the prophylactic mesh increase clinically significant wound events but also it did not decrease the rate of hernia formation [34]. As a result, we recommend against the prophylactic use of biologic mesh as it has not been shown to decrease long-term hernia incidence. A similar study by Pans and colleagues used intraperitoneal polyglactin (rapidly absorbing biosynthetic) mesh and found no difference in hernia rates between two groups [35].

Notably, the use of synthetic mesh in high-risk patients has been associated with lower rates of postoperative hernias. Muysoms and colleagues randomized patients undergoing open abdominal aortic aneurysm repair to receive either a primary fascial closure with a 4:1 SL:WL ratio or a mesh augmented closure [36]. In this study, a lightweight polypropylene mesh was placed in the retro muscular space allowing for 3 cm of overlap in all directions. At 1-year follow-up, the incidence of hernia formation was significantly lower in the mesh group (0% vs 17%, $P = .013$). The mesh group continued to outperform the suture closure group at 2-year follow-up as well (0% vs 28%, $P < .0001$) [36]. Limitations to the adoption of prophylactic mesh utilization based on these results include a small study population ($n = 120$), as well as assessment of hernia formation was based on physical examination only.

Further data supporting prophylactic mesh placement are found in the Prevention of incisional hernia with prophylactic only and subway mesh reinforcement versus primary sure only in midline laparotomies (PRIMA) trial [37]. This multicenter, double-blind, controlled trial evaluated patients undergoing open

Abdominal aortic aneurysm (AAA) repair as well as patients with a BMI greater than 27 kg/m$^2$. Patients were again randomized to receive a sutured fascial closure or a prophylactic mesh augmented closure with mesh in either the sublay position or the onlay position. Similar to Muysoms and colleagues, the PRIMA authors found that prophylactic mesh placement significantly decreased hernia formations rates from 30% in the suture group to 13% and 18% in the onlay and sublay groups, respectively [37]. Notably, there was no significant difference in the rates of hernia between the sublay and onlay mesh groups.

Mesh placement in the sublay and onlay position requires dissection into the abdominal wall which takes additional operative time, opens up potential spaces, and may hinder future hernia repair (such as the gold standard retromuscular operations). Kohler and colleagues evaluated placement of mesh in an intraperitoneal position and found that compared with a large-stitch primary fascial closure, intraperitoneal mesh resulted in a decreased incidence of incisional hernia at 3 years (18.5% vs 7.2%, $P = .3$) without a significant increase in postoperative morbidity [38]. Of note, while rates of SSI were not statistically significant between the two groups, patients with intraperitoneal mesh placement had a longer time to final wound healing.

A meta-analysis conducted by Borab and colleagues found that prophylactic mesh placement decreased incisional hernia formation when compared with a 4:1 SL:WL fascial closure [39]. They also demonstrated that regardless of the location of placement (onlay, sublay, underlay), incisional hernia rates decreased when mesh was used in a prophylactic fashion. However, mesh placed in the preperitoneal (sublay) and onlay positions was associated with an increased incidence of seroma formation [39].

It is important to note that while prophylactic mesh placement was associated with decreased incisional hernia formation rates, the majority of these studies evaluated only patients considered to be at a high risk for hernia development undergoing elective, clean, midline laparotomy incisions. These studies also reveal that the use of prophylactic mesh is not without morbidity, albeit often minimal. What characteristics make a patient "high risk" or "low risk" has yet to be fully delineated, and the potential benefits in "low-risk" patients is yet to be determined. Multiple investigations are ongoing, including the prophylactic use of mesh in clean-contaminated circumstances [40].

Our current clinical practice is to carefully evaluate patient risk factors and to use mesh in select patients at extremely high risk for incisional hernia after a comprehensive discussion with the patient. We recommend using a reduced-weight, macroporous polypropylene mesh placed in the onlay position. This mesh type can be salvaged in the event of wound complications as well as minimizes dissection in the abdominal wall plains that may be used for future hernia repairs [41]. Mesh removal (if necessary) can be done without violating the peritoneal cavity.

*Retention sutures*

Retention sutures, full-thickness bites through all layers of the abdominal wall including the skin, are commonly used in relaparotomies or after a fascial dehiscence. While not routinely used in a primary laparotomy closure, their use may be considered if an incision is under undue tension or if a patient is considered to be at high risk. We do not recommend the use of retention sutures in these circumstances. Complications associated with retention sutures include significant pain, often necessitating early removal and skin breakdown. While there are some data that they decrease the risk of wound dehiscence postoperatively, their use does not decrease the risk of evisceration or postoperative incisional rates [42–44].

*Future directions*

While there is a significant amount of high-quality evidence that suggests a single-layer closure using a slowly absorbable suture with small bites decreases the risk of hernia formation after a midline laparotomy, there are some limitations to the application of this evidence. First, most patients evaluated were patients undergoing elective primary midline laparotomies. In patients who are undergoing emergent surgeries, or those who have had numerous laparotomy incisions before, the data are less conclusive as often these patients were excluded from these studies. Second, the BMI of the patients studied in the numerous randomized controlled trials was approximately 26 kg/m$^2$. Understanding whether the benefits of this closure technique are still seen in a patient population with a higher BMI is essential as there is a significant increase in the rates of obesity worldwide. While the physics of these closures is sound, the ability to technically perform them in populations with a higher BMI has yet to be fully demonstrated. Finally, how these data should be applied to patients with incisional hernias is yet to be determined.

## SUMMARY AND RECOMMENDATIONS

1. Laparotomy incisions should be closed using a slowly absorbable monofilament suture with a small tapered needle.
2. Incisions should be closed with in a continuous fashion with bites of the aponeurosis only.
3. Distance between stitches should be from 5 to 8 mm with stitches 5-8 mm in width to achieve a 4:1 SL:WL ratio.
4. Sutures should be secured with self-locking knots to maximize suture tensile strength.
5. Prophylactic mesh should be used on a case-by-case basis and reserved for patients at high risk of hernia formation.
6. Retention sutures should not be used as they have not been shown to be beneficial.

## CLINICS CARE POINTS

- If there is difficulty identifying the anterior fascia, use a retractor to expose and facilitate fascial only bites.

- Use a small needle (20 mm is best) to ensure small bites and small travel between bites.
- Self-locking knots should be used instead of friction knots.
- When nearing the end of a suture, a self-locking Aberdeen knot should be used, and a new stitch started with a half blood knot instead of tying the two sutures together.
- If a 4:1 SL:WL ratio is not achieved, the fascial closure should be redone.

## Disclosure

Dr Horne is a lecturer for Medtronic Dr Pauli Speaker for Bard Davol, Medtronic and Ovesco Consultant for Boston Scientific, Actuated Biomedical, Baxter, Wells Fargo, Cook Biotech, CMR Surgical, Neptune Medical, Surgimatrix, Boehringer Laboratories Receives royalties from UptoDate and Springer Financial Interests include IHC inc, Contamination Source Identification, SIG Biomedical.

## References

[1] Diener MK, Voss S, Jensen K, et al. Elective midline laparotomy closure: the INLINE systematic review and meta-analysis. Ann Surg 2010;251:843–56.
[2] Fink C, Baumann P, Wente MN, et al. Incisional hernia rate 3 years after midline laparotomy. Br J Surg 2014;101:51–4.
[3] Poulose BK, Shelton J, Phillips S, et al. Epidemiology and cost of ventral hernia repair: making the case for hernia research. Hernia 2012;16:179–83.
[4] Shubinets V, Fox JP, Lanni MA, et al. Incisional hernia in the United States: Trends in hospital encounters and corresponding healthcare charges. Am Surg 2018;84(1):118–25.
[5] Riou JP, Cohen JR, Johnson H Jr. Factors influencing wound dehiscence. Am J Surg 1992;163(3):324–30.
[6] Yahchouchy-Chouillard E, Aura T, Picone O, et al. Incisional hernias. 1. Related risk factors. Dig Surg 2003;20(1):3–9.
[7] Sorenson L, Hemmingsen UB, Kirkeby L, et al. Smoking is a risk factor for incisional hernia. Arch Surg 2005;140(2):119–23.
[8] Millbourn D, Cengiz Y, Israelsson LA. Effect of stitch length on wound complications after closure of midline incisions: a randomized controlled trial. Arch Surg 2009;144(11): 1056–9.
[9] Bucknall TE, Cox PJ, Ellis H. Burst abdomen and incisional hernia: a prospective study of 1129 major laparotomies. Br Med J (Clin Res Ed) 1982;284(6320):931–3.
[10] Israelsson LA, Millbourn D. Prevention of incisional hernias: how to close a midline incision. Surg Clin North Am 2013;93:1027–40.
[11] Millbourn D, Cengiz Y, Israelsson LA. Risk factors for wound complications in midline abdominal incisions related to the size of stitches. Hernia 2011;15(3):261–6.
[12] Cengiz Y, Gislason H, Svanes K, et al. Mass Closure technique: an experimental study on separation of wound edge. Eur J Surg 2001;167:60–3.
[13] Gurusamy KS, Cassar Delia E, Davidson BR. Peritoneal closure versus no peritoneal closure for patients undergoing non-obstetric abdominal operations. Cochrane Database Syst Rev 2013;2013(7):CD010424.
[14] Hugh TB, Nankivell C, Meagher AP, et al. Is closure of the peritoneal layer necessary in the repair of midline surgical abdominal wounds? World J Surg 1990;14(2):231–4.

[15] Deerenberg EB, Harlaar JJ, Steyerberg EW, et al. Small bites versus large bites for closure of abdominal midline incisions (STITCH): a double-blind, multicentre, randomised controlled trial. Lancet 2015;386(10000):1254–60.
[16] Muysoms FE, Antoniou SA, Bury K, et al. European Hernia Society guidelines on the closure of abdominal wall incisions. Hernia 2015;19(1):1–24.
[17] Israelsson LA, Jonsson T. Suture length to wound length ratio and healing of midline laparotomy incisions. Br J Surg 1993;80(10):1284–6.
[18] Seiler CM, Bruckner T, Diener MK, et al. Interrupted or continuous slowly absorbable sutures for closure of primary elective midline abdominal incisions: a multicenter randomized trial (INSECT: ISRCTN24023541). Ann Surg 2009;249(4):576–82.
[19] Sanders RJ, DiClementi D, Ireland K. Principles of abdominal wound closure. I. Animal studies. Arch Surg 1977;112(10):1184–7.
[20] Jenkins TP. The burst abdominal wound: a mechanical approach. Br J Surg 1976;63(11): 873–6.
[21] Cengiz Y, Blomquist P, Israelsson LA. Small tissue bites and wound strength: an experimental study. Arch Surg 2001;136(3):272–5.
[22] Sajid MS, Parampalli U, Baig MK, et al. A systematic review on the effectiveness of slowly-absorbable versus non-absorbable sutures for abdominal fascial closure following laparotomy. Int J Surg 2011;9(8):615–25.
[23] Lewcun JA, Pauli EM, Pameijer C. Incisional hernia formation can be reduced following hyperthermic intraperitoneal chemotherapy with increased suture length to wound length ratio fascial closure. Int J Abdom Wall Hernia Surg 2020;3(4):117.
[24] Van 't Riet M, Steyerberg EW, Nellensteyn J, et al. Meta-analysis of techniques for closure of midline abdominal incisions. Br J Surg 2002;89(11):1350–6.
[25] Henriksen NA, Deerenberg EB, Venclauskas L, et al. Meta-analysis on materials and techniques for laparotomy closure: The MATCH review. World J Surg 2018;42(6):1666–78.
[26] Lau FH, Pomahac B. Wound healing in acutely injured fascia. Wound Repair Regen 2014;22(Suppl 1):14–7.
[27] Velnar T, Bailey T, Smrkolj V. The wound healing process: an overview of the cellular and molecular mechanisms. J Int Med Res 2009;37(5):1528–42.
[28] Bloemen A, van Dooren P, Huizinga BF, et al. Randomized clinical trial comparing polypropylene or polydioxanone for midline abdominal wall closure. Br J Surg 2011;98(5):633–9.
[29] Greenwald D, Shumway S, Albear P, et al. Mechanical comparison of 10 suture materials before and after in vivo incubation. J Surg Res 1994;56(4):372–7.
[30] Osther PJ, Gjøde P, Mortensen BB, et al. Randomized comparison of polyglycolic acid and polyglyconate sutures for abdominal fascial closure after laparotomy in patients with suspected impaired wound healing. Br J Surg 1995;82(8):1080–2.
[31] Trimbos JB, Booster M, Peters AA. Mechanical knot performance of a new generation polydioxanone suture (PDS-2). Acta Obstet Gynecol Scand 1991;70(2):157–9.
[32] Israelsson LA, Jonsson T. Physical properties of self-locking and conventional surgical knots. Eur J Surg 1994;160(6–7):323–7.
[33] Fong ED, Bartlett AS, Malak S, et al. Tensile strength of surgical knots in abdominal wound closure. ANZ J Surg 2008;(78):3164–6.
[34] Sarr MG, Hutcher NE, Synder S, et al. A prospective randomized multicenter trial of Surgisis Gold, a biologic prosthetic, as a sublay reinforcement of the fascial closure after open bariatric surgery. Surgery 2014;156(4):902–8.
[35] Pans A, Elen P, Dewe W, et al. Long-term results of polyglactin mesh for the prevention of incisional hernias in obese patients. World J Surg 1998;22(5):479–83.
[36] Muysoms FE, Detry O, Vierendeels T, et al. Prevention of incisional hernias by prophylactic mesh-augmented reinforcement of midline laparotomies for abdominal aortic aneurysm treatment: a randomized controlled trial. Ann Surg 2016;263(4):638–45.
[37] Jairam AP, Timmermans L, Eker HH, et al. Prevention of incisional hernia with prophylactic onlay and sublay mesh reinforcement versus primary suture only in midline laparotomies

(PRIMA): 2-year-follow-up of a multicenter, double-blind, randomized controlled trial. Lancet 2017;390(10094):567–76.
[38] Kohler A, Lavanchy JL, Lenior U, et al. Effectiveness of prophylactic intraperitoneal mesh implantation for preveniton of incisional hernia in patients undergoing open abdominal surgery: a randomized clinical trial. JAMA Surg 2019;154(2):109–15.
[39] Borab ZM, Shakir S, Lanni MA, et al. Does prophylactic mesh placement in elective, midline laparotomy reduce the incidence of incisional hernia? A systematic review and meta-analysis. Surgery 2017;161(4):1149–63.
[40] Goldwag JL, Wilson LR, Ivatury SJ, et al. Stoma closure and reinforcement (SCAR): A study protocol for a pilot trial. Contemp Clin Trials Commun 2020;19:100582.
[41] Siegal SR, Morrell DJ, Orenstein SB, et al. Mesh salvage following deep surgical site infection. Int J Abdom Wall Hernia Surg 2020;3(1):4–10.
[42] Gislason H, Viste A. Closure of burst abdomen after major gastrointestinal operations—comparisons of different surgical techniques and lateral development of incisional hernia. Eur J Surg 1999;165(10):958–61.
[43] Rink AD, Goldschmidt D, Dietrich J, et al. Negative side-effects of retention sutures for abdominal wound closure: A prospective randomized study. Eur J Surg 2000;166(12):932–7.
[44] Khorgami Z, Shoar S, Laghaie B, et al. Prophylactic retention sutures in midline laparotomy in high-risk patients for wound dehiscence; a randomized controlled trial. J Surg Res 2013;180(2):238–43.

Advances in Surgery 55 (2021) 215–229

ADVANCES IN SURGERY

ELSEVIER
MOSBY

# Can Pancreatic Organoids Help in the Treatment of Pancreatic Cancer?

Toni T. Seppälä, MD, PhD[a,b], Richard A. Burkhart, MD[c,*]

[a]Department of Surgery, Johns Hopkins University, 600 North Wolfe Street, Halsted 612, Baltimore, MD 21287, USA; [b]Department of Surgery, Helsinki University Hospital, Helsinki, Finland; [c]Department of Surgery, Division of Hepatobiliary and Pancreatic Surgery, Johns Hopkins University, 600 North Wolfe Street, Halsted 612, Baltimore, MD 21287, USA

**Keywords**

• Pancreatic cancer • Pancreatic ductal adenocarcinoma • Patient-derived organoid • Organoid • Pharmacotyping

**Key points**

- Organoids are increasingly being used in clinical research and decision-making.
- First Clinical Laboratory Improvement Amendments–certified assays have been presented for individual drug screening and sensitivity testing of solid tumors.
- Most potential is expected for increasing the stratification yield to targeted therapy and drug response prediction.

**Video content accompanies this article at http://www.advancessurgery.com.**

## INTRODUCTION

The potentially curative treatment of patients diagnosed with pancreatic ductal adenocarcinoma (PDAC) relies on complete surgical resection of the primary tumor and the utilization of effective systemic chemotherapeutics. Unfortunately, less than a quarter of patients have localized disease amenable to surgical resection at the time of the diagnosis, and few patients with locally advanced disease are offered surgical exploration after induction chemotherapy. Moreover, even the prognosis of those that undergo surgical resection is heavily

*Corresponding author. *E-mail address:* burkhart@jhmi.edu
Twitter: @Adductor (T.T.S.); @DrRABurkhart (R.A.B.)

https://doi.org/10.1016/j.yasu.2021.05.015
0065-3411/21/

dependent on the systemic control of the disease by adjuvant chemotherapy. Evidence would suggest that effective chemotherapeutics can lead to a doubling of the number of patients surviving long-term [1,2].

There are 2 disparate chemotherapy regimens routinely used in PDAC; gemcitabine/nab-paclitaxel (G/A); and a combination of 5-fluorouracil, leucovorin, irinotecan, and oxaliplatin (FOLFIRINOX). Each regimen has been demonstrated to result in an objective response for just less than one-third of patients with advanced PDAC, a rate that compares favorably against the previous standard-of-care, single-agent gemcitabine [3–5]. Dedicated study in the adjuvant setting, following resection of localized PDAC in a potentially curative paradigm, similarly supported the use of these 2 combination regimens over gemcitabine alone [1,4–6]. To date, however, there are no clinically relevant biomarkers available to distinguish patients with tumors uniquely sensitive to either G/A or FOLFIRINOX. As a result, the selection of a chemotherapy regimen is often guided by individual practitioner bias, with many using patient age and performance status as a marker of the capacity to tolerate chemotherapy-associated toxicity. Historically, FOLFIRINOX has been associated with increased side effects, and these toxicities are at times inferred by some to suggest potentially increased efficacy.

The identification of predictive biomarkers for chemotherapeutic response remains an urgent and unmet need in PDAC. A tailored approach, identifying effective regimens for each patient, has the capacity to improve the durability of surgical cure in this disease. Further, improved chemotherapeutic efficacy may allow for increasing utilization of surgical care in patients initially diagnosed with more advanced disease, through techniques relying on vascular interposition grafts [7], multivisceral resections [8], and even a surgical approach to patients with distant metastases (in a manner similarly used in colorectal cancer) [9].

### Nature of the problem

There is an unmet need to identify predictive biomarkers in pancreatic cancer that enable optimization of systemic therapies. Such a discovery would ultimately lead to increased durable response to patients treated with chemotherapy for advanced disease, increased utilization of surgical exploration after induction therapy for locally advanced disease, and increased disease-free and overall survival following curative resection in patients with resectable and borderline resectable disease.

## SIGNIFICANCE (IN DEPTH ANALYSIS)

### What biomarkers predict treatment response?

In contrast to several other subtypes of malignancy, pancreatic cancer lacks predictive biomarkers available to guide therapeutic selection. In breast cancer, for example, assessment of the hormone receptor status is critical for the identification and selection of an optimal approach to disease management. Similarly, in colorectal cancer, the assessment of a tumor's genetic mutational profile and overall mutational burden can help elucidate unique treatment options.

In PDAC, the potential predictive biomarkers of clinical response are particularly limited. Historically, research aimed at elucidating biomarkers of therapeutic response have focused most prominently on targetable alterations detected in genomic profiling. One solid option in PDAC is represented by the adaption of pan-cancer lessons gleaned from the study of pathogenic germline variants in homologous recombinational repair and mismatch repair genes. In PDAC, the detection of these variants suggest that oncologic outcomes may be improved by selective treatment with PARP and checkpoint inhibitors, respectively. Data supporting this approach have particularly focused on targeted therapeutic administration in the maintenance setting [10,11]. Additional data to support genome profiling in precision medicine approaches to PDAC are provided by early efforts from the "Know your Tumor" program [12,13]. A retrospective review of this largely administrative database identified a relatively small subset of patients with PDAC harboring targetable genomic alterations. In leveraging the overall program to feed patients into targeted therapy trials, outcomes data suggest that patients receiving targeted therapy, when appropriate, have improved survival compared with patients who have the target but receive conventional chemotherapy [13]. Interestingly, however, the program also highlights a unique challenge in PDAC relative to other tumor types. Because of the uniquely paucicellular nature of pancreatic cancer where a fibroblastic cell type and dense stroma can predominate the histopathologic landscape, "Know your Tumor" demonstrates that a conventional molecular workup of the patients can only identify a targetable change in a fraction of tumors [12].

In attempts to move from genotype to phenotype, several translational research groups have focused on defining gene expression patterns with the capacity to define molecular profiles with prognostic or predictive importance [14]. In the first transcriptomic classification, tumor tissue was obtained from 85 untreated patients who underwent surgical resection as the first step in PDAC treatment. Tissues from these resections subsequently underwent epithelial microdissection, and RNA hybridization arrays were used to characterize gene expression and define 3 PDAC subtypes: classical, quasimesenchymal (QM), and exocrine-like. In studying PDAC cell lines derived from both human tumors and humanized mouse models, the classical and QM subtypes seemed to be a promising marker to stratify differential response to conventional cytotoxic chemotherapies. Initial work suggested the classical subtype, characterized by *GATA6* expression and RAS pathway dependency, was more sensitive to erlotinib, whereas the QM subtype was more sensitive to gemcitabine [15]. A second study evaluated 145 primary, untreated PDACs (locally advanced and metastatic) and 61 metastatic PDACs with hybridization array and RNA-seq. This study similarly classified PDAC subtypes according to gene expression profiling, finding the previously reported classical subtype as well as a single, relatively broad cohort termed "basal-like" [16]. Although the basal-like subtype was associated with poorer survival, these patients gained more benefit from adjuvant therapy in an era defined by gemcitabine use as a single agent in the first-line setting. These data were broadly viewed as confirming the findings from the original study, with the QM subtype being more sensitive to therapeutic response with gemcitabine and the naming convention reframed in the context of gene expression in line with basal-cell population. A third study assessed bulk RNA sequencing data from 96 patients with untreated resected, primary PDAC [17] and redefined 4 subtypes: squamous, pancreatic progenitor, aberrantly differentiated endocrine exocrine, and immunogenic. Although initial reports suggested an appreciation of greater underlying nuance to tumors, and these data were eagerly dissected with an eye toward precision medicine approaches in this disease, subsequent limitations arising from methodology and disease biology became apparent. For example, the initial excitement surrounding the immunogenic subtype as one that may benefit from immune modulating therapy quickly retreated, as it was recognized that the data signal was likely driven by the bulk nature of sequencing and, if anything, may indicate that these tumors fail to respond to immune-oncologic agents despite existing immune infiltrate in the tumoral and peritumoral microenvironment. These classifications partially overlap based on common gene expression patterns and prognosis, despite the differences in the molecular techniques used. Squamous, basal-like, and quasimesenchymal subsets are molecularly similar and likely to represent the same subset of PDAC with gene expression that varies somewhat according to the level of "contaminating" nontumor RNA detected by each method [18].

The most critical limitation to using subtyping in precision medicine platforms to date, as discussed earlier, has been the uncertainty, which exists when molecular subclassification is based on RNA sequencing from bulk specimens obtained by clinical laboratory tools. In PDAC, the cancerous ductal component of the specimen is almost always a minor portion of the overall tumor mass. Most of the tumor mass is comprised by the stroma cells and, as a result, molecular profiling tends to highlight gene expression from the stromal cells of the tumor microenvironment rather than the underlying cancer itself. Methods to mitigate these limitations in the research setting, such as tumor microdissection, fresh tumor flow-sorting, or single cell–based bioinformatics approaches, are unwieldy in the clinical environment. One strategy to overcome this barrier, and offer novel approaches to study each patient's tumor, is a tissue culture–based pipeline that leverages the propensity for malignant cells to replicate and divide unchecked, whereas the nonimmortalized components of the tumor microenvironment, such as the stromal cells, undergo cell-cycle arrest, anoikis, and apoptosis. One such tissue culture platform relies on malignant cell growth within a 3-dimensional (3D) model system and is termed an organoid.

## What is an organoid?

Patient-derived organoids (PDOs) are self-organizing, 3D structures that are derived from and cultured after digestion of patient tumor tissues from surgical and diagnostic procedures [19]. By using an artificial extracellular matrix as a scaffold, cells can replicate, divide, expand, and organize into complex 3D structures that replicate those found in vivo, such as cysts and ducts. Success rates for organoid growth, commonly defined as the presence of any cystic or ductal-appearing structures within the culture over a finite period of time, can be as high as 90% in some laboratories. The biomass of an organoid culture is derived from the immortalized malignant stem cell population that maintains the growth and invasiveness of the primary tumor in vivo. As a result, the early culture is maintained as a largely genetically and epigenetically stable replicate in vitro 3D models of their in vivo counterpart tumor from which it was derived. Organoids in early culture have the capacity to recapitulate intratumor and intertumor heterogeneity characteristic of human cancers, allowing studies into heterogeneity of tumor subtype and subclonal evolution of tumors [20]. In addition, organoid co-culture in 3D space with stromal cells and tumor-infiltrating lymphocytes is a promising approach to recapitulate the tumor microenvironment for the study of clinical approaches using targeted agents against the stromal or immune pathways [21].

### Capacity to model human disease

The models used to study PDAC over the past 4 decades have been limited to a relatively small number of patient-derived cells cultured as 2D monolayers, patient-derived murine xenografts, or genetically engineered mouse models. Each model presents unique limitations to our understanding of disease biology. For example, 2D cell lines do not retain tissue-specific architecture, polarized cell-cell interactions among the ductal population of cells, and lack the capacity to model stromal-cancer cell crosstalk. The effect is seen in altered genetic expression in long-standing traditional cell culture models that has impact on the study of stress response, molecular biological study and, likely, therapeutic response. Similarly, mouse models are limited in their capacity to aid in the study of PDAC as well. Owing to the development of a tumor in a syngeneic host, mouse models lack the heterogeneity in genetic and gene expression profile that is otherwise seen in human PDAC. Patient-derived xenograft (PDX) models of disease are more varied than their genetically engineered mouse counterparts but are limited in usefulness due to considerations such as the timeline required to generate each model, associated costs, and the effects of the murine microenvironment on the human tumor model's growth and development [22].

In general, the PDOs derived from PDAC are faithful recapitulations of the in vivo disease. When compared with surgical specimens from which PDOs are often derived, they retain mutation profiles and are genetically stable over early passages. PDOs also retain similar architectural features and protein expression signatures with some specific known exceptions. For example, *TP53* mutations that are present in the primary tumor and PDO both express the *TP53* antibody staining, whereas at times the *SMAD4* expression in *SMAD4*-wt PDOs can be a challenge to detect in a manner similar to the primary tumors [23]. Gene expressional patterns, the principal component of most subtyping schemes, can be detected in a manner similar at the primary tumor tissue when performed from the PDOs by supervised clustering of known profile-related genes [24].

The intratumor heterogeneity present across a tumor's bulk can also be recapitulated by organoid cultures. In perhaps the most classic example of this, Roerink and colleagues established colorectal adenocarcinoma organoids from different sections of a tumor and showed that the organoids shared the genomic alterations with the tissues of the same geography from where they were derived. Although all 5 organoids per patient established from the normal mucosa were alike, organoids from geographically remote tumor sections displayed a diversity of morphologies. Oncogenic mutations were absent in normal organoids but such drivers were always shared by the organoid and their geographically correlated tumor section [25]. These findings were supported by similar data from single-cell RNA sequencing approaches in early organoid growth, showing the presence of 28 different cell types in CRC-derived organoids [26].

Romero-Calvo and colleagues studied organoid models of pancreatic tumors derived from single patients with comparison against multiple parallel methods including murine xenograft and 2D cell lines. They confirmed the phenotypic resemblance of the organoid with the primary tumor, as well as exploring the somatic genome in each model. Although a somatic analysis of the primary tumor can often be limited by the paucicellular nature of the specimen, the mutant allele frequencies are often enriched after establishment of tumor models such as organoids and 2D cell lines. Reassuringly, the mutations specific to individual patients, including *CDKN2A*, *NALCN*, *ZBTB16*, and *PARP1*, were readily detectable in corresponding tumor models, and copy number alterations were retained (eg, diploid karyotype when the primary tumors remain chromosomally stable) [23,27,28].

Although heterogeneity can be retained in early passages, when passaged in bulk, the growth advantages of one clone can often outpace its brethren. For example, Fujii led the effort to label paired cultures of CRC organoids with unique identifying fluorescent markers and establish a mixed cell population for bulk passaging over the course of more than 1 month. In each instance, the culture became dominated by single populations, indicating dynamic alteration of clonal occupancy during culture [29].

### How to make use of the pure ductal cancer cell population?

In a manner similar to the colorectal work performed earlier, studies with pancreatic cancer have verified that a dominant clone emerges during bulk passage in PDAC-derived organoids as well. When investigating the somatic mutational profile using a Clinical Laboratory Improvement Amendments (CLIA)-certified laboratory, early genomic heterogeneity is progressively lost, as a single clone predominates in a bulk sequencing approach [24]. Importantly, the organoid culture technique is able to reveal this early heterogeneity in a manner that is superior to that done when sequencing using clinical formalin-fixed paraffin-embedded (FFPE) specimens alone. In one example, a minor allele (*KRAS* G12R) was present at only 1% frequency at the first PDO passage but became the dominant clone later in passage 4, as seen in the primary tumor sequencing [24] (Fig. 1). These data are analogous to work performed with CRC organoids [30].

The potential value in using organoids for genotyping in the current clinical care of patients is grounded in 3 facts. First, PDAC is a tumor dominated by stroma and with a relatively paucicellular malignant component making primary tumor sequencing a unique technologic challenge relative to other cancer types. Second, an established organoid retains the genetic and molecular features of the primary tumor during early passage. Third, organoid technology is a uniquely rapid technique for the isolation and expansion of the purely malignant cell component. With these advantages in mind, an organoid approach to PDAC clinical molecular characterization may actually be superior to a sequencing approach from primary tumor tissues by a CLIA-certified laboratory. Early data suggest that lower-frequency variant subpopulations are present and more easily detectable in the organoid sequencing than sequencing of bulk FFPE-derived tumor DNA. Similarly, when planning a framework for the adoption of RNA sequencing–based PDAC subtyping, such as the ones proposed by Moffit and colleagues, an organoid approach is likely superior as well. Both lower-frequency mutation burden, subtle gene expression profiling differences, and the effects and extent of intratumoral heterogeneity

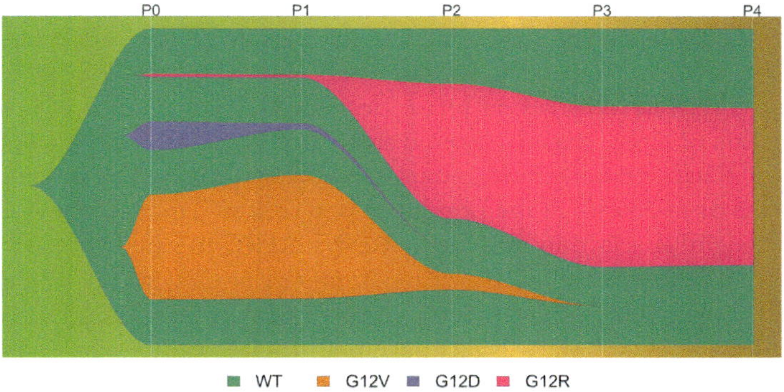


| Passage | Position | Nucleotide change | Codon change | Alleles | % (MAF) |
|---|---|---|---|---|---|
| P0 | 12b | G→T/ G→A | GTT/GAT | G12V/G12D/G12R | 33/9/1 |
| P1 | 12b | G→T/ G→A | GTT/GAT | G12V/G12D/G12R | 39/2/1 |
| P2 | 12b/12a | G→T/ G→C | GTT/CGT | G12V/ G12R | 5/43 |
| P3 | 12a | G→C | CGT | G12R | 51 |
| P4 | 12a | G→C | CGT | G12R | 50 |

**Fig. 1.** Clonal heterogeneity of a patient-derived organoid. The *KRAS* variant G12R evolves into a dominant clone over culture and becomes the only clone noted on CLIA testing of the primary tumor.

between the epithelial cells that are composed in many cases of both classical and basal-like subtypes are likely more readily detected in an organoid framework [31]. Especially relevant are recent single-cell RNA sequencing studies suggesting that classical and basal-like subtypes are heterogeneously maintained in an early organoid culture and may be recapitulated by the enriched epithelial compartment [32,33].

### Success rates in organoid establishment protocols

One fundamental difference between PDO, PDX, and 2D cell lines is the timeline and success rates at which they can be established as patient-specific tumor model of PDAC. Sometimes referred to in the literature as a patient "avatar," the time required to create a 2D model of a patient's tumor typically exceeds 8 to 12 weeks [22]. Success rates in the generation of 2D cell lines are generally limited to only those with features, often remaining undefined, that are conducive to adhesive propagation along the top of a plastic surface. Historically in our hands, for example, success rates in 2D line generation can be expected between 30% and 50% of the time. Similarly, when creating an in vivo model in PDX, at least 6 to 8 months [34] from a tumor biopsy are typically required and successful growth can be precarious. In contrast to the experience in 2D lines and PDX, organoids can be established and propagated to a characterizable biomass in as few as 2 to 6 weeks. Success rates, too, are dramatically higher, with most high-volume laboratories now reporting establishment in as many as 80% of samples processed [24,35].

The definition of success in PDO generation can vary somewhat depending on the purpose and goal for clinical and/or translational research initiatives. We have previously proposed a classification schema for PDO culture maturation to describe 3 clinically relevant phases: establishment, expansion, and characterization [24]. The *establishment* phase describes the emergence and biomass accumulation of viable ductal organoid structures. Typically, this phase is highlighted by a balance between biomass preservation in the ductal component and anoikis or apoptosis of the nonductal population. This balance is directed by the thoughtful selection of growth factors added to establishment culture medium that supports those cells of most interest at the expense of other cell types. Typically, the establishment culture media can vary from one tumor type to the next, as the growth factors supporting the tumor stem cells reflect the underlying organ of tumor origin. Throughout the establishment phase in pancreas-derived biopsies, the culture may contain biomass originating from either normal ducts, PDAC, or both. The establishment phase is generally short, requiring days to weeks under the right conditions. The *expansion* phase is characterized by increasing biomass accumulation and the elimination of "nonductal contamination." The result is a culture that is clean in visual appearance and reflects a biomass that is relatively pure with ductal cells. The expansion phase varies the most in duration, as each PDO culture has a unique growth rate likely based on regulatory mechanisms that remain relatively poorly understood. The *characterization* phase is a descriptor used to infer that a critical biomass has been reached allowing for molecular characterization or phenotypic analysis. Depending on the primary purpose for the PDO generation, the amount of biomass required to successfully characterize can also vary. For example, a PDO generated only for genetic study can be characterized at a time point with quite limited biomass. Alternatively, a PDO earmarked for pharmacotyping against a wide variety of potential therapies would require a significantly greater amount of biomass. Although in most cases portions of the expanded biomass can be sacrificed at any of the phases for limited characterization, it is important to keep in mind that reaching the expansion phase generally leads to the best results for capturing a pure epithelial population and providing continued biomass available for the propagation of the PDO culture if needed.

There are several pitfalls to keep in mind when leveraging PDOs for the use in clinical care of patients. For simplicity, these pitfalls can be divided into the phases of PDO culture growth. Most obstacles in the establishment phase are related to initial or postshipping quality of the biopsy cores or surgical specimen. These include specimens that are nonviable, infected, or comprised only of noncancerous tissues. Most pitfalls in this phase can be overcome with meticulous planning in specimen collection, the investment of a highly experienced pathologist in specimen selection for organoid growth and a commitment to optimal logistic processes. The expansion phase offers most room for study and improvement. Culture time needed for expansion varies and depends highly on the culture conditions; this includes a recognition of the effect of the media and the identification of appropriate supplemental factors to support PDAC growth, minimize the growth of normal ductal cells, and preserve clonal heterogeneity where appropriate in culture.

## How are pancreatic ductal adenocarcinoma organoids used currently in research?

Organoids are widely used in PDAC research for their capability to form, maintain, and expand a living biobank of patient-specific tumors for continuing experiments, technical repetition, and validation work. In general, PDOs are collected, maintained, and cryopreserved to generate large repositories of a wide variety of tumor examples in a singular living biobank. These are accumulated with an eye toward representation across a spectrum of disease subtypes and heterogeneity to facilitate downstream research and drug discovery or validation.

PDOs can be used for studying the genomic hallmarks that lead to tumor development and evolution in PDAC carcinogenesis. The consequences of specific individual mutations on tumor development and behavior can be explored, recorded, and altered, both in the primary culture as well as after transplantation [36]. Manipulation can also take place by microorganism injections, or as co-culture of a microorganism and PDAC PDO, to study the effects of microbiota on tumor cells phenotype, metabolism, and microenvironmental crosstalk.

One area of increasing interest involves the rapid establishment and characterization of PDOs for patient-specific drug sensitivity testing. In this manner, clinician scientists aim to demonstrate a correlation between the in vitro patient-specific assay and clinical response to chemotherapy. Methods in using PDO models to study pharmacologic sciences may be divided into 3 approaches: (1) drug discovery and efficacy screening; (2) rational study of the mechanisms of drug synergy, antagonism, and combination; and (3) drug delivery and administration strategy research. In classical pharmacotyping for compound efficacy testing, organoids are dissociated into single cells and plated on a multiwell (eg, 384-well) assay plate in 10% Matrigel. After a 48-hour recovery period, chemotherapeutics are administered using a semiautomated dispenser platform (online Video 1). Chemotherapeutics are tested across a logarithmically designed and clinically relevant dose range to explore drug response for each PDO. Methods to explore chemotherapeutic combinations can include either simplistic fixed ratios or similar designed ranges of multiple agents to detect synergy or antagonism. The readouts can be constructed to basic dose response as sigmoid curves, or illustrate the combinations in 2D combination index matrices, or even 3D surface plots indicating the most optimal dose-response ranges to find synergistic regimens in vitro (online Video 2) [37]. Individualized PDO profiles can be viewed in the context of a broader population distribution, generated from existing biobank studies, to subgroup patients into likely-resistant, intermediate, or sensitive tumors (Fig. 2) [24]. Another novel method of drug discovery recently being explored leverages microfluidic platforms to control flow, concentration, and duration of exposure of therapeutic agents through bioengineered channels lined with PDOs. This technology aims to mimic clinical therapeutic delivery with temporal variation, the adaptation of combination chemotherapeutics through parallel channels, and the capacity to expose the culture to other stressors of the tumor microenvironment (ie, hypoxia or hypoglycemia). Using these culture-based technologies, the PDOs can be viewed and recorded in real time with live-cell imaging to document apoptosis without compromising biomass collection for downstream studies in medium-to-high throughput [38].

PDOs can be manipulated by gene editing techniques to discover key molecular nodes that control therapeutic sensitivity and explore engineered vulnerabilities for novel or existing therapies. Deconstructing the carcinogenic process into single genetic elements by engineering cancer genes in untransformed human organoids is a powerful approach for investigating how individual genetic aberrations contribute to cancer phenotypes [27]. In organoid technology, the genetic and epigenetic features of tissues are preserved during initial passages, and with co-culture techniques, even mechanisms that facilitate interactions in the tumor microenvironment can be mimicked [19]. Research investigating the use of PDOs in co-culture together with the other components of tumor microenvironment for in vitro testing of oncoimmunotherapeutic agents is ongoing. PDO models can also be used to study the spatial interactions that occur as

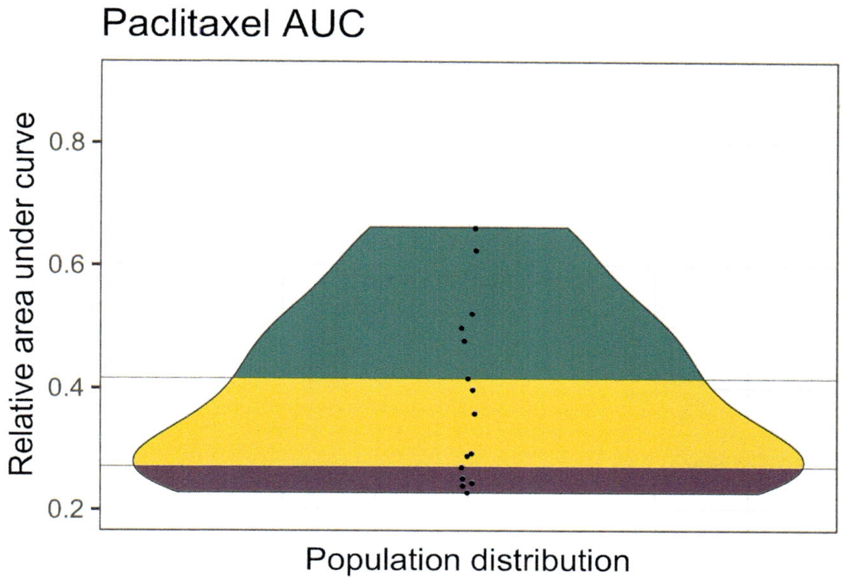


**Fig. 2.** Organoids show a variable population distribution of sensitivity to standard-of-care chemotherapeutics.

tumor cells approximate other components of the tumor microenvironment in real time using labeled live-cell imaging technologies.

Another potential indication for PDO use is to leverage them as a transitional step over 1 to 2 passages to rapidly expand the ductal component of the PDAC to increase the originally low epithelium-stromal ratio and overcome the paucicellular limitations posed in current CLIA-certified pipelines. This will enable the utilization of novel translational tools with increasingly more pure tumor material, for example, single cell transcriptomics, proteomics, secretomics, and whole-genome sequencing.

## Proposed frameworks of care

A clinical framework, in which PDOs are efficiently generated from surgical specimens or endoscopic biopsies and characterized by pharmacotyping, can be established at academic medical centers with integrated research facilities with appropriate CLIA approval [24]. In generating PDOs and expanding the malignant biomass available for study, the integration of additional techniques for molecular characterization becomes more straightforward. This clinical practice integration may rationally follow diagnostic EUS with core biopsies, surgical resection of the primary tumor, and even biopsy or excision of metastases. Strategies for potential molecular characterization in PDAC could include molecular RNA subtyping, therapeutic target identification to enable precision stratification into targeted clinical trials and novel treatment strategies, patient-specific responses to conventional cytotoxic agents for therapeutic selection, and even patient-specific drug discovery (Fig. 3). Advantages to these precision approaches include reduced morbidity from ineffective treatments and a reduced need to allow patients to fail or relapse before entertaining new therapeutic approaches. In selected cases, especially after good response to neoadjuvant therapy, PDOs could be used to improve the diagnostic sensitivity of standard somatic tumor testing by next-generation panel sequencing and molecular methods targeting microsatellite instability assessment.

## Barriers to clinical implementation today and strategies for the future

There are factors, both regulatory and biologic, that currently limit the clinical use of PDOs. From a regulatory standpoint, the utilization of cancer tumor models in direct study for clinical feedback is an emerging area with many unknown factors. Unlike the ubiquity of clinical testing with bacterial culture methods, there remains uncertainty regarding the rigor and broad reproducibility of malignant tissue culture in laboratory environments. Further, the capacity of an in vitro model to be reliably interpreted as a direct and clinically accurate model of the original tumor has yet to be definitively tested. With this in mind, prospective clinical data validation of PDO pharmacotyping and in vivo outcomes of the patient are needed to definitively justify clinical decisions being made in response to in vitro data. Most data currently available are retrospective and may be subject to bias in interpretation [39,40]. Data are expected soon in this regard, as prospective studies are ongoing as an integrated translational research component of a multicenter randomized clinical trial (NCT03563248). The impact of technical standards on molecular data obtained during PDO has also yet to be fully characterized. There are multiple options as a base for the 3D culture matrix, intervals between culture passage

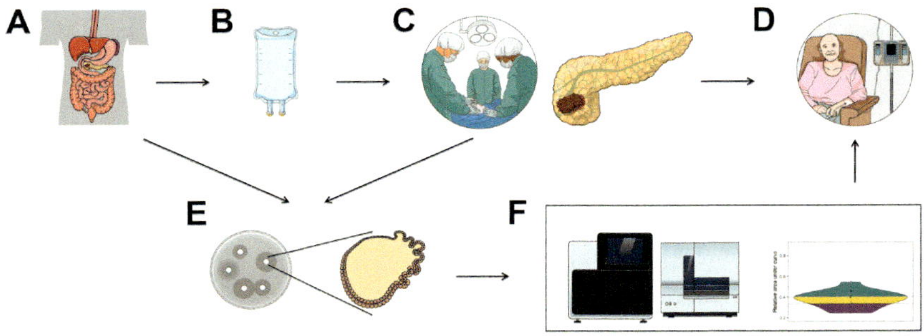


**Fig. 3.** Frameworks of care. (*A*) A core needle biopsy is acquired guided by endoscopic ultrasound. (*B*) Patient undergoes neoadjuvant or induction chemotherapy for locally advanced PDAC before (*C*) surgical resection of the primary tumor. (*D*) PDOs are established and expanded from the pretreatment or posttreatment specimen or both. (*E*) Characterization of the organoids can be performed by histopathological and molecular methods. Drug discovery, sensitivity, and resistance studies can be performed on time before the patient enters (*F*) adjuvant chemotherapy that can be advised by the results for dose and regimen selection.

or manipulation, media supplementation, and the possible selection bias over the medium and long term for highly tumorigenic subclones. Thirdly, although most robust research platforms can facilitate a highly efficient primary tumor culture, the co-culture platforms are still being developed; this clearly limits the adaptation of this technology in work exploring agents targeting the tumor microenvironment such as fibroblast targeting agents and immunotherapeutics. Lastly, organoid culture platforms are still limited by the price and complexity of media creation protocols relying on conditioned media protocols and recombinant protein technologies. Large institutions with vast clinical and academic resources can be equipped with organoid core facilities that obtain suitable experience and volumes in practical handling of the fresh tumor tissue sample and logistics and greatly benefit from synergistic efforts and co-operation.

## SUMMARY

PDOs provide a promising tool for individual diagnostics, discovery of unique tumor vulnerabilities, and therapeutic response prediction. PDOs recapitulate the genomic and transcriptomic properties of the primary tumor and may facilitate the characterization of tumor-specific host immune responses as clarified in future research endeavors.

## CLINICS CARE POINTS

- Organoids are increasingly being used in translational research in wide-ranging work spanning from basic science laboratories to those with an eye toward adaptation to clinical decision-making.
- The first CLIA-certified assays are being developed through both academic and commercial pipelines for trials of individual drug screening and sensitivity testing for several solid tumors, including PDAC.
- The greatest area of anticipated clinical impact is in defining the genetic makeup of these otherwise paucicellular tumors and in identifying individualized therapeutics with maximized therapeutic windows.

## DISCLOSURE

Toni T. Seppälä: CEO and co-owner of Healthfund Finland.

Richard A. Burkhart: Nothing to disclose.

## SUPPLEMENTARY MATERIAL

Supplementary data to this article can be found online at https://doi.org/10.1016/j.yasu.2021.05.015.

## References

[1] Oettle H, Post S, Neuhaus P, et al. Adjuvant chemotherapy with gemcitabine vs observation in patients undergoing curative-intent resection of pancreatic cancer: a randomized controlled trial. JAMA 2007;297(3):267–77.

[2] Sinn M, Striefler JK, Sinn BV, et al. Does long-term survival in patients with pancreatic cancer really exist? Results from the CONKO-001 study. J Surg Oncol 2013;108(6):398–402.
[3] Von Hoff DD, Ervin T, Arena FP, et al. Increased survival in pancreatic cancer with nab-paclitaxel plus gemcitabine. N Engl J Med 2013;369(18):1691–703.
[4] Neoptolemos JP, Palmer DH, Ghaneh P, et al. Comparison of adjuvant gemcitabine and capecitabine with gemcitabine monotherapy in patients with resected pancreatic cancer (ESPAC-4): a multicentre, open-label, randomised, phase 3 trial. Lancet 2017;389(10073):1011–24.
[5] Conroy T, Hammel P, Hebbar M, et al. FOLFIRINOX or gemcitabine as adjuvant therapy for pancreatic cancer. N Engl J Med 2018;379(25):2395–406.
[6] Conroy T, Desseigne F, Ychou M, et al. FOLFIRINOX versus gemcitabine for metastatic pancreatic cancer. N Engl J Med 2011;364(19):1817–25.
[7] Kasumova GG, Conway WC, Tseng JF. The role of venous and arterial resection in pancreatic cancer surgery. Ann Surg Oncol 2018;25(1):51–8.
[8] Giuliani T, López Rubio M, Montalvá Oron E, et al. Extended distal pancreatectomy with thoracic wall resection after neoadjuvant FOLFIRINOX: is there a limit of resection for pancreatic cancer after downstaging? Ann Hepatobiliary Pancreat Surg 2020;24(1):90.
[9] Sakaguchi T, Valente R, Tanaka K, et al. Surgical treatment of metastatic pancreatic ductal adenocarcinoma: a review of current literature. Pancreatology 2019;19(5):672–80.
[10] Golan T, Hammel P, Reni M, et al. Maintenance olaparib for germline BRCA-mutated metastatic pancreatic cancer. N Engl J Med 2019;381(4):317–27.
[11] Le DT, Uram JN, Wang H, et al. PD-1 blockade in tumors with mismatch-repair deficiency. N Engl J Med 2015;372(26):2509–20.
[12] Pishvaian MJ, Bender RJ, Halverson D, et al. Molecular profiling of patients with pancreatic cancer: initial results from the know your tumor initiative. Clin Cancer Res 2018;24(20):5018–27.
[13] Pishvaian MJ, Blais EM, Brody JR, et al. Overall survival in patients with pancreatic cancer receiving matched therapies following molecular profiling: a retrospective analysis of the know your tumor registry trial. Lancet Oncol 2020;21(4):508–18.
[14] Von Hoff DD, Stephenson JJ, Rosen P, et al. Pilot study using molecular profiling of patients' tumors to find potential targets and select treatments for their refractory cancers. J Clin Oncol 2010;28(33):4877–83.
[15] Collisson EA, Sadanandam A, Olson P, et al. Subtypes of pancreatic ductal adenocarcinoma and their differing responses to therapy. Nat Med 2011;17(4):500–3.
[16] Moffitt RA, Marayati R, Flate EL, et al. Virtual microdissection identifies distinct tumor- and stroma-specific subtypes of pancreatic ductal adenocarcinoma. Nat Genet 2015;47(10):1168–78.
[17] Bailey P, Chang DK, Nones K, et al. Genomic analyses identify molecular subtypes of pancreatic cancer. Nature 2016;531(7592):47–52.
[18] Mizrahi JD, Surana R, Valle JW, et al. Pancreatic cancer. Lancet 2020;395(10242):2008–20.
[19] Tuveson D, Clevers H. Cancer modeling meets human organoid technology. Science 2019;364(6444):952–5.
[20] Bleijs M, Wetering M, Clevers H, et al. Xenograft and organoid model systems in cancer research. EMBO J 2019;38(15):1–11.
[21] Neal JT, Li X, Zhu J, et al. Organoid modeling of the tumor immune microenvironment. Cell 2018;175(7):1972–88.e16.
[22] Knudsen ES, Balaji U, Mannakee B, et al. Pancreatic cancer cell lines as patient-derived avatars: genetic characterisation and functional utility. Gut 2018;67(3):508–20.
[23] Driehuis E, Van Hoeck A, Moore K, et al. Pancreatic cancer organoids recapitulate disease and allow personalized drug screening. Proc Natl Acad Sci U S A 2019;116(52):26580–90.

[24] Seppälä TT, Zimmerman JW, Sereni E, et al. Patient-derived organoid pharmacotyping is a clinically tractable strategy for precision medicine in pancreatic cancer. Ann Surg 2020;272(3):427–35.
[25] Roerink SF, Sasaki N, Lee-Six H, et al. Intra-tumour diversification in colorectal cancer at the single-cell level. Nature 2018;556(7702):437–62.
[26] Chen KY, Srinivasan T, Lin C, et al. Single-cell transcriptomics reveals heterogeneity and drug response of human colorectal cancer organoids. Proc Annu Int Conf IEEE Eng Med Biol Soc EMBS 2018;2018:2378–81.
[27] Fujii M, Clevers H, Sato T. Modeling human digestive diseases with CRISPR-Cas9–modified organoids. Gastroenterology 2019;156(3):562–76.
[28] Li X, Francies HE, Secrier M, et al. Organoid cultures recapitulate esophageal adenocarcinoma heterogeneity providing a model for clonality studies and precision therapeutics. Nat Commun 2018;9(1):1–13.
[29] Fujii M, Shimokawa M, Date S, et al. A colorectal tumor organoid library demonstrates progressive loss of niche factor requirements during tumorigenesis. Cell Stem Cell 2016;18(6): 827–38.
[30] Yan HHN, Siu HC, Ho SL, et al. Organoid cultures of early-onset colorectal cancers reveal distinct and rare genetic profiles. Gut 2020;69(12):2165–79.
[31] Juiz N, Elkaoutari A, Bigonnet M, et al. Basal-like and classical cells coexistence in pancreatic cancer revealed by single cell analysis. bioRxiv 2020; https://doi.org/10.1101/2020.01.07.897454.
[32] Juiz N, Elkaoutari A, Bigonnet M, et al. Basal-like and classical cells coexist in pancreatic cancer revealed by single-cell analysis on biopsy-derived pancreatic cancer organoids from the classical subtype. FASEB J 2020;34(9):12214–28.
[33] Krieger T, LeBlanc-Soto S, Jabs J, et al. Single-cell analysis of patient-derived PDAC organoids reveals cell state heterogeneity and a conserved developmental hierarchy. Christian Conrad bioRxiv 2020.
[34] Hidalgo M, Bruckheimer E, Rajeshkumar NV, et al. A pilot clinical study of treatment guided by personalized tumorgrafts in patients with advanced cancer. Mol Cancer Ther 2011;10(8):1311–6.
[35] Tiriac H, Bucobo JC, Tzimas D, et al. Successful creation of pancreatic cancer organoids by means of EUS-guided fine-needle biopsy sampling for personalized cancer treatment. Gastrointest Endosc 2018;87(6):1474–80.
[36] Lau HCH, Kranenburg O, Xiao H, et al. Organoid models of gastrointestinal cancers in basic and translational research. Nat Rev Gastroenterol Hepatol 2020;17(4):203–22.
[37] Ianevski A, Giri AK, Aittokallio T. SynergyFinder 2.0: visual analytics of multi-drug combination synergies. Nucleic Acids Res 2020;48(W1):W488–93.
[38] Schuster B, Junkin M, Kashaf SS, et al. Automated microfluidic platform for dynamic and combinatorial drug screening of tumor organoids. Nat Commun 2020;11(1):1–12.
[39] Tiriac H, Belleau P, Engle DD, et al. Organoid profiling identifies common responders to chemotherapy in pancreatic cancer. Cancer Discov 2018;8(9):1112–29.
[40] Aberle MR, Burkhart RA, Tiriac H, et al. Patient-derived organoid models help define personalized management of gastrointestinal cancer. Br J Surg 2018;105(2):e48–60.

Advances in Surgery 55 (2021) 231–250

ADVANCES IN SURGERY

# Necrosectomy in the Management of Necrotizing Pancreatitis

Amy Y. Li, MD[a], John R. Bergquist, MD, MS[a], Brendan C. Visser, MD[b,*]

[a]Department of Surgery, Section of Surgical Oncology, Stanford University School of Medicine, 300 Pasteur Drive, Room H3591, Stanford, CA 94305, USA; [b]Department of Surgery, Section of Surgical Oncology, Stanford University School of Medicine, 300 Pasteur Drive, H3680, Stanford, CA 94305-5655, USA

**Keywords**

• Necrotizing pancreatitis • Walled-off pancreatic necrosis
• Pancreatic debridement • Necrosectomy • Step-up approach
• Video assisted retroperitoneal debridement (VARD)
• Minimally invasive retroperitoneal pancreatectomy (MIRP)
• Transgastric necrosectomy (TGN)

**Key points**

- Percutaneous or endoscopic drainage can be performed to bridge critically ill patients to definitive debridement (surgical and endoscopic step-up approaches).
- Anatomic location of walled-off pancreatic necrosis can dictate treatment:
  - Retrogastric collections are amenable to transgastric interventions (endoscopic or surgical drainage/debridement).
  - Collections located in the paracolic gutter are appropriate for retroperitoneal percutaneous drainage and/or debridement.
- Surgical transgastric necrosectomy is an effective single-stage debridement procedure, with creation of a large cystgastrostomy that allows ongoing internal auto-debridement.

Disclosures
The authors have no financial disclosures or conflicts of interest to disclose.
Financial support: None.

*Correspondence to: Associate Professor of Surgery, Department of Surgery, Section of Surgical Oncology, Stanford University School of Medicine, 300 Pasteur Dr., H3680, Stanford, CA 94305-5655. *E-mail address:* bvisser@stanford.edu

https://doi.org/10.1016/j.yasu.2021.05.016
0065-3411/21/

**Video content accompanies this article at http://www.advancessurgery.com.**

## INTRODUCTION

Necrotizing pancreatitis and walled-off pancreatic necrosis (WOPN) is a devastating condition, occurring in approximately 20% of patients diagnosed with pancreatitis [1–3]. Infected necrosis confers an associated mortality reported as high as 30% to 40% [1,2]. Management of this disease process has evolved substantially over the past three decades, and multidisciplinary decision-making for WOPN is an essential element in the modern care of pancreatitis [1].

Owing to varying patterns of disease, there is no single ideal approach for management of WOPN. Instead, interventions are tailored individually to each patient based on clinical status, anatomy, and nature of WOPN contents [2,4,5]. The purpose of this review is to provide an overview on the evolution of surgical debridement as well as the latest practices and techniques for the management of pancreatic necrosis.

## BACKGROUND AND DEFINITIONS

Necrotizing pancreatitis is a disease spectrum with respect to the maturity, quality, and sterility of any given collection [6,7]. These characteristics vary from patient to patient in the development of WOPN, necessitating a variable approach to management. It is critical that the vocabulary used to describe necrotizing pancreatitis be precisely defined because the terminology impacts clinical data interpretation and, therefore, management. If a collection is erroneously labeled a "pseudocyst" on an imaging report but is in fact semi-solid necrosis, this error may have substantial clinical significance.

The most recent revision of the Atlanta classification for acute pancreatitis defines four major categories of acute pancreatitis based on clinical symptoms, severity, and radiographic findings [6] (Fig. 1). *Acute peripancreatic fluid collection* is defined as peripancreatic fluid present in the early stage of acute (<4 weeks) interstitial edematous pancreatitis, without evidence of necrosis, pseudocyst, or pancreatic extension. This peripancreatic fluid is described as homogenous fluid density without a defined wall on computed tomography (CT) imaging. When the peripancreatic fluid collection persists beyond 4 weeks and develops a well-defined mature wall, the well-circumscribed homogenous fluid collection is now called a pancreatic pseudocyst. These collections are predominantly comprised of fluid, without a solid component and associated with minimal necrosis [6].

A heterogenous collection of fluid and solid pancreatic and/or peripancreatic necrosis is an *acute necrotic collection*. These collections develop early (<4 weeks) in the course of necrotizing pancreatitis and have not yet matured a well-defined wall. The major distinction between acute peripancreatic fluid collection and acute necrotic collection is the presence of pancreatic and/or

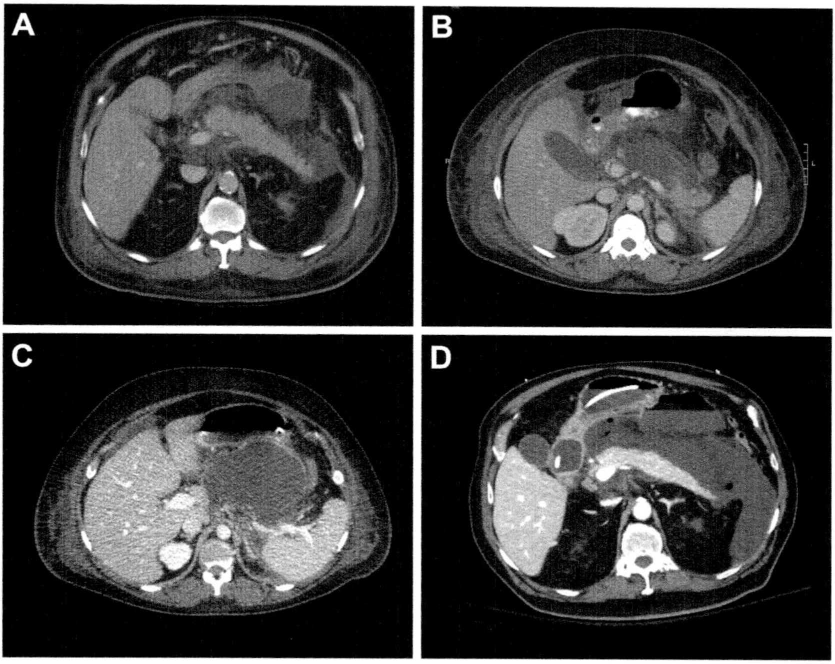


**Fig. 1.** Stages of necrotizing pancreatitis. Computed tomography (CT) imaging depicting the stages of necrotizing pancreatitis. (*A*) Acute pancreatitis with *peripancreatic fluid collection*; (*B*) necrotizing pancreatitis with an *acute necrotic collection* and a viable pancreatic tail; (*C*) necrotizing pancreatitis with *walled-off necrosis* abutting the posterior wall of the stomach; (*D*) necrotizing pancreatitis with gas bubbles throughout the collection, indicative of *infected necrosis*.

peripancreatic necrosis that is absent in the former [6]. An acute necrotic collection that persists beyond 4 weeks develops into *walled-off necrosis*, after maturation of a well-defined enhancing wall that encapsulates the pancreatic and/or peripancreatic necrosis. The presence of gas within necrotizing pancreatitis on imaging or clinical deterioration can be used to diagnose *infected necrosis* [6]. While CT is widely used in the diagnosis, staging and treatment of necrotizing pancreatitis, MRI is superior in evaluating walled-off necrosis for the quantity for solid debris versus liquid contents as well as pancreatic duct integrity [4,8–11] (Fig. 2). Because of MRI's advantage in detecting solid debris, unstable anatomy, and extent of pancreatic necrosis over CT imaging, MRI is a tool that can aid in directing treatment toward debridement over percutaneous drainage for a collection with solid necrosis [10,11].

## INDICATIONS AND TIMING FOR NECROSECTOMY

Confirmed infected pancreatic necrosis usually requires intervention, in the form of drainage and/or pancreatic debridement [1,4,5]. Necrosectomy is

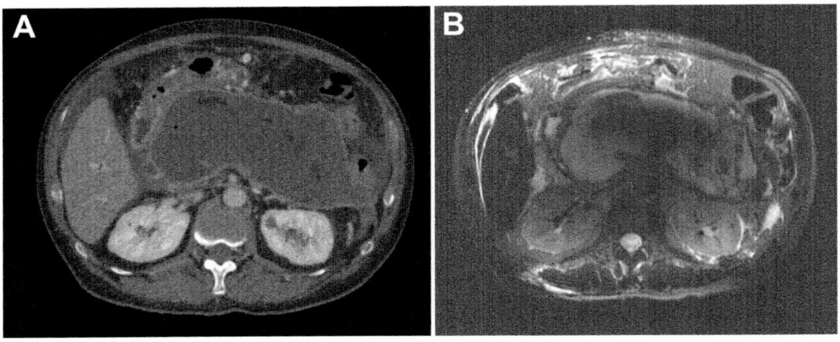


**Fig. 2.** Necrotizing pancreatitis CT versus MRI. Comparison of (*A*) computed tomography imaging, in contrast to (*B*) MRI. The MRI T2 weighted phase is the best modality for visualizing the heterogeneity of solid debris and liquid necrosis present in walled-off pancreatic necrosis.

recommended for cases with clinical suspicion of infected necrosis as well as necrotizing pancreatitis with deteriorating or persistent organ failure in the absence confirmed infection [1,4,12]. Routine fine needle aspiration is rarely required for diagnosis of infected necrosis, as clinical symptoms of deterioration or persistent sepsis and radiologic findings are generally adequate [1,4,5,12–14].

Additional indications for necrosectomy include:

- "Persistent unwellness," a constellation of symptoms first described by Andrew Warshaw [15], consisting of persistent pain, inability to tolerate diet resulting in weight loss/nutritional failure, and/or low-grade systemic illness [1,4,5].
- Unstable anatomy (disconnected duct syndrome), a phenomenon that manifests when necrosis occurs in the pancreatic neck or body, disrupting the pancreatic duct. This results in complete transection and discontinuity of the pancreatic duct, with a persistent pancreatic fistula at the pancreatic remnant [1,4,5,16].
- In rare cases, WOPN (infected or sterile) may be associated with abdominal compartment syndrome, acute bleeding, bowel ischemia, and obstructive symptoms due to mass effect, requiring urgent or emergent intervention [1,4].

A small number of patients will have limited infected necrosis that is not anatomically accessible through percutaneous, endoscopic or surgical means for drainage and/or debridement. In these cases, antibiotics alone may be adequate in management of infected WOPN in clinically stable patients [1,12,17–20]. This typically requires a prolonged recovery period with long duration of antibiotic therapy. The mean duration of antibiotics ranges from 27 to 56 days across multiple retrospective studies [19,20]. In addition, intervention is not required for asymptomatic WOPN, as these collections will typically resolve without intervention. Prior studies have noted that 45% to 70% of patients will remain asymptomatic, and complete regression can be expected in 30% to 68% after a mean period of 6 months [21–23].

There is consensus that intervention should be delayed until approximately 4 weeks after the onset of pancreatitis whenever possible [1,4,5,12]. This allows for liquification of the necrotic collection and development of a mature wall [6,24]. Occasionally, intervention may be necessary within 4 weeks, such as the emergency scenarios outlined previously or early infected necrosis with clinical deterioration despite optimized medical therapy. Early intervention is associated with worse clinical outcomes, specifically for open necrosectomy [1,5,25–27]. However, earlier intervention by percutaneous or endoscopic means may be acceptable source control [28], and there is currently a prospective trial evaluating early drainage of WOPN [29].

The Dutch Pancreatitis Study Group is currently conducting the POINTER trial to better define the ideal timing of intervention by randomizing patients to immediate (early) versus delayed percutaneous drainage of necrotizing pancreatitis [29]. The authors recruited 104 patients (55 immediate, 49 delayed drainage). There was approximately 1-day delay between randomization and drainage in the immediate drainage arm, as opposed 9 days in the delayed drainage cohort. Preliminary results noted no significant difference in new-onset organ failure, morbidity, and mortality between the two cohorts. However, 39% of patients in the postponed cohort did not require any drainage intervention, and patients who underwent immediate drainage required an increased number of interventions [30]. This study supports the notion that delayed intervention is preferred, but if early intervention is absolutely necessary, drainage is feasible.

## APPROACHES TO NECROSECTOMY

While open necrosectomy has traditionally been considered the "gold standard," the approach to interventional management of WOPN has evolved

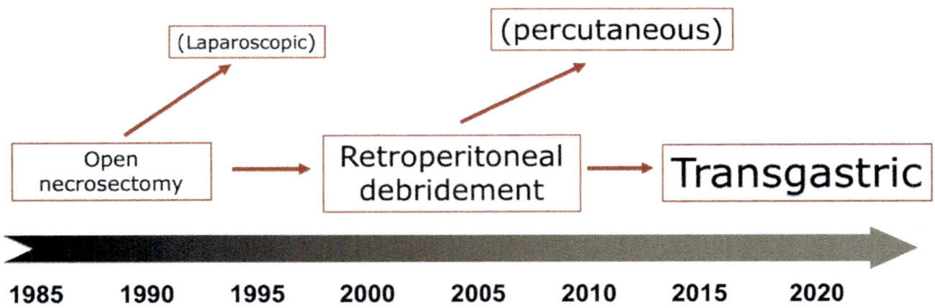


**Fig. 3.** Timeline and evolution of necrosectomy. Open necrosectomy was the traditional gold standard for debridement of walled-off pancreatic necrosis. Laparoscopic debridement was explored as an alternative technique that resulted in less surgical trauma, but this technique was limited. Attention turned to retroperitoneal debridement, combining percutaneous drainage and surgical debridement into the step-up approach for retroperitoneal collections. The transgastric approach, surgical debridement in particular, gained recognition as a single-stage procedure for retrogastric collections and circumvents the need for percutaneous drains.

**Box 1: Anatomic considerations**

Location of pancreatic necrosis is a key factor in guiding management:

- Collections involving the pancreatic tail that extend into the paracolic gutter would most benefit from retroperitoneal approach, with percutaneous drainage, followed by minimally invasive retroperitoneal pancreatic debridement (MIRP) or video-assisted retroperitoneal debridement (VARD) if necessary.
- Collections contained within the lesser sac that interface with the posterior gastric wall can be approached in a transgastric fashion – either open, laparoscopic or endoscopic.
- Collections isolated to the root of the mesentery may not be accessible percutaneously and instead, may require traditional open necrosectomy or laparoscopic transperitoneal approach
- Patients with limited collections should be considered for antibiotics alone. While this commits the patient to a prolonged course of antibiotics, this would potentially avoid the high risk of morbidity associated with formal necrosectomy.
- Patients with isolated tail remnants are best managed by surgical as opposed to endoscopic methods.

considerably over time [12] (Fig. 3). Percutaneous, endoscopic, and laparoscopic approaches have been explored as minimally invasive options with the objective of reducing morbidity and mortality associated with open necrosectomy [1,4,5]. Owing to the heterogeneity of the disease process, there is no "one-size fits all" treatment. Treatment should be tailored toward each individual patient, based on clinical status, anatomic location (Box 1), as well as quality (solid vs liquid) of pancreatic necrosum [2,4,5] (Fig. 4). The remainder of this review will focus on the approaches and evolution of necrosectomy for walled-off pancreatic necrosis.

## Open necrosectomy

A variety of open necrosectomy techniques have been described, usually including repeated trips to the operating room and complex irrigation/drainage systems [31–33]. However, these approaches were associated with significant physiologic stress and subsequent morbidity including pancreatic insufficiency, pancreatic fistula, and incisional hernia [1,34–36]. Historically, the rate of morbidity after open necrosectomy approached 60% to 90%, while mortality has previously ranged from 25% to 60% [25,35–38]. Modern series have demonstrated improvement in mortality, now ranging from 4% to 18% [36,39,40]. A large contemporary series from University of Indiana reported outcomes of 116 patients who underwent open necrosectomy between 2006 and 2018, including 74% open debridement and 26% open transgastric necrosectomy. Morbidity ranged from 48% to 88% (for elective and urgent/emergent cases, respectively), and mortality was approximately 2%. The authors

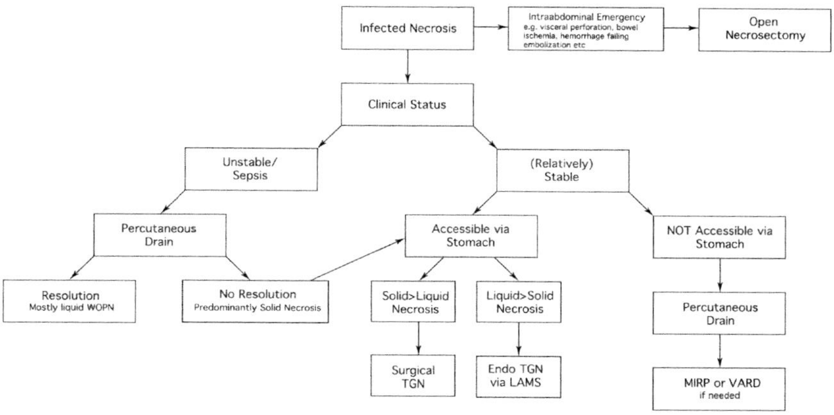


**Fig. 4.** Algorithm of Treatment Management for Walled-off Pancreatic Necrosis. Management is tailored individually to each patient based on clinical status, anatomic location of necrosis (accessible via the stomach or not), the maturity of the necrosis, quality of contents (from largely liquid to largely solid) and the state of infection (from sterile to profound sepsis). *Abbreviations:* LAMS, lumen-apposing metal stent; MIRP, minimally invasive retroperitoneal pancreatectomy; TGN, transgastric necrosectomy; VARD, video-assisted retroperitoneal debridement.

cited better understanding of the disease process and improvements in critical care of severe disease leading to decreased mortality [36].

With technological advances in laparoscopic and endoscopic techniques, open debridement has faded into the background. While minimally invasive techniques have largely replaced open surgery, there remain instances where open surgery is unavoidable. Laparotomy may be required in cases of associated intraabdominal emergencies, such as abdominal compartment syndrome, perforation of a visceral organ, and hemorrhage that cannot be controlled with angiography [24]. In addition, there is a small subset of patients who fail minimally invasive management and thus require a "salvage" open debridement for ongoing organ failure and infection [36].

## Laparoscopic necrosectomy

It has been established that less invasive approaches result in less profound inflammatory response and decreased physiologic stress [1,5]. Laparoscopic transperitoneal debridement of WOPN was explored as a minimally invasive alternative in an effort to mitigate the postoperative morbidity and mortality associated with open necrosectomy [41]. The components of this strategy are described in the following steps [41–46]:

1. Pneumoperitoneum is established, and diagnostic laparoscopy is performed.
2. An additional 2 to 3 trocars are placed under direct vision.
3. For WOPN involving the head and/or body of the pancreas, the gastrocolic ligament is opened, and the retroperitoneum is exposed to access the necrosum.

4. For collections located in the tail of the pancreas, the mesocolon is opened at the root of the mesentery, to the left of the middle colic artery adjacent to the ligament of Treitz.
5. The necrotic collection is bluntly debrided with laparoscopic graspers or spoon forceps and the necrosum evacuated in an endoscopic specimen bag.
6. The pancreatic cavity is irrigated, and drains are left for postoperative lavage.

Retrospective cohort studies report morbidity of approximately 20% and mortality from 4% to 18% [12,42,44,45,47,48]. Among the largest series published, Tan and colleagues compared laparoscopic approach (n = 25) to a historical cohort (n = 51) and found that although operative time was significantly longer (157 min vs 127 min), there was less morbidity in the laparoscopic cohort [45]. The literature supporting this technique is limited to retrospective case series.

Laparoscopic necrosectomy is limited by several factors: the rigidity of laparoscopic instruments which is difficult working with in a cavity; the size of laparoscopic spoon forceps can make debriding solid necrosis tedious; laparoscopic suction devices are susceptible to obstruction when evacuating semi-solid and/or viscous liquid necrosis; and inability to control bleeding or hemorrhage. In addition, laparoscopic transperitoneal debridement risks potentially "un-walling off" (unroofing) the previously walled-off necrosis and an inadequate debridement would potentially disseminate the infection into the abdominal cavity [24,46]. In addition, this approach commits the patient to several weeks to months of multiple drains and irrigations, impacting patient quality of life.

This technique has largely fallen out of favor. Nonetheless, there may occasionally be a patient with infected necrosis that is not accessible via the gastric lumen or percutaneously (very centrally in the root of the mesentery) for which selecting this approach may be most appropriate [24].

### Retroperitoneal debridement

Around the same time in the 2000s, transcutaneous retroperitoneal surgical debridement was explored as an alternative minimally invasive approach. Several techniques arose from this period, which all follow similar basic

**Box 2: Surgical pearls for retroperitoneal debridement**

Principles of performing retroperitoneal debridement:

- This technique targets retroperitoneal collections involving the tail, localized in between the spleen and kidney, as well as right sided collections, located behind the pancreatic head.
- Preoperative percutaneous drain placement creates a tract that is serially dilated or upsized for surgical instruments to traverse during surgical debridement.
- Patients may require multiple trips to the operating room for repeat debridements. Drains remain in place until complete resolution (clearance) of walled-off necrosis.

principles of establishing and performing debridement through a percutaneous tract into the WOPN [12] (Box 2). These techniques vary based on entry into the retroperitoneum:

- *Minimally invasive retroperitoneal pancreatectomy* (MIRP) first involved percutaneous drain placement into the collection of pancreatic necrosis. This tract is then serially dilated under radiologic guidance—typically to 30 Fr, which allows the use of an operating nephroscope through a 30 Fr Amplatz sheath. The nephroscope contains two channels, which allows debridement with small forceps and irrigation [24,49–51] (Fig. 5). However, debridement is slow because of the size limitations imposed by the nephroscopic instruments and the sheath. For very large collections, we use a two-trocar technique. This requires two percutaneous drains placed under radiographic guidance with insertion sites separated by approximately 3 to 4 cm. One drain is dilated to 30 Fr to allow the use of a nephroscope, similar to MIRP, while a wire is placed through the other. Using fluoroscopy and water irrigation via the nephroscope, a tract is created connecting to the wire. Under direct vision of the nephroscope, the drains are replaced with Versastep (Medtronic) trocars along the wire to ensure trocar placement into the collection. The nephroscope is then switched out for a laparoscope, the cavity is insufflated with carbon dioxide, and debridement can proceed more efficiently with 10-mm laparoscopic stone forceps [24,52,53].
- *Video-assisted retroperitoneal debridement* (VARD) similarly requires percutaneous drain placement that is upsized to 18 Fr. A 3- to 5-cm flank incision is created over the drain insertion site, and the drain tract is followed into the walled-off necrosis, guided by a laparoscope. Renal vein retractors can be used for exposure. Debridement is performed using ring forceps and suction [54,55].

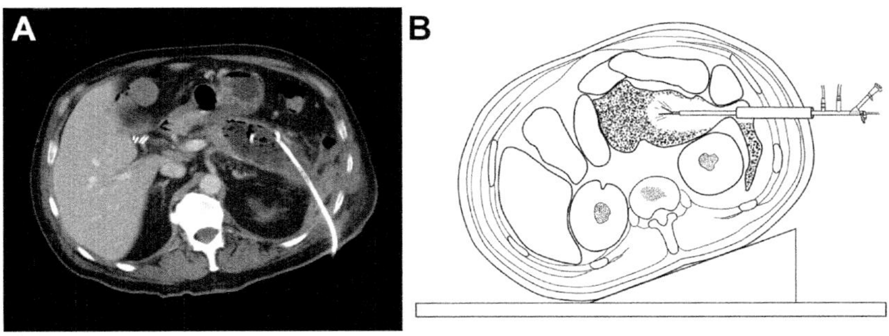


**Fig. 5.** Minimally invasive retroperitoneal pancreatectomy. (*A*) Computed tomographic axial imaging of walled-off pancreatic collection that does not have any contact with the stomach. There is a percutaneous drain entering the collection from the retroperitoneum. (*B*) During a minimally invasive retroperitoneal pancreatic necrosectomy (MIRP), the drain is replaced with a sheath, through which a nephroscope with two working channels (light source and forceps) can be placed for debridement.

These techniques generally require multiple trips to the operating room for repeat debridement, with several cohort studies reporting an average of 3 interventions. In addition, these studies found that retroperitoneal debridement seemingly resulted in decreased morbidity (10%–20%) and mortality (0%–20%, and even as high as 40% in one series) compared with historic series of open debridement [35,49,54,56–59].

In 2010, the Dutch Pancreatitis Study Group published the landmark PANTER study comparing their "Step-Up" approach (percutaneous drainage, followed by VARD as necessary) versus open necrosectomy. In this trial, 378 patients were enrolled, and 88 underwent randomization, of which 45 patients underwent primary open necrosectomy, while 43 patients were treated with the step-up approach. While neither mortality nor length of stay differed between groups, morbidity was reduced in the step-up arm, specifically incisional hernia and new-onset diabetes. Notably, 35% of patients who underwent initial percutaneous drainage improved without requiring any surgical intervention.

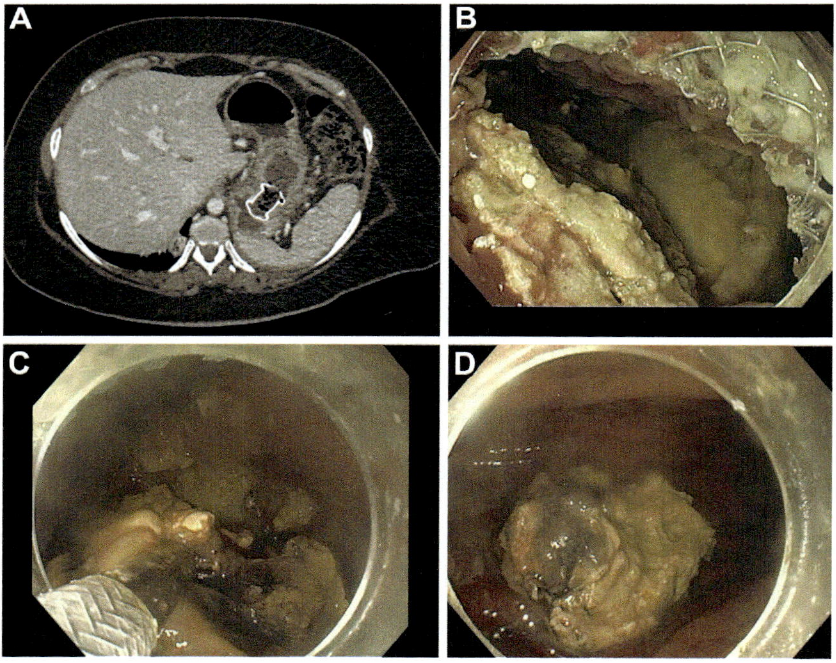


**Fig. 6.** Endoscopic transgastric necrosectomy. (*A*) Computed tomographic imaging of an AXIOS (Boston Scientific) lumen-apposing metal stent (LAMS) placed transmurally across the posterior gastric wall into the walled-off pancreatic necrosis. (*B*) Endoscopic view of the walled-off pancreatic necrosis through the LAMS. (*C,D*) Debridement of the white necrotic pancreatic tissue and evacuation of purulence is performed through the stent.

Overall, given the reduced morbidity of the step-up approach, this strategy was considered to be superior to traditional open necrosectomy [54].

### Endoscopic transgastric drainage and necrosectomy

Shortly thereafter, endoscopic (transluminal) drainage gained recognition as an alternative minimally invasive nonsurgical approach for retrogastric WOPN. This technique entails endoscopic access to the stomach and transmural intervention into the necrotic collection through the posterior stomach or duodenal wall (under ultrasound assistance) [12,24]. The tract is dilated so pigtail drains or lumen-apposing metal stents (LAMS) can be placed to create a cystgastrostomy [60,61] (Fig. 6). Through this channel, debridement and lavage can be carried out with a variety of endoscopic instruments, such as forceps, balloons, baskets, irrigation, and suction catheters [12,24].

Then, the Dutch Pancreatitis Study Group evaluated an endoscopic step-up approach (initial endoscopic catheter drainage with two 7 Fr pigtail stents and one nasocystic drain, followed by endoscopic transluminal necrosectomy if no clinical improvement) head-to-head with the surgical step-up approach (percutaneous drainage, followed by VARD, if necessary) in the TENSION trial. Of the 418 patients screened, 98 patients were enrolled into the study, of which 47 were assigned to the previously established step-up arm, and the remaining 51 patients were randomized to the endoscopic step-up approach. Only 1 of 4 patients screened were enrolled, indicating that this is a highly selected group of patients with WOPN that was anatomically feasible for both endoscopic and retroperitoneal approaches [55].

The authors found no difference in major morbidity, mortality, or number of interventions. However, there was a lower rate of pancreatic fistula and shorter postoperative hospital stay (by 16 days, 53 vs 69 days) in the endoscopic cohort. Similar to the PANTER trial, there was a subset of patients within each cohort that did not require additional necrosectomy after initial drainage (51%). This randomized controlled trial confirmed prior observational studies' findings that endoscopic transgastric drainage resulted in fewer complications (namely, pancreatic fistula) and shorter hospitalizations than surgical and step-up approaches [55].

It should be noted that pigtail drains are limited in their ability to fully drain thick, viscous fluid or solid debris, and stents are susceptible to solid debris clogging the channel lumen. However, the technology is improving. Presently, 20 mm is the largest lumen size for the current existing AXIOS (Boston Scientific) LAMS approved for endoscopic transgastric necrosectomy [62]. In addition to traditional endoscopic instruments, the EndoRotor (Interscope Medical) is a novel mechanical instrument that combines the use of a rotating cutting blade and suction for tissue dissection and resection [63,64]. However, endoscopic debridement typically requires multiple sessions to achieve complete debridement if there is a significant quantity of true solid necrosis (rather than largely liquid contents with a limited solid component). While the clinical trials found a median of 3 (IQR 2–6 in both series) interventions necessary, a systematic review found an average of 4 interventions from 14 retrospective studies, which ranged from as low as 1 intervention to as high as 15 endoscopic reinterventions [65]. It should be noted that patients who undergo endoscopic LAMS placement must undergo at least one additional endoscopy for stent removal. Currently, the European Society of Gastrointestinal Endoscopy recommends LAMS retrieval within 4 weeks [14,66], but there is limited evidence on optimal timing as removal timing ranges between 1 to 20 weeks across multiple studies [66]. While endoscopic drainage is an appealing approach that allows internal debridement without requiring a drain or risk of pancreatic fistula, this technique remains limited in its ability to resolve large, solid collections and the necessity for multiple endoscopic interventions.

### Surgical transgastric necrosectomy

A solution to the limitations of endoscopic necrosectomy is surgical transgastric debridement with the creation of a larger cystgastrostomy, allowing for a more efficient debridement. Surgical transgastric necrosectomy (TGN) can be performed via laparoscopy or laparotomy, with the same fundamental principles of debridement [67–69] (Box 3).

*Open transgastric necrosectomy* is performed through a short upper midline laparotomy. Intraoperative ultrasound remains a critical component in identifying the extent of necrosis and planning gastrotomy. Anterior and posterior gastrostomies are created with electrocautery or ultrasonic shears. Debridement is performed with a combination gentle, blunt dissection, and irrigation. It is worth noting that debridement should be focused on necrosis that is loose and can be easily freed. The anterior gastrostomy is sutured closed. If indicated, a cholecystectomy can be performed before or after the debridement [67,68].

**Box 3: Surgical pearls for transgastric debridement**

Principles of performing transgastric necrosectomy:

- This technique requires a large area of contact between the collection of walled-off pancreatic necrosis and the posterior gastric wall.
- Use intraoperative ultrasound against the posterior wall of the stomach to localize the area of walled-off pancreatic necrosis. Confirmation of necrosum can be performed with needle aspiration prior to creation of cystgastrostomy.
- Cystgastrostomy can be performed with the LigaSure (Covidien) and reinforced with staples or suture, to promote hemostasis in the setting of varices as well as adherence between the stomach and walled-off pancreatic necrosis.
- Delaying transgastric debridement by approximately 4 weeks from onset of necrotizing pancreatitis will allow for development of a mature wall around the necrosum. This also promotes adherence of the necrosum to the posterior wall of the stomach and ease in creation of cystgastrostomy.
- Surgical transgastric debridement allows for single stage necrosectomy with ongoing internal drainage of remaining necrosum through wide surgical cystgastrostomy.

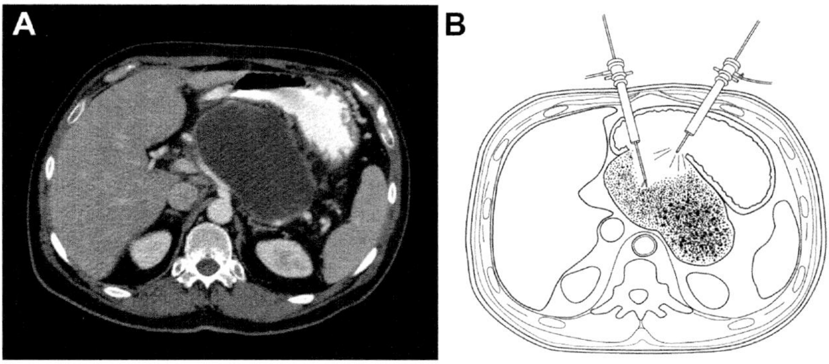


**Fig. 7.** Surgical transgastric necrosectomy. (*A*) Computed tomography axial imaging of a large retrogastric walled-off pancreatic collection with a large area of contact with the posterior gastric wall. (*B*) During laparoscopic transgastric necrosectomy, after obtaining pneumoperitoneum, the stomach is insufflated to achieve contact between the anterior stomach and abdominal wall so that radially dilating trocars can be placed directly into the stomach. A laparoscope and other instruments are used to proceed with debridement.

The "MIS" correlate, *laparoscopic transgastric necrosectomy*, is performed by the following steps [68,69] (Fig. 7, Video 1):

1. Endoscopic gastroscopy is performed first, then the abdomen is accessed laparoscopically through the umbilicus, and potential sites for transgastric trocars are identified.
2. The stomach is maximally insufflated with the endoscope, and intraabdominal insufflation is lowered to allow contact between the abdominal wall and anterior gastric wall.
3. Under direct laparoscopic and endoscopic vision, 2 to 3 Versastep (Medtronic) trocars are placed through the anterior abdominal wall and anterior gastric wall to access the gastric lumen.
4. The insufflation is transferred from the intraperitoneal trocar to an intragastric trocar. The peritoneal insufflation is released so that the stomach can be insufflated.
5. The laparoscopic ultrasound probe is used to locate the collection of pancreatic necrosis, then confirmed with laparoscopic needle aspiration.
6. A posterior gastrotomy is created with electrocautery and extended with LigaSure (Covidien) and/or laparoscopic vascular stapler. A wide gastrotomy will help facilitate adequate intraoperative debridement as well as ongoing postoperative internal auto-debridement.
7. Debridement of necrosis is performed with laparoscopic graspers (with hand-over-hand technique, for solid debris) and suction (for liquid necrosis). Necrosis can be pulled into the stomach and/or pushed into the duodenum.
8. After completing debridement, the intragastric trocar sites are closed individually.

We published our initial series of laparoscopic TGN in 2014, reporting 21 patients [69]. Most patients recovered without complications (43%) or minor complications (29%), with major complications in 6 patients (29%). No additional drainage/debridement were needed, and no patients developed fistula. Our ongoing experience since those initial publications has continued to demonstrated that laparoscopic TGN provides effective debridement in a single operation with low rate of complications overall (with no fistulas) [68].

A larger multicenter retrospective study of 178 patients evaluated surgical transgastric management (combined open and laparoscopic series) of pancreatic necrosis across three institutions (including 43 patients from our institution) recently reported morbidity of 38% and mortality of 2%. The rate of pancreatic fistula was only 4%, and only three patients required additional necrosectomy (1.7%) [70]. The postoperative median length of hospital stay was a mere 8 days (as compared to prolonged hospitalizations of 50+ days for endoscopic and surgical step-up patients in the Dutch trials [54,55,70]). It is worth noting that 39% of patients from this multicenter cohort were confirmed to have infected necrosis [70], while the Dutch trials' rigorous guidelines selected for patients with confirmed or suspected infected pancreatitis necrosis [54,55]. Nonetheless, this publication confirmed that surgical TGN, whether open or laparoscopic, is an excellent and durable single-stage surgical option for patients with retrogastric walled-off necrosis.

The MISER trial was a single-center randomized controlled trial that compared minimally invasive surgery (n = 23 laparoscopic cystgastrostomy, 9 VARD) to endoscopic step-up approach (transluminal drainage with or without necrosectomy, n = 34) [71]. The authors did not find a difference in mortality between cohorts (8.8% in endoscopic cohort, 6.3% in surgical group), but there was a higher number of complications in the surgical group, particularly fistulas in the surgery arm (28% vs 0% in endoscopic). However, there was no significant difference in reinterventions performed for lack of clinical improvement (38% vs 44%), the number of interventions performed per patient (median 1 intervention [IQR 1–2] in both arms), or postprocedural hospital length of stay (18.5 vs 14 d) [71]. This is the only randomized trial examining surgery against endoscopic step-up approach, but the inclusion of VARD into the surgical arm begs the question of whether these patients are anatomically equivalent to those who underwent endoscopic treatment. The authors noted that of the 8 patients with postoperative pancreatic fistula, four patients underwent VARD, and an additional four "who underwent percutaneous catheter placement at laparoscopic debridement" (This is difficult to understand and not typical of the surgical transgastric strategy.). This may have led to an elevated incidence of this complication in the MISER trial, and indeed, when pancreatic fistula is excluded, the trial composite endpoint was similar for both treatment arms [72]. Finally, it is notable that the same center was conducting an overlapping randomized trial of endoscopic pigtails against LAMS [73], suggesting that there may have been some selection bias in accrual to competing trials. Thus, the MISER trial has not yet clarified the relative role of the surgical and endoscopic approaches.

In contrast, in our own single-center retrospective study, Dua and colleagues reviewed 74 patients who underwent transgastric intervention for necrotizing pancreatitis, of which 40 underwent laparoscopic TGN and 34 endoscopic cystgastrostomy [74]. In this study, there were no postprocedural pancreatic fistulas, despite 29% of patients found to have disconnected duct syndrome (13 in laparoscopic cohort, 9 endoscopic). Of these patients, only two (both from the endoscopic cohort) required future resection in the form of distal pancreatectomy [74], whereas resection has traditionally been performed for up to 45% of patients with unstable anatomy [16]. There were no differences in other morbidity. The endoscopic cohort required an average of 2.5 debridements. Although this study is limited by its sample size and patient selection, these findings suggest that creation of an internal fistula via cystgastrostomy through laparoscopic or endoscopic means can adequately drain an isolated tail remnant, without requiring resection of healthy pancreatic tissue [74]. Surgical cystgastrostomy, in particular, is an effective transgastric strategy that leads to resolution with the index procedure.

Taken together, the data described previously demonstrate that the transgastric approach, whether endoscopic or surgical, is a very effective strategy overall, avoiding in particular the need for prolonged drains. We have found that the surgical approach provides an effective debridement with a single operation and expedites patients' return to prepancreatitis health without the need for repeat debridement and drains [68]. The endoscopic approach is improving with larger LAMS and better instrumentation, so there is clearly a wide overlap in the application of these techniques. The decision regarding which to perform (surgical or endoscopic) must be individualized to patient and should be made based on local expertise, the nature of the WOPN (relative quantity of solid vs liquid necrosis), and the clinical status of the patient.

## Percutaneous drainage

Percutaneous drainage acts as a bridge to definitive debridement in septic patients. However, in a subset of patients, percutaneous drainage alone may adequately treat WOPN. As noted previously in the Dutch trials, 35% of step-up patients in the PANTER trial and 51% in the TENSION trial did not require surgical debridement after primary percutaneous drainage [54,55]. While systematic reviews have reported successful primary percutaneous drainage in approximately 55% of patients in the pooled data [75,76], individual studies' success rates range widely from 10% to 90% [2,75–79]. This wide variation may be due to the heterogeneity in disease severity as well as patient selection study to study. It is also possible that the quality of pancreatic necrosis may be a determinant factor in the success of drainage alone, especially with largely liquid collections.

Nonetheless, even though percutaneous drainage alone may be effective in select patients, catheter drainage is not benign, and there are shortcomings in this treatment strategy. The major morbidity associated with percutaneous drainage are pancreatic fistulas, which have been reported in up to 50% of patients [75,76]. In addition, patients experience pain and discomfort from the drainage catheter. Often, patients are committed to prolonged duration with a drain and may require several additional drain exchanges. These drawbacks should be weighed against operative morbidity in management of necrotizing pancreatitis.

## SUMMARY

The approach to management of walled-off pancreatic necrosis has evolved considerably over the past three decades, transforming the landscape of surgery from open debridement to laparoscopic options to development of step-up approaches that combine percutaneous/endoscopic drainage and minimally invasive debridement. However, there is no one ideal approach for all patients, as patients vary widely in clinical status, contents of the pancreatic collection (liquid vs solid), and anatomic location. Owing to heterogeneity of the disease process, the timing and specific treatment strategies are tailored toward each individual patient, focusing on minimizing morbidity and mortality. Our current approach is percutaneous drainage followed by minimally invasive retroperitoneal debridement with a two-trocar technique for collections located in the paracolic gutters. We advocate for laparoscopic transgastric necrosectomy for retrogastric collections with a significant solid component, particularly for patients with disconnected duct and isolated tail remnant, as this results in an effective debridement in one operation and frees patients from the morbidity associated with a percutaneous drain. Given the improvements in mortality with better data and understanding in the management of necrotizing pancreatitis, therapeutic focus should be trained on returning the patient to prepancreatitis wellness.

## CLINICS CARE POINTS

- Asymptomatic walled-off pancreatic necrosis does not warrant intervention, and these patients can be safely monitored.
- Percutaneous or endoscopic drainage can be performed to bridge critically ill patients to definitive debridement (surgical and endoscopic step-up approaches).
- Anatomic location of walled-off pancreatic necrosis can dictate treatment: Retrogastric collections are amenable to transgastric interventions (endoscopic or surgical drainage/debridement); collection locations in the paracolic gutter are appropriate for retroperitoneal percutaneous drainage and/or debridement.
- Surgical transgastric necrosectomy is an effective single-stage debridement procedure, with the creation of a large cystgastrostomy that allows ongoing internal auto-debridement.
- A patient with isolated tail remnants is best managed by surgical as opposed to endoscopic methods, as a surgical cystgastrostomy is durable and allows for ongoing internal drainage without requiring additional interventions.

## Acknowledgments

The authors thank Jeanne Koelling for her excellent original illustrations created for this work.

## SUPPLEMENTARY DATA

Supplementary data to this article can be found online at https://doi.org/10.1016/j.yasu.2021.05.016.

## References

[1] Trikudanathan G, Wolbrink DRJ, van Santvoort HC, et al. Current concepts in severe acute and necrotizing pancreatitis: an evidence-based approach. Gastroenterology 2019;156(7):1994–2007.e3.
[2] Roch AM, Maatman T, Carr RA, et al. Evolving treatment of necrotizing pancreatitis. Am J Surg 2018;215(3):526–9.
[3] Rashid MU, Hussain I, Jehanzeb S, et al. Pancreatic necrosis: complications and changing trend of treatment. World J Gastrointest Surg 2019;11(4):198–217.
[4] Working Group IAP/APA Acute Pancreatitis Guidelines. IAP/APA evidence-based guidelines for the management of acute pancreatitis. Pancreatology 2013;13(4 Suppl. 2): e1–15.
[5] Baron TH, DiMaio CJ, Wang AY, et al. American Gastroenterological Association Clinical Practice Update: Management of Pancreatic Necrosis. Gastroenterology 2020;158(1): 67–75.e1.
[6] Banks PA, Bollen TL, Dervenis C, et al. Classification of acute pancreatitis - 2012: Revision of the Atlanta classification and definitions by international consensus. Gut 2013;62(1): 102–11.
[7] Dua MM, Worhunsky DJ, Amin S, et al. Getting the dead out: modern treatment strategies for necrotizing pancreatitis. Dig Dis Sci 2014;59(9):2069–75.
[8] Dhaka N, Samanta J, Kochhar S, et al. Pancreatic fluid collections: What is the ideal imaging technique? World J Gastroenterol 2015;21(48):13403–10.
[9] Morgan DE, Baron TH, Smith JK, et al. Pancreatic fluid collections prior to intervention: Evaluation with MR imaging compared with CT and US. Radiology 1997;203(3):773–8.
[10] Colvin SD, Smith EN, Morgan DE, et al. Acute pancreatitis: an update on the revised Atlanta classification. Abdom Radiol 2020;45(5):1222–31.
[11] Shyu JY, Sainani NI, Anik Sahni V, et al. Necrotizing pancreatitis: diagnosis, imaging, and intervention. Radiographics 2014;34(5):1218–40.
[12] Bugiantella W, Rondelli F, Boni M, et al. Necrotizing pancreatitis: a review of the interventions. Int J Surg 2016;28:S163–71.
[13] Leonard-Murali S, Lezotte J, Kalu R, et al. Necrotizing pancreatitis: a review for the acute care surgeon. Am J Surg 2020;0(0).
[14] Arvanitakis M, Dumonceau JM, Albert J, et al. Endoscopic management of acute necrotizing pancreatitis: European Society of Gastrointestinal Endoscopy (ESGE) evidence-based multidisciplinary guidelines. Endoscopy 2018;50(5):524–46.
[15] Warshaw AL. Pancreatic necrosis: To debride or not to debride - That is the question. Ann Surg 2000;232(5):627–9.
[16] Maatman TK, Roch AM, Lewellen KA, et al. Disconnected pancreatic duct syndrome: spectrum of operative management. J Surg Res 2020;247:297–303.
[17] Runzi M, Niebel W, Goebell H, et al. Severe Acute Pancreatitis: Nonsurgical Treatment of Infected Necroses. Pancreas 2005;30(3):195–9.
[18] Garg PK, Sharma M, Madan K, et al. Primary conservative treatment results in mortality comparable to surgery in patients with infected pancreatic necrosis. Clin Gastroenterol Hepatol 2010;8(12):1089–94.e2.

[19] Lee JK, Kwak KK, Park JK, et al. The efficacy of nonsurgical treatment of infected pancreatic necrosis. Pancreas 2007;34(4):399–404.
[20] Wysocki AP, McKay CJ, Carter CR. Infected pancreatic necrosis: minimizing the cut. ANZ J Surg 2010;80(1–2):58–70.
[21] Rana SS, Sharma RK, Gupta P, et al. Natural course of asymptomatic walled off pancreatic necrosis. Dig Liver Dis 2019;51(5):730–4.
[22] Wroński M, Cebulski W, Pawłowski W, et al. Walled-Off Necrosis: Safety of Watchful Waiting. Dig Dis Sci 2015;60(4):1081–6.
[23] Jagielski M, Smoczyński M, Studniarek M, et al. Spontaneous regression of asymptomatic walled-off pancreatic necrosis. Arch Med Sci 2019;15(5):1278–87.
[24] Javadi C, Dua M, Visser B. A modern approach to complicated pancreatitis. In: Davis KA, Coimbra R, editors. Surgical decision making in acute care surgery. 1st ed. New York: Thieme Medical Publishers; 2020. p. 160–71.
[25] Mier J, Luque-De León E, Castillo A, et al. Early versus late necrosectomy in severe necrotizing pancreatitis. Am J Surg 1997;173(2):71–5.
[26] Van Santvoort HC, Bakker OJ, Bollen TL, et al. A conservative and minimally invasive approach to necrotizing pancreatitis improves outcome. Gastroenterology 2011;141(4): 1254–63.
[27] Reddy MS, Jindal R, Gupta R, et al. Outcome after pancreatic necrosectomy: trends over 12 years at an indian centre. ANZ J Surg 2006;76(8):704–9.
[28] Trikudanathan G, Tawfik P, Amateau SK, et al. Early (<4 Weeks) versus standard (≥ 4 Weeks) endoscopically centered step-up interventions for necrotizing pancreatitis. Am J Gastroenterol 2018;113(10):1550–8.
[29] van Grinsven J, van Dijk SM, Dijkgraaf MG, et al. Postponed or immediate drainage of infected necrotizing pancreatitis (POINTER trial): study protocol for a randomized controlled trial. Trials 2019;20(1):239.
[30] Besselink MG. Timing of intervention in necrotizing pancreatitis: POINTER trial results. In: American College of Surgeons Clinical Congress. 2020.
[31] Rodriguez JR, Razo AO, Targarona J, et al. Debridement and closed packing for sterile or infected necrotizing pancreatitis: Insights into indications and outcomes in 167 patients. Ann Surg 2008;247(2):294–9.
[32] Harris HW, Barcia A, Schell MT, et al. Necrotizing pancreatitis: A surgical approach independent of documented infection. HPB 2004;6(3):161–8.
[33] Maatman TK, Zyromski NJ. Open pancreatic debridement in necrotizing pancreatitis. J Gastrointest Surg 2020;1–2.
[34] Ashley SW, Perez A, Pierce EA, et al. Necrotizing pancreatitis: Contemporary analysis of 99 consecutive cases. Annals of surgery, vol. 234. Philadelphia: Lippincott, Williams, and Wilkins; 2001. p. 572–80.
[35] Connor S, Alexakis N, Raraty MGT, et al. Early and late complications after pancreatic necrosectomy. Surgery 2005;137(5):499–505.
[36] Maatman TK, Flick KF, Roch AM, et al. Operative pancreatic debridement: Contemporary outcomes in changing times. Pancreatology 2020;20(5):968–75.
[37] Rattner DW, Legermate DA, Lee MJ, et al. Early surgical débridement of symptomatic pancreatic necrosis is beneficial irrespective of infection. Am J Surg 1992;163(1):105–10.
[38] Rau B, Bothe A, Beger HG. Surgical treatment of necrotizing pancreatitis by necrosectomy and closed lavage: Changing patient characteristics and outcome in a 19-year, single-center series. Surgery 2005;138(1):28–39.
[39] Howard TJ, Patel JB, Zyromski N, et al. Declining morbidity and mortality rates in the surgical management of pancreatic necrosis. In: Journal of Gastrointestinal Surgery, vol. 11. New York: Springer; 2007. p. 43–9.
[40] Parikh PY, Pitt HA, Kilbane M, et al. Pancreatic necrosectomy: North American mortality is much lower than expected. J Am Coll Surg 2009;209(6):712–9.

[41] Fink D, Soares R, Matthews JB, et al. History, goals, and technique of laparoscopic pancreatic necrosectomy. J Gastrointest Surg 2011;15(7):1092–7.
[42] Zhu JF, Fan XH, Zhang XH. Laparoscopic treatment of severe acute pancreatitis. Surg Endosc 2001;15(2):146–8.
[43] Pamoukian VN, Gagner M. Laparoscopic necrosectomy for acute necrotizing pancreatitis. J Hepatobiliary Pancreat Surg 2001;8(3):221–3.
[44] Mathew MJ, Parmar AK, Sahu D, et al. Laparoscopic necrosectomy in acute necrotizing pancreatitis: Our experience. J Minim Access Surg 2014;10(3):126–31.
[45] Tan J, Tan H, Hu B, et al. Short-term outcomes from a multicenter retrospective study in china comparing laparoscopic and open surgery for the treatment of infected pancreatic necrosis. J Laparoendosc Adv Surg Tech 2012;22(1):27–33.
[46] Wani SV, Patankar RV, Mathur SK. Minimally invasive approach to pancreatic necrosectomy. J Laparoendosc Adv Surg Tech 2011;21(2):131–6.
[47] Parekh D. Laparoscopic-assisted pancreatic necrosectomy: A new surgical option for treatment of severe necrotizing pancreatitis. Arch Surg 2006;141(9):895–902.
[48] Zhou ZG, Zheng YC, Shu Y, et al. Laparoscopic management of severe acute pancreatitis. Pancreas 2003;27(3).
[49] Carter CR, McKay CJ, Imrie CW. Percutaneous necrosectomy and sinus tract endoscopy in the management of infected pancreatic necrosis: An initial experience. Ann Surg 2000;232(2):175–80.
[50] Logue JA, Carter CR. Minimally invasive necrosectomy techniques in severe acute pancreatitis: role of percutaneous necrosectomy and video-assisted retroperitoneal debridement. Gastroenterol Res Pract 2015;2015.
[51] Connor S, Ghaneh P, Raraty M, et al. Minimally invasive retroperitoneal pancreatic necrosectomy. Dig Surg 2003;20(4):270–7.
[52] Horvath KD, Kao LS, Ali A, et al. Laparoscopic assisted percutaneous drainage of infected pancreatic necrosis. Surg Endosc 2001;15(7):677–82.
[53] Horvath KD, Kao LS, Wherry KL, et al. A technique for laparoscopic-assisted percutaneous drainage of infected pancreatic necrosis and pancreatic abscess. Surg Endosc 2001;15(10):1221–5.
[54] van Santvoort HC, Besselink MG, Bakker OJ, et al. A step-up approach or open necrosectomy for necrotizing pancreatitis. N Engl J Med 2010;362(16):1491–502.
[55] van Brunschot S, van Grinsven J, van Santvoort HC, et al. Endoscopic or surgical step-up approach for infected necrotising pancreatitis: a multicentre randomised trial. Lancet 2018;391(10115):51–8.
[56] Raraty MGT, Halloran CM, Dodd S, et al. Minimal access retroperitoneal pancreatic necrosectomy: Improvement in morbidity and mortality with a less invasive approach. Ann Surg 2010;251(5):787–93.
[57] Gambiez LP, Denimal FA, Porte HL, et al. Retroperitoneal approach and endoscopic management of peripancreatic necrosis collections. Arch Surg 1998;133(1):66–72.
[58] Castellanos G, Piñero A, Serrano A, et al. Infected pancreatic necrosis: Translumbar approach and management with retroperitoneoscopy. Arch Surg 2002;137(9):1060–3.
[59] Bakker OJ, Van Santvoort HC, Van Brunschot S, et al. Endoscopic transgastric vs surgical necrosectomy for infected necrotizing pancreatitis: A randomized trial. JAMA 2012;307(10):1053–61.
[60] Siddiqui AA, Kowalski TE, Loren DE, et al. Fully covered self-expanding metal stents versus lumen-apposing fully covered self-expanding metal stent versus plastic stents for endoscopic drainage of pancreatic walled-off necrosis: clinical outcomes and success. Gastrointest Endosc 2017;85(4):758–65.
[61] Chen Y-I, Yang J, Friedland S, et al. Lumen apposing metal stents are superior to plastic stents in pancreatic walled-off necrosis: a large international multicenter study. Endosc Int Open 2019;07(03):E347–54.

[62] Weilert F, Binmoeller KF. Specially designed stents for translumenal drainage. Gastrointest Interv 2015;4(1):40–5.
[63] Van Der Wiel SE, Poley JW, Grubben MJAL, et al. The EndoRotor, a novel tool for the endoscopic management of pancreatic necrosis. Endoscopy 2018;50(9):E240–1.
[64] van der Wiel SE, May A, Poley JW, et al. Preliminary report on the safety and utility of a novel automated mechanical endoscopic tissue resection tool for endoscopic necrosectomy: a case series. Endosc Int Open 2020;08(03):E274–80.
[65] Van Brunschot S, Fockens P, Bakker OJ, et al. Endoscopic transluminal necrosectomy in necrotising pancreatitis: A systematic review. Surg Endosc 2014;28(5):1425–38.
[66] De Angelis CG, Venezia L, Cortegoso Valdivia P, et al. Lumen-apposing metal stents in management of pancreatic fluid collections: The nobody's land of removal timing. Saudi J Gastroenterol 2019;25(6):335–40.
[67] Zyromski NJ, Nakeeb A, House MG, et al. Transgastric pancreatic necrosectomy: how I do it. J Gastrointest Surg 2016;20(2):445–9.
[68] Dua MM, Worhunsky DJ, Malhotra L, et al. Transgastric pancreatic necrosectomy—expedited return to prepancreatitis health. J Surg Res 2017;219:11–7.
[69] Worhunsky DJ, Qadan M, Dua MM, et al. Laparoscopic transgastric necrosectomy for the management of pancreatic necrosis. J Am Coll Surg 2014;219(4):735–43.
[70] Driedger M, Zyromski NJ, Visser BC, et al. Surgical transgastric necrosectomy for necrotizing pancreatitis: a single-stage procedure for walled-off pancreatic necrosis. Ann Surg 2020;271(1):163–8.
[71] Bang JY, Arnoletti JP, Holt BA, et al. An endoscopic transluminal approach, compared with minimally invasive surgery, reduces complications and costs for patients with necrotizing pancreatitis. Gastroenterology 2019;156(4):1027–40.e3.
[72] Garg PK, Zyromski NJ, Freeman ML. Infected necrotizing pancreatitis: evolving interventional strategies from minimally invasive surgery to endoscopic therapy—evidence mounts, but one size does not fit all. Gastroenterology 2019;156(4):867–71.
[73] Bang JY, Navaneethan U, Hasan MK, et al. Non-superiority of lumen-apposing metal stents over plastic stents for drainage of walled-off necrosis in a randomised trial. Gut 2019;68(7): 1200–9.
[74] Dua MM, Jensen CW, Friedland S, et al. Isolated pancreatic tail remnants after transgastric necrosectomy can be observed. J Surg Res 2018;231:109–15.
[75] Ke L, Li J, Hu P, et al. Percutaneous catheter drainage in infected pancreatitis necrosis: a systematic review. Indian J Surg 2016;78(3):221–8.
[76] Van Baal MC, Van Santvoort HC, Bollen TL, et al. Systematic review of percutaneous catheter drainage as primary treatment for necrotizing pancreatitis. Br J Surg 2011;98(1): 18–27.
[77] Besselink MG, De Bruijn MT, Rutten JP, et al. Surgical intervention in patients with necrotizing pancreatitis. In: British Journal of Surgery, vol. 93 2006;. 2006. p. 593–9.
[78] Shenvi S, Gupta R, Kang M, et al. Timing of surgical intervention in patients of infected necrotizing pancreatitis not responding to percutaneous catheter drainage. Pancreatology 2016;16(5):778–87.
[79] Horvath K, Freeny P, Escallon J, et al. Safety and efficacy of video-assisted retroperitoneal debridement for infected pancreatic collections: A multicenter, prospective, single-arm phase 2 study. Arch Surg 2010;145(9):817–25.

Advances in Surgery 55 (2021) 251–271
ADVANCES IN SURGERY

# Vascular Reconstruction for Traumatic Injuries

Ali Khalifeh, MD, Todd E. Rasmussen, MD*
Division of Vascular and Endovascular Surgery, Mayo Clinic, 200 First Street Southwest, Rochester, MN 55905, USA

**Keywords**

• Vascular trauma • Hemorrhagic shock • Extremity ischemia • Blood vessel repair • Traumatic vascular injuries • Vascular reconstructions • Endovascular repair

**Key points**

- Traumatic vascular injury is a leading cause of mortality and morbidity.
- Mechanism of injury and anatomic location present with variable clinical presentations.
- If a patient presents with hard signs of vascular injury, prompt operative intervention is mandated.
- Familiarity with different exposures facilitates obtaining vascular control.
- Endovascular repair is useful in certain torso injuries as well as in obtaining balloon vascular occlusion.

## INTRODUCTION

Exsanguination and/or ischemia resulting from vascular injury are leading causes of disability and death in military and civilian settings [1–3]. Due to anatomic proximity, these injuries frequently involve both arteries and veins and often are associated with damage to other important structures, such as bones, nerves, and viscera. Death from exsanguination can be prevented if the vascular disruption is recognized rapidly and managed appropriately. Surgeons should be familiar with the kinetics of the different types of wounding mechanisms to retain an appropriate index of suspicion when the injury is not immediately obvious. In the polytrauma patient, surgeons should establish a logical treatment sequence but maintain focus on the vascular injury as a top priority to be addressed in a timely manner. This may include ligation of the

*Corresponding author. *E-mail address:* Rasmussen.Todd@mayo.edu

https://doi.org/10.1016/j.yasu.2021.05.017
0065-3411/21/

vessel as a damage control maneuver or use of a temporary shunt to restore flow quickly. In some circumstances, open reconstruction is appropriate, whereas in other cases endovascular techniques can be used to fix the problem. Experience and technological advances stemming from decades of military and civilian collaboration in this area have resulted in decreased fatality rates, better limb salvage, and the ability to improve the functional recovery of patients having sustained vascular trauma. This article provides an overview of the diagnosis and management of vascular trauma and aims to expand the readers' knowledge base as they prepare to tackle this daunting injury pattern.

## DIAGNOSIS AND INITIAL MANAGEMENT

The lifesaving concepts taught as part of the American College of Surgeons (ACS) Advanced Trauma Life Support program are crucial when treating a patient with major vascular injury. After securing the patient's airway and ability to breathe, attention must be turned immediately to circulation and taking steps to apportion and restore blood volume and central aortic pressure properly. Obvious sites of exsanguination should be managed with immediate manual pressure, with use of a tourniquet if possible and/or packing to create tamponade. In some instances, control of external hemorrhage takes priority over establishing an airway, using a CABC approach, in which the initial "C" stands for "control of catastrophic bleeding" before addressing airway, breathing and circulation."

As a lesson from the Iraq and Afghanistan wars, tourniquets are an effective means to save lives from extremity hemorrhage. In response to the epidemic of shootings in the United States, the ACS has teamed with private and public partners in a major initiative called Stop the Bleed [4]. The goal of this global initiative is to "build resilience by better preparing the public to save lives by raising awareness of basic actions to stop life threatening bleeding following everyday emergencies and man-made and natural disasters" (bleeingcontrol.org).

Other immediate steps to stabilize patents with vascular trauma include use of blood component–based resuscitation, the principle of permissive hypotension, tranexamic acid, and in some instances resuscitative endovascular balloon occlusion of the aorta (REBOA) [5,6]. Patients with major vascular injury should be kept warm to reduce the likelihood of coagulopathy, and those with a deformed and ischemic extremity should have the fracture pulled to length or reduced to restore flow through the axial vessels. Signs of a cervical vascular injury should alert the surgeon to potential airway compromise and to other aerodigestive injuries. Prehospital personnel and emergency medical services units (eg, ambulances) should be enabled to triage and transport patients with suspected vascular injuries to an ACS verified trauma center. If a level 1 trauma center is too far from the injury scene, patients should be transported to the closest capable facility to be stabilized and then transferred quickly to a higher level of care, ideally one with the range of capabilities needed to manage this challenging type of injury.

## Mechanism of Injuries and Diagnosis

Vascular injury can be caused by blunt or penetrating mechanisms and can occur in the extremities; the cervical region; the torso, which consists of thorax, abdomen, and pelvis; or the junctional regions between the extremities and the torso (eg, axillary and femoral regions). Just like different blood vessels present with different signs and symptoms after injury, certain injury mechanisms are associated with distinct clinical presentations. The breadth of anatomic patterns of injury and clinical presentations require the astute surgeon to apply objective means of diagnosis as well as a high index of suspicion in order to avoid morbidity and mortality from vascular trauma.

Penetrating trauma is more likely to transect the wall of the vessel contacted by the projectile (ie, fragmentation or munition) or knife. Depending on the degree of vessel transection, bleeding may ensue, or the vessel may just be contused. If the projectile contacts the artery or vein directly, it often destroys a longer segment, a situation that requires removal of all of the damaged vessel and replacement with an interposition or bypass graft. Even if penetrating munitions or fragments do not contact an artery or vein directly, they can be associated with kinetic energy that, if great enough, can result in concussive waves that directly damage vessels leading to thrombosis or disruption. In contrast, damage associated with a stab injury depends on the direction and depth of the blade and often results in a focal, or clean, vessel injury that is amenable to primary repair.

Blunt trauma mechanisms result in acceleration-deceleration and or crush injury to the vasculature. Blunt injury often is associated with fractured bones that stretch and, in some instances, penetrate arteries or veins. Certain patterns of orthopedic injury (eg, fractures or dislocations) are associated with distinct vascular injuries. In these situations, although the vascular component may be less obvious at the time of presentation, the surgeon should recognize the association and perform vascular-specific testing to confirm or exclude arterial and venous injury. Motor vehicle crashes are the most common cause of blunt vascular injury in the civilian setting whereas penetrating mechanisms are more common in the combat environment. Blunt vascular injury resulting from motor vehicle crashes also is associated frequently with injuries to solid organs (eg, liver, kidney, and spleen), bones, and or nerves.

Physical examination and the primary survey are the initial steps in confirming or excluding the presence of a vascular injury and forming an index of suspicion. Exposure of the whole patient can be overlooked amidst all that accompanies the primary survey but is a critically important maneuver in identifying all injuries, including open wounds, hematomas, and fractures. Examination of extremity pulses and assessment for symmetry of color (or pallor), along with the presence of large bruises can alert the surgeon to a vascular injury. The hard and soft signs of vascular injury are listed in Table 1 and should be considered when evaluating a patient and considering next diagnostic and therapeutic steps [7,8]. For the most part, hard signs of vascular injury, such as major external bleeding and an obviously ischemic

**Table 1**
Clinical manifestations and signs of arterial injury

| Hard signs | Soft signs |
|---|---|
| Arterial bleeding | Report of exsanguination on trauma scene |
| Loss of pulse | Diminished pulses |
| Expanding hematoma | Moderate hematoma |
| Bruit or thrill | Proximity of injury to vessel or long bone |
| Signs of ischemia | Ipsilateral neurologic deficit |

limb, require expeditious transport of the patient to the operating room. As an example of a soft sign, proximity of a penetrating wound, long bone fracture, or dislocation near a major vessel should prompt vascular-specific testing, such as measurement of the injured extremity index using continuous-wave Doppler, duplex ultrasonography, or computed tomographic angiography (CTA). Familiarity with the mechanisms of injury also is important in determining which and in what order further diagnostic tests should be obtained.

Following primary and secondary survey, several adjuncts to the physical examination can confirm or refute the presence of a significant vascular injury. Plain chest radiographs are a useful initial examination to evaluate for blunt thoracic aortic injury (BTAI). A widened mediastinum, apical cap, and inferior displacement of the left main bronchus and/or hemothorax point toward major thoracic injuries, including BTAI. Multiple rib or vertebral body fractures are signs of a high kinetic energy trauma and predict the probability of vascular disruption. Trauma providers who are experienced in ultrasonography can detect several types of injuries on a focused assessment with sonography for trauma examination. These may include abdominal and retroperitoneal hemorrhage, pericardial effusion, and pleural effusion. Continuous-wave Doppler alone or in conjunction with pressure measurements (eg, injured extremity index) using a manual blood pressure cuff is an extremely useful tool with which to assess perfusion. An injured extremity index of less than 0.9 is highly predictive of a flow-limiting injury to the more proximal arteries of the arm or leg. Continuous-wave Doppler is a particularly useful adjunct with which to evaluate for vascular injury because it can be easily used at the bedside and repeated multiple times at various stages of care (eg, resuscitation room, operating room, intensive care unit [ICU], and so forth) [9,10].

In most level 1 trauma centers, CTA is readily available and largely has replaced the need for traditional, catheter-directed diagnostic angiography. In addition to early recognition of vascular injuries, CTA can delineate other concomitant visceral, solid organ, and bony injuries. If CTA is not readily available, or the patient needs to go first to the operating room, then traditional, catheter-directed angiography remains a great diagnostic tool. As discussed previously, patients with less acute or soft signs may benefit from duplex ultrasound to assess for vascular injury. Magnetic resonance angiography is time consuming and utilized less frequently may be helpful, however, in a stable patient [8].

## Operating Room and Setup

Setting up the operating room is crucial for the effective management of vascular injury. Recently, many trauma centers have established hybrid operating rooms, which combine fixed imaging units and the capability to perform the spectrum of open operations [11]. In most instances, the presence of a hybrid room eliminates the time and risk associated with transporting patients to and from otherwise separately located imaging suites (eg, interventional radiology suite) and operating rooms [12]. Studies have shown that the use of hybrid operating rooms have reduced time to definitive hemorrhage control, and use of blood products and resulted in better patient outcomes. If a hybrid operating room is not available, the surgeon should make sure that the operating table is C-arm compatible and have a radiology technician available to assist, if needed. The surgeon, operating room staff, nurses, and surgical technologists should be familiar with both endovascular and open vascular instruments. Open operating instrument sets as well as endovascular catheters, wires, sheaths, stents, and stent grafts should be available either in the operating room or in a nearby center core or storage area to facilitate swift and uncomplicated angiographic studies and endovascular interventions.

The surgeon and operating room team should prepare the patient widely and anticipate the need to have open access for proximal vascular control. Injured extremities should be prepped circumferentially. In addition, anticipating other anatomic sites that may be needed as part of the operation (eg, lower extremity for saphenous vein harvest), saves time when it comes to performing the reconstruction. Surgeons should anticipate that vascular injuries in contaminated operative fields may require extra-anatomical bypass and be prepared to do so. A main tenet of vascular injury management is establishing proximal and distal control when readying to explore and repair the injury. As such, prepping and draping of anatomic inflow and outflow regions should be ensured as adequate. Devitalized and infected tissues must be débrided, and arterial repairs or bypasses covered by healthy soft tissue, muscle flaps, or omental flaps, depending on the anatomic region.

Communication with the anesthesiology team regarding blood loss and clamp and reperfusion times is important to avoid preventable causes of intraoperative shock and even death. In the lead up to and at the start of the operation, the surgeon should maintain a big picture view as it relates to the patient's physiologic condition. Working with anesthesia to understand the degree of the physiologic derangement helps with prudent decisions that pertain to the need for and sequence of different operative approaches to vascular trauma. For example, patients who are multiply injured and have adverse physiologic measures are likely to be best served with quick, damage control maneuvers, such as vessel ligation or placement of a temporary vascular shunt, rather than performance of a time-consuming vascular reconstruction. In addition to communicating with anesthesiology, the treating surgeon often needs to plan the type and timing of vascular repair with other specialties, such as orthopedics, neurosurgery, and others.

### Temporary Vascular Shunts

Temporary intraluminal shunts have been used as a standard part of carotid artery and other types of elective cardiovascular surgery for some time. Their use as an adjunct to quickly restore perfusion in the setting of vascular injury, however, has gained increasing acceptance over the past couple of decades, a phenomenon greatly accelerated by the wartime experiences in Iraq and Afghanistan [13]. Shunting is valuable as a damage control maneuver when immediate repair or reconstruction of the injured vessel is not feasible due to lack of experience or resources or the need to tend to other life-threatening injuries. Vascular shunts also can be used as a temporizing measure in contaminated fields or in situations in which a patient's condition cannot tolerate additional time in the operating room. Vascular shunts serve as a temporizing bridge for perfusion until a definitive maneuver can be performed, be it ligation or reconstruction.

Temporary shunts remain patent without systemic anticoagulation for at least 4 hours to 6 hours, especially in more proximal, high-flow vessels. In some extreme circumstances, shunts remain patent for up to 24 hours, but these situations are fraught with shunt-related complications resulting from the accumulation and embolization of thrombus. Venous flow also can be bridged with shunts, although veins are prone to higher rates of thrombosis because of their inherently lower flow rates. The redundant nature of arterial perfusion in the leg and forearm means that shunts are required less commonly when small arteries in these areas are injured. If multiple tibial or forearm arteries are injured simultaneously and a shunt is placed, it can be effective despite lower patency compared with a shunt placed in larger, more proximal vessel. In other words, although shunts in the more distal vessels have a higher rate of thrombosis, if clotting does occur, it does not preclude performing a thrombectomy and completing a successful small vessel reconstruction for limb salvage. Overall, the use of temporary shunts has expanded the window of limb salvage in the most severely injured of patients, helping transform an older paradigm of life over limb to one in which both life and limb can be saved.

There are multiple types of commercially available shunts. Although they come in different lengths, shapes, and designs, they have equal efficacy as pertaining to patency and limb salvage. Some shunts have distal and proximal balloons, or bulbs that secure them in place, whereas others come with specialized clamps. In the setting of trauma, it is most common to secure an intralumenal shunt with heavy silk ties as a matter of expediency. The more frequently used shunts are the Javid (Bard Peripheral Vascular, Tempe, Arizona), the Argyle (Kendall Healthcare Products, Mansfield, Massachusetts) and the Sundt (Integra, Health Management, Cyprus). Shunts are available in different diameters and should be thought of as either straight, or in-line, or in a longer and looped configuration.

Before placing a shunt, proximal and distal control of the injured vessel must be obtained and the thrombus removed from the inflow and outflow portions diligently. If this step is overlooked or performed inadequately, the shunt is likely to be fail because of clot that was associated with the original injury. Flushing of diluted heparin (ie, heparinized saline) in the proximal and distal portions of the vessel to be shunted is another useful maneuver to optimize flow through the shunt as it is placed. If commercial shunts are not available, other types of sterile tubing of appropriate diameter can be used (eg, small thoracostomy or nasogastric or intravenous tubing), although blunt or frayed edges of these makeshift devices should be avoided.

### Endovascular Balloon Occlusion of The Aorta

Extrapolating from experience with ruptured abdominal aortic aneurysms, REBOA has been extended to circumstances of severe injury and shock as means to stem the bleeding and rapidly restore central aortic pressure and perfusion to the heart and brain. First described as an operative adjunct for shock during the Korean War, balloon occlusion of the aorta has transformed, first with large-caliber, over-the-wire, compliant balloons to expand endografts, to a modern era of small-caliber, semicompliant REBOA balloons designed to be used in trauma and emergency settings.

Initially, REBOA for trauma and shock was performed using standard, large-diameter over-the-wire catheters, such as Coda (Cook Medical, Bloomington, Indiana), Reliant (Medtronic, Minneapolis, Minnesota), or GORE Molding & Occlusion Balloon (GORE, Newark, Delaware). These devices are designed to be used under x-ray guidance by endovascular specialists in well-equipped operating rooms, however, and the sheath sizes (10F–14F) required for their insertion make them impracticable for emergency situations. Driven by the military's need for new approaches to noncompressible hemorrhage in resource-limited settings, the first trauma-specific REBOA device was approved by the Food and Drug Administration (FDA) in 2015. The ER-REBOA catheter (Prytime Medical, Boerne, Texas) is a 7F, single-pass device with a trauma and fluoroscopy-free indication. The ER-REBOA also has a small wire inside the catheter (ie, hypotube design) that obviates using a long, cumbersome guide wire.

The evolution of REBOA has included morphometric study and definition of aortic target zones for occlusion depending on a patient's injury pattern and the source of bleeding. Zone I extends from the origin of the left subclavian to the takeoff of the celiac artery and is the desired location for REBOA in the setting of subdiaphragmatic hemorrhage and shock. Zone II is the paravisceral segment of the aorta and as of now is thought to be an area that should not be covered by balloon occlusion. REBOA in distal zone III occurs between the lowest renal artery and the aortic bifurcation and is applicable to pelvic and junctional femoral hemorrhage.

REBOA has been popularized over the past several years with mostly favorable reports, although the optimal timing and patient population(s) (ie, indications) for its use still are being defined. Not to be overlooked, REBOA is associated with a 3% to 5% rate of femoral access-site complications, a small percentage of which can be limb-threatening. Prolonged complete REBOA beyond 20 minutes to 30 minutes can result in life-threatening reperfusion and hypotension when the balloon is deflated, a limitation that has driven various approaches to partial aortic occlusion (ie, partial REBOA) as a strategy to mitigate distal ischemia. Current limitations of REBOA notwithstanding, as experience is gained and as new, small-caliber, partial occlusion technologies are developed, it is likely that this approach will play an important role in the management of certain scenarios of injury and shock.

### Other Types of Balloon Occlusion

The balloon tip of Fogarty thromboembolectomy catheters (Edwards, Irvine, California) also is useful in controlling bleeding. Fogarty catheters range from 2F to 7F, with corresponding balloon diameters from 2 mm to 9 mm. When placed into the orifice of a bleeding vessel and inflated with a 1-mL tuberculin syringe, appropriately sized Fogarty balloons stop bleeding. Hands-free Fogarty balloon control can be continued with a 3-way stopcock that is closed to maintain the balloon inflation and position. This handy maneuver can be performed to allow visualization, further dissection, and clamp placement, or it can serve as the sole mechanism of bleeding control (inflow and/or outflow). Fogarty balloon occlusion can also be utilized electively in situations when the surgeon wants to avoid clamping and risk injury to a heavily calcified/diseased vessel. Given the utility of Fogarty balloon occlusion as a bail-out maneuver, the surgeon is well served in knowing the exact catheter and corresponding balloon sizes of Fogarty devices as well as the technical aspects of how to place and maintain their intralumenal position.

### Endovascular Repair of Vascular Trauma

Endovascular approaches to specific patterns of injury are discussed later but suffice it to say catheter-based technologies provide an effective and less-invasive approach to treat several types of vascular trauma. Studies of large national registries show that the use of endovascular methods to manage vascular injury increased at a rapid rate, between 2000 and 2020, propelled largely by improvements in sheath, coil, and stent graft technology and promulgation of the endovascular skill set.

Most striking is the transformation in the management of blunt aortic injury, which, prior to 2000, was managed solely with open operation and today is treated effectively with endografts in more than 90% of cases. Similar changes in practice have effected the management of great vessel injury (eg, subclavian, carotid, and axillary) as well as many patterns of solid organ bleeding [14]. The use of catheter-directed methods to control bleeding from the internal iliac arteries and their branches has transformed the management of pelvic injuries. When preceded by zone III REBOA, catheter-directed embolization of bleeding from pelvic fracture provides an intuitive sequence of endovascular steps to stabilize shock and bleeding from a major cause of death. Outcomes data from national registries and reports from individual trauma centers show that, on the whole, morbidity is less with endovascular approaches and, in many cases, survival is better as well. Although less applicable for peripheral arterial injuries, the use of endovascular techniques, such as covered stents, coils, and plugs, also has been reported effective in the management of select cases of extremity trauma [15].

Based on concerns that endovascular repairs might not last or that they might be prone to infection in the setting of penetrating injury, calls have been made for better long-term or outcomes data on their durability. Although large longitudinal studies still are lacking, 10 years to 15 years into endovascular repair there is a paucity of experience or published studies showing that these techniques are not durable. Catheter-based management of certain types of vascular injury works and provides a lasting solution for complex patients, and the lack of long-term data for this approach is no more notable than the lack of similar data for other trauma-related interventions (resuscitation strategies, open revascularization, and so forth) [16].

## Conduits for Vascular Reconstruction

Repair or reconstruction of a vascular injury can be approached using several different techniques. Simple primary, or suture, repair can be used for focal injuries to healthy vessels in which there has been little to no loss of the vessel itself or damage to a length of the artery or vein. Patch angioplasty can be used to repair injuries that are not circumferential or those that are partial thickness to vessels that are diseased with atherosclerosis. More severe forms of vascular trauma require replacement or bypass of the injured segment using a biologic or synthetic patch material or tubelike conduit.

Numerous types of conduits (ie, grafts) and patch materials are available, and surgeons should be familiar with their use and propensity to result in a good outcome in each injury situation. These materials can be considered as autografts, allografts, xenografts, synthetic, or bioengineered (Table 2). Sometimes, a bioengineered material or conduit is referred to as a regenerative medicine product. The ideal conduit should resemble in size the injured vessel and be readily available and easy to handle and sew. For injuries in which wound contamination is an issue, the vascular reconstruction material, be it for a patch or an interposition or bypass graft, should be resistant to infection and ideally incorporated by the recipient patient.

The most used autograft (ie, autologous conduit) is one of the patient's own superficial veins, most commonly the great saphenous. In most instances, the great saphenous is accessible, comes in adequate diameter and length, is relatively resistant to infection, and is likely to be incorporated, even in open and contaminated wounds. The great saphenous has demonstrated superior patency as a conduit compared with other types of materials, such as xenografts or synthetics [17]. Other superficial extremity veins, such as the cephalic

**Table 2**
Conduits for vascular reconstructions

| Conduit type | | Examples | Anatomic sites used | Advantages | Disadvantages |
|---|---|---|---|---|---|
| Autologous | Superficial vein | GSV, SSV, basilic and cephalic veins | Extremities<br>Cervical<br>Visceral vessels | Accessible<br>Low morbidity harvest<br>Infection resistant | Size mismatch<br>Limited availability in some patients |
| | Deep vein | FV, hypogastric vein, internal jugular vein | Aorta and iliac vessels<br>Cervical<br>Portal vein | Larger vessel reconstruction<br>Infection resistant<br>Useful multiple sites | Limited availability<br>Morbid harvesting<br>Limited length |
| | Arteries | Radial, hypogastric, SFA | Iliac vessels<br>Cervical<br>Extremity | Similar thickness for arterial reconstruction<br>Infection resistant | More morbid harvesting<br>Limited by length and donor site |
| Bioprosthetic | Cryopreserved venous allograft | Cryopreserved Saphenous vein | Extremities | Infection resistant<br>Good for bailout | Size limit<br>Lower patency rates<br>Biodegradation<br>Expensive<br>Thaw time |
| | Cryopreserved arterial allograft | Cryolife DTA, AOI, SFA-Pop | Aorta and iliac vessels<br>Extremities<br>Cervical<br>Visceral vessels | Vessel wall integrity<br>Variable diameters<br>Infection resistant | Expensive<br>Thaw time |
| | Cryopreserved xenografts | Bovine carotid artery | Extremities<br>Cervical<br>Visceral | Vessel wall integrity<br>Medium-size diameter<br>Infection resistant | Expensive<br>Thaw time |
| | Biosynthetic grafts | Omniflow<br>HAV | Extremities | Good for bailout<br>Infection resistant | Expensive<br>Low patency rates (historical)<br>Aneurysmal degeneration<br>No long-term follow-up |
| Prosthetic | PTFE<br>Dacron | Gore-Tex<br>Hemashield | Aorta and iliac vessels<br>Extremities<br>Visceral bypasses | Off the shelf availability<br>Multiple lengths, diameters, and configuration<br>Less morbidity on patient | Lower patency infrainguinal/ infragenicular compared with autologous<br>Infection prone |

*Abbreviations:* AOI, aortoiliac; DTA, descending thoracic aorta; FV, femoral vein; GSV, greater saphenous vein; SFA, superficial femoral artery; SFA-Pop, superficial femoral artery and popliteal; SSV, superficial saphenous vein.

and basilic and even the small saphenous, can be used when they are of appropriate diameter and able to be harvested. Deep veins, such as the femoral may be more suitable for reconstructing larger-caliber injuries but harvesting and preparing this conduit require more skill and experience. Deep vein harvest also is associated with a greater degree of venous hypertension and thus with higher rates of morbidity. Less commonly used autologous conduits include internal iliac and superficial femoral artery. In addition to inconsistent size and quality, and the time that it takes to harvest and prepare them, autologous veins require long extremity incisions, which themselves can become a problem.

Prosthetic materials have been used in elective vascular reconstruction for many decades. Expanded polytetrafluorethylene (PTFE) and Dacron come in different sizes, have predictable and uniform contour, and are available off the shel". Used as a patch or tube conduit, synthetic materials obviate the time it takes to harvest and prepare vein and spare the added morbidity associated with vein harvest incisions. The main drawback of synthetics is their propensity to become infected when used in the setting of open or contaminated wounds. Short of overt infection, synthetic materials often fail to become incorporated by the patient and are surrounded by a chronic biofilm or seroma. Despite years of research and development, synthetic materials do not become coated with a patient's own cells (ie, endothelialized) and thus they remain a functional foreign body for as long as they are in the patient.

Cryopreserved xenografts and cadaveric allografts have gained popularity over the past couple of decades and are readily available in some specialty medical centers. These biologic conduits are easy to handle and come in different lengths and diameters, and, although difficult to prove, it stands to reason that they are more resistant to infection than synthetics. Unfortunately, most xenografts and cadaveric allografts are more expensive than synthetics and in many health care systems they must be ordered individually or on a case-by-case basis. As discussed previously, in certain scenarios in which there is limited vessel damage xenograft material, such as bovine pericardium or autologous vein, can be used to patch the injury (ie, patch angioplasty).

The newly developed Human Acellular Vessel (HAV) (Humacyte, Durham, North Carolina) is a biologic conduit undergoing regulatory clinical study. A compelling regenerative medicine innovation, the HAV is composed of biologically silent human extracellular matrix derived from aortic smooth muscle cells grown to desired length and diameter in an organ chamber. This biologic product performed well in phase I and phase II clinical studies as a dialysis conduit and showed feasibility and reasonable durability as a bypass conduit for patients with peripheral arterial disease (PAD). Additional human study is being performed on the HAV as a conduit for use in vascular injury and the product is being studied in a wide range of real-world use cases under FDA expanded access provisions [18]. As a biologic, the HAV has the unique potential to be populated or incorporated by the patient's own cells and thus be more resistant to infection and prone to better patency. The predictable contour and size of the HAV, its potential to be off the shelf, and the fact that it avoids the morbidity and time associated with vein harvest all are appealing feature of this innovative product.

### Anticoagulation and Antiplatelet Use

Although it may sound counterintuitive to systemically anticoagulate exsanguinating patients, thrombosis in vascular injuries can be detrimental. Not all patients can be anticoagulated systemically and, as such, this decision should be individualized. When even small doses of systemic anticoagulation are contraindicated, flushing the involved vessel with heparinized saline and frequent back and fore bleeding can prevent vessel thrombosis. Data from multiple large multi-institutional studies present conflicting outcomes regarding anticoagulation and patency [19,20]; however, the authors' preference is to give the minimal amount of systemic anticoagulation, if possible. If possible, trauma patients who have undergone vascular reconstruction ideally are placed on a low-dose aspirin for antiplatelet therapy as well as deep vein thrombosis mechanical and pharmacologic prophylaxis. The traumatic inflammatory response has been widely recognized to promote thrombosis, whether anastomotic or deep venous [21].

## ANATOMIC REGIONS

### Extremity injuries

Extremity trauma requiring vascular reconstruction often is readily identifiable from physical examination. More proximal vasculature entering the chest, or the pelvis can be more challenging to identify and may fall within the realm of torso vascular injuries rather than peripheral. The goals of management should be hemorrhage control first and foremost, revascularization of the ischemic extremity, and limb salvage with minimal future disability. If a patient presents with hard signs of vascular injury (see Table 1), immediate surgical exploration in the operating room with the availability of endovascular approach should be adopted. Soft signs of vascular injuries may allow time for further diagnostic imaging prior to proceeding to the operating room. Decisions for immediate repair or reconstruction versus temporary shunting are dictated by the patient's overall physiologic status in the presence of other devastating injuries. Depending on length of ischemic time or the presence of crush injury, the surgeon should decide whether the patient requires an extremity fasciotomy prior to leaving the operating room. If fasciotomies are not performed, the patient should be monitored closely for signs of developing compartment syndromes after reperfusion. If a patient's neurologic status does not permit early detection of compartment syndrome, it is recommended that prophylactic fasciotomies are performed, especially in long ischemic times and combined arterial and venous reconstructions. Ligation of the deep venous system also should prompt prophylactic fasciotomies because compartment syndrome can develop from outflow obstruction.

Reconstruction of the vascular disruption in the extremity is highly dependent on the extent of the injury, location, and arterial branches. Small focal injuries may be amenable to primary repair. Slightly larger injuries may require extension of the arteriotomy or venotomy with a patch angioplasty. If neither is feasible, and the length of the injury is small, an end-to-end anastomosis should be performed. Débridement of the vessel edges in addition to proximal and distal mobilization with spatulating both ends aid in this end-to-end anastomosis. This should be done without tension on the anastomosis with the full range of motion of the extremities. If the extent of the injury prevents all of these, then a bypass is employed with an autogenous vein preferably. The proximal and distal targets of a bypass are dictated by the extent of the injury. For example, injury to the proximal axillary artery or proximal common femoral artery necessitates further central access to the subclavian artery or external iliac arteries. In certain scenarios, to avoid longer incisions or more morbid exposures, proximal balloon occlusion can be employed for proximal control. Venous injuries ideally should be repaired, especially if it involves the deep venous system of the extremity. Vascular shunts also could be used to stage the repair or bypass. Ligation of deep veins can have high morbidity and should be performed only in situations where reconstruction is not feasible.

*Upper extremity*

The axillary artery starts at the lateral margin of the first rib and extends to the lateral edge of the teres major muscle. It can be susceptible to penetrating traumatic injuries as well as blunt injuries associated with shoulder trauma. Proximal exposure may be required via an infraclavicular and supraclavicular incisions to gain control. If more proximal subclavian artery control is required, the patient will require access to the thoracic cavity unless balloon occlusion is feasible. The mid to distal axillary artery can be approached through an infraclavicular incision. While exposing the axillary artery or vein, great caution should be taken to avoid brachial nerve injuries. Missed or iatrogenic brachial plexus nerve injuries can have devastating functional outcomes.

The brachial artery starts at the lower margin of the teres major and runs in the anterior compartment of the arm alongside with the median nerve. The basilic and brachial veins accompany and often cross over the artery. This artery can be injured in both penetrating traumas as well as a blunt trauma causing humeral fractures. Frequently, the brachial arteries main proximal branch the profunda brachii can provide significant perfusion to the distal upper extremity if it remains intact.

Both the radial and ulnar arteries are terminal branches of the brachial artery with variable points of bifurcations among patients. Radial artery travels in the anterior compartment until it runs deep into the deep palmar arch. Ulnar arteries usually are the larger terminal artery and once at the wrist forms the superficial palmar arch joining the deep palmar arch. The standard blood pressure cuff or a tourniquet usually can be used for proximal control. If both these arteries are injured, the priority is to repair at least 1, usually the ulnar dominant artery. If the patient has intact deep and superficial arches, a single arterial runoff should be sufficient for distal perfusion. Superficial veins of the upper extremities can be ligated if the injuries are devastating. They also can be used as a conduit for bypass if they are of adequate quality and diameter. The use of covered stents for repair of subclavian-axillary artery injuries remains controversial and used only in highly selective scenarios [22,23].

*Lower extremity*

Traumatic injury of the femoral artery constitutes 20% of all traumatic arterial injuries, supracondylar femur and tibial plateau fractures are associated with superficial femoral and popliteal injuries. For proximal femoral control on initial evaluation, digital pressure against the femur head can control exsanguination. For more distal injuries, appropriately applied tourniquets do the job. Both the assistant's hand and the tourniquet can be prepped into the operative field.

Exposure of the femoral artery involves a longitudinal incision over the anterior aspect of the thigh, through the soft tissue and opening the femoral sheath. This incision can be extended proximally with division of the inguinal ligament for an extraperitoneal exposure of the external iliac arteries. Through that incision, the surgeon can access the profunda and superficial femoral arteries. For superficial femoral artery exposure, a medial incision over the length of the Sartorius muscle is made, and, if extended distally, it allows supragenicular access of the popliteal artery. Below the knee access of the popliteal artery is performed through medial leg incision retracting the gastrocnemius and soleus muscles posteriorly. This incision also gives access to the takeoff of the anterior tibial artery in addition to the tibioperoneal trunk and posterior tibial arteries. For isolated popliteal vascular injuries, a soft bump is placed under the flexed knee with hip slightly externally rotated. This allows for below and above the knee access to the popliteal vessels through medial incisions. Completion angiography is recommended in most situations to evaluate tibial outflow. Simple repair, patch angioplasty, or interposition grafts are mainstays for femoropopliteal arteries. Although vein conduit generally is preferred, prosthetic graft can be used when necessary. This is useful especially when dealing with larger-diameter arteries with adequate muscle coverage above the knee joint. Arterial ligation should be avoided when possible because it is associated with high rates of amputations. Repair and bypass for deep venous injuries also should be performed when feasible using contralateral saphenous vein. Again, the use of covered stents for management of isolated femoropopliteal arterial injury remains controversial with anecdotal reports [23].

Single terminal artery injury can be ligated in an otherwise healthy patient without peripheral vascular disease. Anterior tibial artery can be accessed for repair or bypass through a lateral leg incision if necessary while the posterior tibial and peroneal arteries through a medial incision.

## Cervical

The neck traditionally is divided into 3 zones to identify which arteries and structures are at risk of injury. Zone I is from the thoracic inlet to the cricoid cartilage, zone II is between the cricoid and the angle of the mandible, and zone III is above the angle of the mandible to the base of the skull. The carotid and vertebral arteries are at risk of injury in all 3 zones [24], and hard signs of vascular injury should prompt immediate exploration. Along with the cervical arteries, the jugular veins, vagus and hypoglossal nerves, and aerodigestive tracts can be injured through the same mechanisms.

Zone II injuries are the most common in penetrating neck traumas, with approximately 20% vascular injuries. If there are no hard signs of vascular injury, patients can be evaluated by CT angiograms prior to operative intervention with very high sensitivity and specificity [25–27]. Exploration of these injuries is best obtained through a lateral neck incision along the anterior border of the sternocleidomastoid muscle. Occasionally, a collar incision can be utilized if both sides of the neck are involved by the injury. Zone I injuries with hard signs may indicate great vessel injury, necessitating a median sternotomy for proximal control and repair. Zone III injuries are more difficult to expose using an open approach and may require subluxation of the mandible or mandibulotomy. Endovascular or hybrid strategies can be lifesaving in high injuries inaccessible to open repair [28].

Exposure with proximal and distal control of the carotid artery should be performed expeditiously. The internal carotid artery always should be repaired because there is a high reported mortality with ligation (up to 45%) [29]. Stab wounds often can be repaired primarily or with a patch as dictated by the degree of vessel disruption. Ballistic injuries typically require segmental resection with an interposition graft. Greater saphenous vein should be used as conduit whenever possible. Heparinization with or without shunting is utilized during these repairs unless major contraindications exist in the multi-injured trauma patient. The external carotid artery can be ligated without significant consequence. It is imperative to look for possible dissection flaps in the internal carotid artery. This can be performed via intraoperative ultrasonography if available. Missed dissection flaps may lead to thrombosis and devastating strokes. The internal jugular vein can be ligated in an emergent setting but, if possible, should be repaired, especially if injury is bilateral.

Zone III injuries are more difficult to expose using an open approach and can require subluxation of the mandible or mandibulotomy. Endovascular or hybrid strategies can be lifesaving in high injuries inaccessible to open repair. For common carotid and internal carotid artery repair patch with vein with or bovine carotid patch can be performed for focal injuries. If bypass is required, autogenous vein graft usually is preferred. If the vein graft is not of adequate diameter, then other autogenous or bioprosthetic can be used (see Table 2). It is highly encouraged to use either vein or bio prosthetic specially in scenarios where there is contamination from aerodigestive injury, in addition to obtaining muscular cutaneous coverage for the graft.

Vertebral artery injuries often are associated with cervical spine transverse process fractures, subluxations, or penetrating injuries to the back of the neck. Open exposure is similar to that for the common carotid artery however more lateral and often requires the ligation of the vertebral vein. After the sternocleidomastoid and anterior scalene muscles are mobilized, the vertebral artery can be isolated and ligated proximally after its takeoff from the subclavian artery. Control of the foraminal or extradural portions, is more challenging in open approach and may require compression against transverse foramina. In this procedure, care must be taken to avoid injury to the phrenic nerve and thoracic duct. When feasible and available, proximal and distal control of a more distal vertebral artery injury may be facilitated by endovascular techniques as with a zone III carotid injury. In a recent review of the contemporary management of combat-related vertebral artery injuries, injuries included occlusion, pseudoaneurysms, dissection, and arteriovenous fistula. Injury was most commonly in the V2 segment, and treatment included coils and covered stents [30].

Blunt cerebral vascular injury (BCVI) includes both carotid and vertebral injuries. Although BCVI represents less than 1% of admissions for blunt trauma, these injuries can lead to mortality rates from 23% to 28% with 48% to 58% of survivors having permanent severe neurologic deficits. Given the high morbidity of unrecognized BCVI in the asymptomatic patient, many screening protocols recommend screening CTA in trauma patients presenting with petrous bone fractures, diffuse axonal injury, Glasgow Coma Scale score less than 8, complex C1 to C2 cervical fractures, and Le Fort II or III facial fractures. Treatment is dictated by the severity of the injury as defined by the Biffl grading score [31,32] (Table 3). Although no prospective data exist to define optimal treatment regiments, low-grade injuries should be treated with antithrombotic agents such as aspirin or heparin. Grade III injuries rarely resolve with observation and medical therapy alone; therefore, surgical therapy should be considered. Patients presenting with severe deficits generally do not improve with revascularization. Injury severity of carotid artery correlated with stroke risk in contrast to vertebral artery injury where grade severity was independent from stroke risk.

### Torso

The difficulty in managing torso vascular injuries lies in that these present as noncompressible hemorrhage, which carries a high rate of mortality [1,33]. Initial management is dictated by the patient's hemodynamics. Patient with profound hemodynamic collapse or witnessed cardiac arrest need more aggressive surgical exploration, such as a resuscitative thoracotomy. This exposure can provide the surgeon with the release of possible tamponade, control of massive air leaks if present, thoracic aortic clamping, and internal cardiac massage. The thoracotomy incision can be extended to the contralateral side to become a high clamshell thoracotomy. This usually is performed at the level of the inframammary crease around the fourth intercostal space. Attention should be taken not to injure the phrenic nerve while opening the pericardium longitudinally. Injuries to zone I of the neck or subclavian arteries also require either clamshell thoracotomy or median sternotomy for proximal control.

*Thoracic cavity*

Patients with vascular traumatic injury to the aortic arch and its major branches often present in hemorrhagic shock requiring immediate surgical intervention. Unstable patients would require immediate tube thoracostomies, resuscitative thoracotomy, or median sternotomy. Penetrating thoracic cavity trauma that caused vascular traumatic injuries usually is associated with multiple other injuries. In that scenario, median sternotomy provides the widest versatile exposure for these arch vessels with the exception of the proximal left subclavian artery, which is best approach via left anterior lateral thoracotomy. Ligation of the innominate vein may facilitate rapid exposure of the ascending aorta and pericardium for repair of any possible cardiac injury. It is wise to involve cardiothoracic surgery if such an injury is suspected, which may require hypothermic circulatory arrest for repair. The descending thoracic aorta and pulmonary hilum can be approached via left anterolateral thoracotomy. If the patient is stable, a left posterolateral thoracotomy would be ideal.

For blunt thoracic aortic injuries management is dictated by the radiological grading of the injury if the patient is hemodynamically stable. Injury commonly occurs at the site of the descending thoracic aorta distal to the ligamentum arteriosum and can range from small intimal tear, intramural hematoma, contained pseudoaneurysm, or ruptured pseudoaneurysm. Ruptured or contained pseudoaneurysm, grade III and grade IV injury, dictates immediate surgical repair. This has shifted over the past 2 decades toward endovascular repair [14,34]. If necessary, the origin of the left subclavian artery can be covered with the thoracic endograft [34]. If the patient develops postoperative left upper extremity ischemia, a carotid subclavian bypass can be performed subsequently. For small intimal tears or intramural hematomas, grades I and grade II, the patient should be admitted to the ICU. These patients require very close blood pressure and heart rate control preventing shear stress from extending the injury. The patients should undergo reimaging within 24 hours to 48 hours if they are hemodynamically stable to determine whether the injury has evolved or remained stable. If the patient is unstable for endovascular repair, or not possible, then open repair with an interposition graft should be performed. Great venous injuries also should be repaired or patched if possible. There have been more reports as well in managing isolated subclavian artery injuries via endovascular covered stents.

*Abdomen and retroperitoneum*

Abdominal vasculature traditionally has been divided into intra-abdominal and retroperitoneal. The retroperitoneal is further divided into 4 surgical zones. Zone I is centrally located containing the aorta and its major branches as well as the inferior vena cava (IVC). This is divided further into the

**Table 3**
Biffl grading score of blunt cerebral vascular injury and prognosis

| Grade | Description | Stroke Risk: Carotid (%) | Stroke Risk: Vertebral (%) |
|---|---|---|---|
| I | Luminal irregularity, dissection with <25% narrowing | 8 | 6 |
| II | Dissection or IMH with >25% thrombus, intraluminal thrombus or raised intimal flap | 14 | 38 |
| III | Pseudoaneurysm, AV fistula | 26 | 27 |
| IV | Occlusion | 50 | 28 |
| V | Transection with free extravasation | 100 | — |

*Abbreviations:* AV, arteriovenous; IMH, intramural hematoma.

supramesocolic and inframesocolic areas. Zone II involves the left and the right retroperitoneum, which contains the kidneys and the renal vasculature. Zone III contains the pelvis and injuries in that area largely involve the iliac vessels. Zone IV includes the perihepatic vasculature and retrohepatic IVC.

When abdominal or retroperitoneal vascular injury is suspected, the abdomen should be opened through a midline incision from xiphoid to pubic symphysis to permit unhindered access to all 4 quadrants. Initial packing of all 4 quadrants obtains initial hemostasis and permits further resuscitation. In penetrating traumas, all retroperitoneal hematomas should be explored with the exception of zone IV retrohepatic IVC injuries. In blunt trauma zone I, hematomas should be opened. Proximal control should be obtained from the supraceliac aorta at the diaphragmatic hiatus. If the hematoma extends to the diaphragmatic hiatus, then either open thoracic aortic clamp should be utilized or placement of aortic occlusive balloon, such as the ER-REBOA catheter (Prytime Medical, Boerne, TX). Supramesocolic bleeding should be explored via wide left medial visceral rotation mobilizing the left colon, spleen, tail of pancreas, and left kidney (Mattox maneuver). If IVC bleeding is suspected in that area, right medial visceral rotation should be performed (Cattell-Braasch maneuver). Zone II injuries likely involve the kidney and the renal arteries. If there is a devastating injury to the renal hilum or renal parenchyma, a nephrectomy may be required. Zone III injuries should be explored if there are any signs concerning for a large vessel injury, such as expanding hematomas. Zone IV injuries should not be explored unless there is exsanguination, and shunting usually is required for repair. These injuries notoriously carry high mortality rates, even in level 1 trauma centers. Intra-abdominal mesenteric hematomas should be explored if there is ischemic bowel and to rule out injuries to the superior mesenteric artery. The porta hepatis can be explored as well if there is evidence of hepatic ischemia.

Reconstruction of any major vessel should utilize autogenous vein, typically the greater saphenous vein, especially in the presence of contaminated field. If there is no adequate diameter vein, then cryograft can be utilized. In the setting of damage control surgery, large vasculature can be shunted while the patient returns to the ICU for further resuscitation. Small venous injuries can be ligated; however, larger veins should be repaired whenever possible. Aortic injuries can be repaired primarily if feasible, patch angioplasty or interposition graft. In cases of abdominal contamination, femoral vein usually is an adequate conduit. For iliac artery and vein injuries, primary repair or patch angioplasty is performed when feasible. If intact, the hypogastric artery can be used as an interposition conduit to repair large common iliac injuries. When in-line reconstruction is not possible, extra-anatomic reconstruction can be performed.

Endovascular repair of abdominal blunt traumatic injuries also is emerging as a possible treatment option in very specific scenarios. Isolated aortic pseudoaneurysms and iliac artery pseudoaneurysms or dissections, can be managed with endovascular covered stents in stable patients. Furthermore, endovascular coil embolization of seecond-order and third-order order pelvic vasculature has changed the management of zone III bleeding greatly.

## SUMMARY

Vascular injury remains the leading cause of morbidity and mortality in civilian and military settings. Torso injuries are especially dangerous as they are not immediately compressible and can quickly lead to shock and death. Survival is dependent on proximity to care provided by a team versed in the principles of bleeding control, resuscitation, diagnosis, and operative management. Familiarity with operative exposure and open vascular reconstruction is instrumental for good outcomes, although there is an expanding role for less invasive endovascular approaches for resuscitation and repair. While definitive management may be best provided at a well-resourced, high volume medical center, the importance of prehospital care, early resuscitation and damage control surgery cannot be overstated as key factors in the survival and recovery of patients with vascular trauma.

## CLINICS CARE POINTS

- If a patient has evidence of exsanguination from extremities, direct pressure or properly placed tourniquets can be lifesaving as well as limb saving
- If a patient is manifesting signs of noncompressible hemorrhagic injuries, aortic occlusive balloons can be placed by trained practitioners
- Patients presenting with signs of high kinetic energy injuries (facial fractures, rib fractures, and so forth), should undergo imaging evaluation for blunt vascular injuries.

- If hard signs of vascular injury are present, it is essential to promptly take the patient to an operating room.
- Patients who have multiple other injuries and are hypothermic, coagulopathic, and acidotic benefit from temporary vascular shunts and delayed repairs or reconstructions
- In cases of need for a vascular reconstruction, autogenous veins are the preferred.
- If autogenous vein is not adequate or available, bioprosthetics (allografts or xenografts) can be used.

## References

[1] Eastridge BJ, Mabry RL, Seguin P, et al. Death on the battlefield (2001-2011): Implications for the future of combat casualty care. J Trauma Acute Care 2012;73:S431–7.
[2] Mattox KL, Feliciano DV, Burch J, et al. Five thousand seven hundred sixty cardiovascular injuries in 4459 patients. Epidemiologic evolution 1958 to 1987. Ann Surg 1989;209(6):698–705 [discussion: 6–7].
[3] White JM, Stannard A, Burkhardt GE, et al. The epidemiology of vascular injury in the wars in Iraq and Afghanistan. Ann Surg 2011;253(6):1184–9.
[4] Bulger EM, Kuhls DA, Campbell BT, et al. Proceedings from the Medical Summit on Firearm Injury Prevention: A Public Health Approach to Reduce Death and Disability in the US. J Am Coll Surg 2019;229(4):415–430 e12.
[5] Brenner M, Teeter W, Hoehn M, et al. Use of resuscitative endovascular balloon occlusion of the aorta for proximal aortic control in patients with severe hemorrhage and arrest. JAMA Surg 2018;153(2):130–5.
[6] Das JM, Anosike K, Waseem M. Permissive Hypotension (2020). *StatPearls [Internet].*
[7] Sise M. Diagnosis of vascular injury. In: Todd Rasmussen NT, editor. Rich's vascular Trauma. 3rd edition. Philadelphia: Elsevier; 2016. p. 35–43.
[8] Dawson D. Imaging for the evaluation and treatment of vascular trauma. In: Todd Rasmussen NT, editor. Rich's vascular trauma. 3rd edition. Philadelphia: Elsevier; 2016. p. 44–55.
[9] Frykberg ER. Advances in the diagnosis and treatment of extremity vascular trauma. Surg Clin North Am 1995;75(2):207–23.
[10] Frykberg ER, Dennis JW, Bishop K, et al. The reliability of physical examination in the evaluation of penetrating extremity trauma for vascular injury: results at one year. J Trauma 1991;31(4):502–11.
[11] Loftus TJ, Croft CA, Rosenthal MD, et al. Clinical impact of a dedicated trauma hybrid operating room. J Am Coll Surg 2020;232(4):560–70.
[12] Kirkpatrick AW, Vis C, Dube M, et al. The evolution of a purpose designed hybrid trauma operating room from the trauma service perspective: the RAPTOR (Resuscitation with Angiography Percutaneous Treatments and Operative Resuscitations). Injury 2014;45(9): 1413–21.
[13] Polcz JE, White JM, Ronaldi AE, et al. Temporary intravascular shunt use improves early limb salvage after extremity vascular injury. J Vasc Surg 2020;73(4):1304–13.
[14] Neschis DG, Scalea TM, Flinn WR, et al. Blunt aortic injury. N Engl J Med 2008;359(16): 1708–16.
[15] White R, Krajcer Z, Johnson M, et al. Results of a multicenter trial for the treatment of traumatic vascular injury with a covered stent. J Trauma 2006;60(6):1189–95 [discussion: 95–6].
[16] Chopra A, Modrall JG, Knowles M, et al. Uncertain patency of covered stents placed for traumatic axillosubclavian artery injury. J Am Coll Surg 2016;223(1):174–83.

[17] Nguyen KP, Moneta G, Landry G. Venous conduits have superior patency compared with prosthetic grafts for femorofemoral bypass. Ann Vasc Surg 2018;52:126–37.
[18] Gutowski P, Gage SM, Guziewicz M, et al. Arterial reconstruction with human bioengineered acellular blood vessels in patients with peripheral arterial disease. J Vasc Surg 2020;72(4):1247–58.
[19] Maher Z, Frank B, Saillant N, et al. Systemic intraoperative anticoagulation during arterial injury repair: Implications for patency and bleeding. J Trauma Acute Care Surg 2017;82(4):680–6.
[20] Loja MN, Galante JM, Humphries M, et al. Systemic anticoagulation in the setting of vascular extremity trauma. Injury 2017;48(9):1911–6.
[21] Barrera LM, Perel P, Ker K, et al. Thromboprophylaxis for trauma patients. Cochrane Database Syst Rev 2013;3:CD008303.
[22] Gill H, Jenkins W, Edu S, et al. Civilian penetrating axillary artery injuries. World J Surg 2011;35(5):962–6.
[23] Desai SS, DuBose JJ, Parham CS, et al. Outcomes after endovascular repair of arterial trauma. J Vasc Surg 2014;60(5):1309–14.
[24] Nunez DB Jr, Torres-Leon M, Munera F. Vascular injuries of the neck and thoracic inlet: helical CT-angiographic correlation. Radiographics 2004;24(4):1087–98 [discussion: 99–100].
[25] Inaba K, Munera F, McKenney M, et al. Prospective evaluation of screening multislice helical computed tomographic angiography in the initial evaluation of penetrating neck injuries. J Trauma 2006;61(1):144–9.
[26] Munera F, Soto JA, Nunez D. Penetrating injuries of the neck and the increasing role of CTA. Emerg Radiol 2004;10(6):303–9.
[27] Munera F, Soto JA, Palacio D, et al. Diagnosis of arterial injuries caused by penetrating trauma to the neck: comparison of helical CT angiography and conventional angiography. Radiology 2000;216(2):356–62.
[28] Cohen JE, Ben-Hur T, Rajz G, et al. Endovascular stent-assisted angioplasty in the management of traumatic internal carotid artery dissections. Stroke 2005;36(4):e45–7.
[29] du Toit DF, van Schalkwyk GD, Wadee SA, et al. Neurologic outcome after penetrating extracranial arterial trauma. J Vasc Surg 2003;38(2):257–62.
[30] Greer LT, Kuehn RB, Gillespie DL, et al. Contemporary management of combat-related vertebral artery injuries. J Trauma Acute Care Surg 2013;74(3):818–24.
[31] Biffl WL, Moore EE, Offner PJ, et al. Blunt carotid arterial injuries: implications of a new grading scale. J Trauma 1999;47(5):845–53.
[32] Biffl WL, Moore EE, Ryu RK, et al. The unrecognized epidemic of blunt carotid arterial injuries: early diagnosis improves neurologic outcome. Ann Surg 1998;228(4):462–70.
[33] Kotwal RS, Montgomery HR, Kotwal BM, et al. Eliminating preventable death on the battlefield. Arch Surg 2011;146(12):1350–8.
[34] Skripochnik E, Novikov D, Bilfinger TJ, et al. Short-term results of left subclavian artery salvage in blunt thoracic aortic injury with short proximal landing zones. J Vasc Surg 2018;68(4):985–90.

Advances in Surgery 55 (2021) 273–297
ADVANCES IN SURGERY

# Evolution of Point-Of-Care Ultrasound in Surgical Management

William A. Teeter, MD[a,*], Thomas Scalea, MD[b]

[a]Department of Emergency Medicine, University of Maryland School of Medicine, Program in Trauma and Critical Care, R Adams Cowley Shock Trauma Center, 22 S. Greene Street, T1R51, Baltimore, MD 21201, USA; [b]R Adams Cowley Shock Trauma Center, University of Maryland Medical System, Program in Trauma, University of Maryland School of Medicine, 22 S. Greene Street, T1R51, Baltimore, MD 21201, USA

**Keywords**

• Echocardiography • Focused assessment with sonography for trauma (FAST) • Focused rapid echocardiographic examination (FREE) • Ultrasound • Resuscitation

**Key points**

- The focused assessment with sonography for trauma (FAST) examination is now common practice in the initial evaluation of trauma patients.
- Inclusion of thoracic imaging in the extended FAST (eFAST) examination improves sensitivity and specificity for the detection of clinically significant pneumothorax.
- The FAST examination includes 4 major views, specifically cardiac, left upper quadrant, right upper quadrant, and pelvic. The eFAST examination includes thoracic views.
- Bedside echocardiography includes the parasternal long and short views, the apical 4 and 5 chamber views, and assessment of the inferior vena cava.
- Bedside echocardiography allows for assessment of fluid responsiveness, fluid overload, and estimation of hemodynamic indices.

## FOCUSED ASSESSMENT WITH SONOGRAPHY FOR TRAUMA

The first use of ultrasound for the diagnosis of intraabdominal injury was described by Kristensen [1] in 1972 with subsequent work by Asher and colleagues [2] in 1976, demonstrating a sensitivity of 80% in the detection of splenic injury in blunt trauma. The technique then fell out of favor until

*Corresponding author. *E-mail address:* william.teeter@som.umaryland.edu

https://doi.org/10.1016/j.yasu.2021.05.018
0065-3411/21/

1991 when Kimura and colleagues demonstrated that ultrasound can detect hemoperitoneum following blunt abdominal trauma with a specificity of 86.7% and sensitivity of 100%. Further, Tso and colleagues [3] demonstrated similar results in 1992 with a sensitivity of 69% specificity of 99% of the detection of "clinically significant hemoperitoneum." The use of POCUS for the detection of intraperitoneal fluid after trauma was subsequently developed into the focused assessment with sonography for trauma (FAST) examination [4–6]. Eventually, the FAST examination was included in the Advanced Trauma Life Support training course in 1996 and is now used widely in the evaluation of trauma patients with about 90% sensitivity for detecting any intraperitoneal free fluid. A "high-quality" examination reliably detects about 200 mL of free intraperitoneal fluid [7], with sensitivity improving with the inclusion of its multiple examination sites [8] (Table 1). Subsequently in 2004, Kirkpatrick and colleagues [9] proposed the inclusion of thoracic imaging in the extended FAST (eFAST) examination, improving sensitivity (95.3%) and specificity (91.1%) for the detection of clinically significant pneumothorax over plain radiographs, with a reported negative predictive value of 100% [10]. The eFAST examination is now common practice in the initial evaluation of trauma patients.

## PATIENT PLACEMENT

As virtually every seriously injured trauma patient arrives for evaluation to the trauma bay supine, the eFAST examination has naturally been studied and validated in this position. However, variations in patient position can improve ultrasonographic windows, such as placing the patient in the left lateral decubitus position for parasternal and apical views of the heart or placing the patient in Trendelenburg for intraabdominal views of the eFAST. However, although placing the patient in these alternate positions may improve the sensitivity of the examination overall, any view of the pericardial space can effectively rule

**Table 1**
Components, probe placement, and probe selection of extended focused assessment for sonography for trauma examination

| Examination | Probe placement | Preferred probe |
|---|---|---|
| Pericardium | Subcostal | Phased array, curvilinear |
| Morison's's pouch | Right upper quadrant | |
| Splenorenal recess | Left upper quadrant | |
| Pouch of Douglas | Pelvic | Curvilinear, phased array |
| Lung apex | Bilateral midclavicular lines near ICS 2 | Linear probe |
| Lung base | Bilateral midaxillary lines at diaphragmatic recesses | |

*Abbreviation:* ICS, intercostal space.
Phased array and curvilinear, low-frequency probes (1–5 MHz); linear, high frequency (~10 MHz).

out a significant pericardial tamponade, and the complete examination has a sensitivity that is virtually 100% for detecting volumes of intraperitoneal hemorrhage that are capable of causing shock and thus requiring emergent laparotomy in the supine position [5,6].

## EVALUATION OF THE HEART AND PERICARDIUM

### Subxiphoid view

To evaluate the heart and pericardium one may use either the phased array or the curvilinear probes that are relatively low-frequency, allowing easier resolution of tissue and fluid. The probe is placed immediately below the xiphoid process, angling up approximately 20° to 45° and pointing through the heart toward the left shoulder (Fig. 1). Downward pressure may need to be applied in the protuberant abdomen to obtain a satisfactory view. Fig. 2 demonstrates the major cardiac structures, including the right ventricle (RV), left ventricle (LV), intraventricular septum (IVS), pericardium, and pericardial space. Fig. 3 shows a subxiphoid view with evident pericardial effusion. Blue star shows collapsed RV free wall. Red line indicates normal position of free wall.

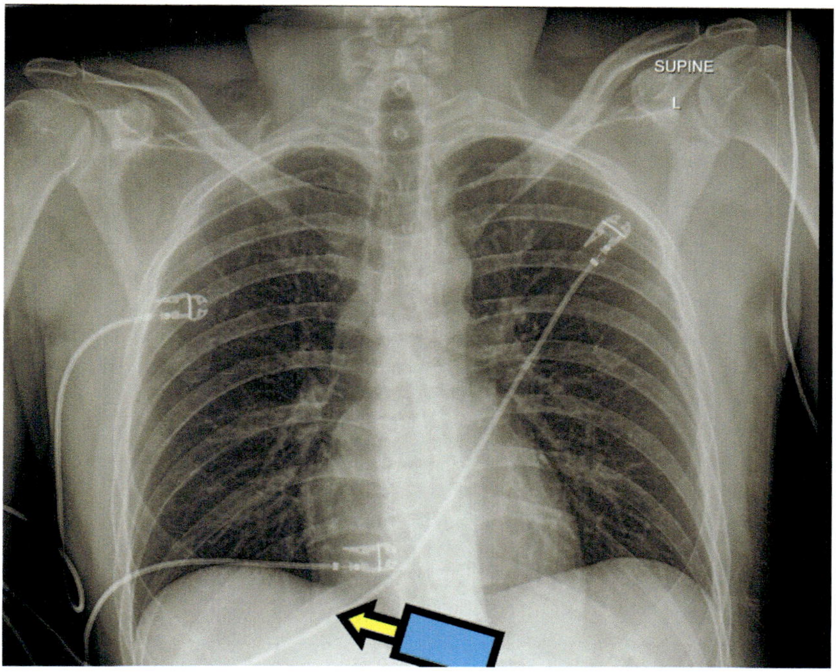


**Fig. 1.** Placement of phased array (or curvilinear) ultrasound probe (blue box) for subxiphoid view as part of the FAST, with indicator pointed to the patients right (*yellow arrow*) overlayed on a chest radiograph.

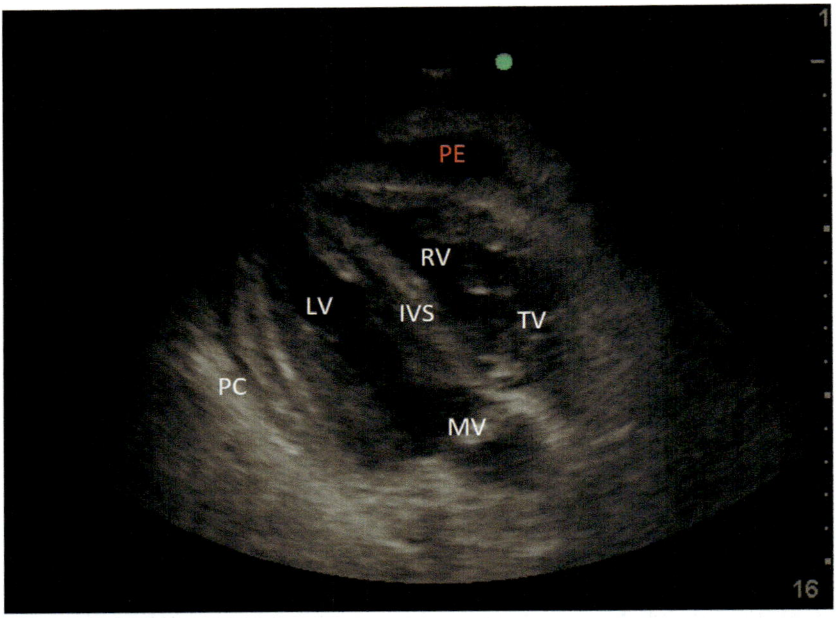


**Fig. 2.** Subxiphoid view of the heart for FAST showing cardiac structures with pericardial effusion (PE).

The following figure shows a subxiphoid view of the heart with near total end-diastolic right ventricular collapse (blue arrowhead) consistent with pericardial tamponade (Fig. 4).

### Parasternal long view

If the subxiphoid view cannot be achieved, one may instead examine the heart in the parasternal long window. To achieve this view, place the probe (blue box) in the second intercostal space at the left parasternal border with the indicator pointing toward the right shoulder (yellow arrow, Fig. 5), then moving inferiorly (black arrow) early until the cardiac structures can be identified (Fig. 6). When evaluating the heart and pericardium using ultrasound, one must note that an anterior fat pad on the cardiac surface can give the impression of a pericardial effusion but will be lacking on the posterior border of the heart.

## MORISON'S'S POUCH

To evaluate the right upper quadrant and Morison's pouch, with the patient supine, a low-frequency probe is placed longitudinally in the seventh or eighth intercostal space (sometimes as low as the 11th) at the midaxillary line below the diaphragmatic recess and probe marker cephalad, which will allow visualization of the kidney and liver and the hepatorenal space named Morison's pouch. One may need to fan anteriorly and posteriorly to identify the

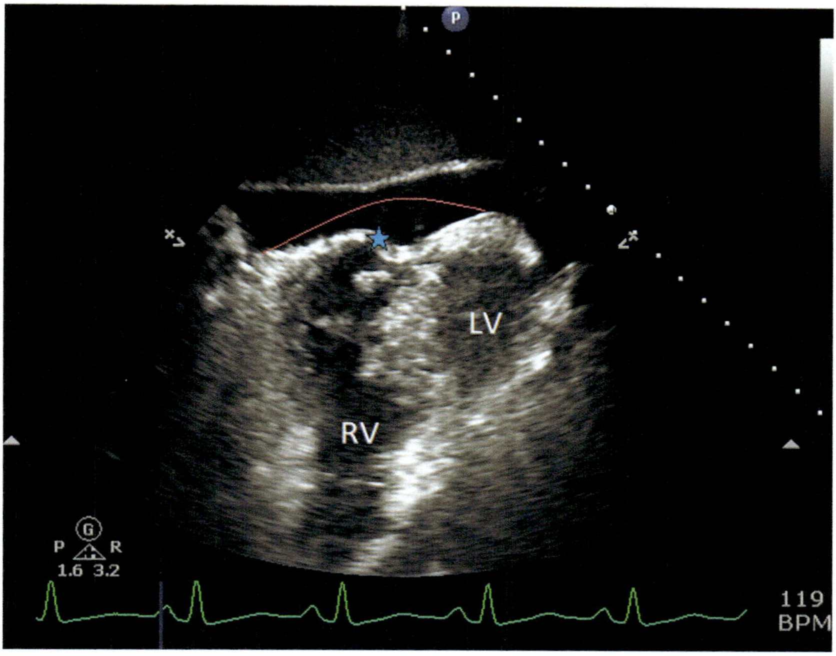


**Fig. 3.** Subxiphoid view of the heart for FAST showing large pericardial effusion (PE). Note: normal anatomy is distorted by tamponade physiology.

structures, usually moving the probe posterior on the flank or caudally to identify the caudal tip of the liver (blue arrow, Fig. 7). The following figures show a normal right upper quadrant examination on the left and the presence of free fluid in Morison's pouch, which will appear an anechoic or black stripe (Fig. 8). One must visualize the caudal tip of the liver to be a diagnostic examination.

## SPLENORENAL RECESS

To evaluate the left upper quadrant for intraperitoneal hemorrhage, a low-frequency probe is placed longitudinally in the sixth or seventh intercostal space of the midaxillary line (can be as low as the nineth intercoastal space) with the marker probe cephalad, visualizing the left kidney and spleen and fanning anteriorly and posteriorly to identify the splenorenal space. Fig. 9 shows the a normal-appearing left upper quadrant FAST examination on the left and the anechoic, black strip of free fluid found on a pathologic scan on the right (Fig. 10).

## POUCH OF DOUGLAS

To visualize the pelvic view of the eFAST examination and fluid in the pouch of Douglas, 2 views must be obtained to increase the chances of detecting free

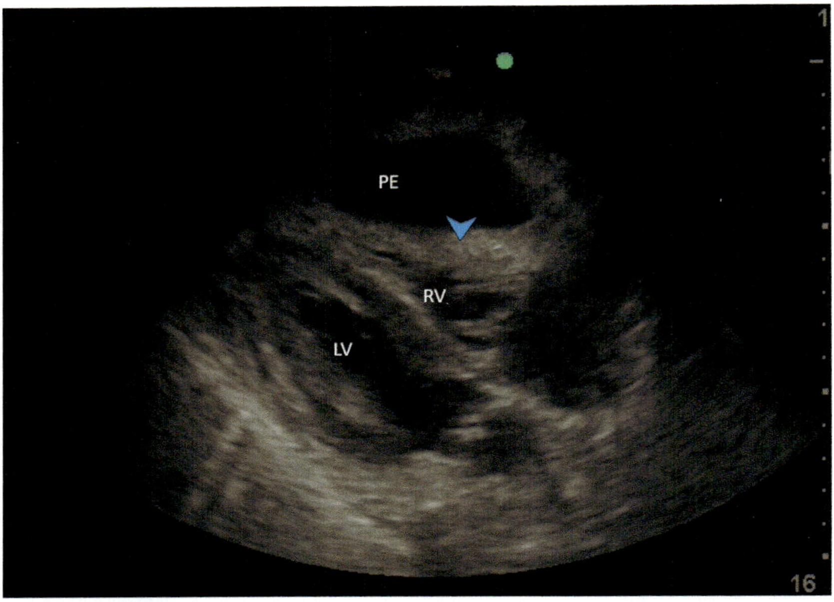


**Fig. 4.** Subxiphoid view of the heart for FAST showing large pericardial effusion (PE) and tamponade physiology.

fluid. For this view, a curvilinear probe is prefered but can be easily done with the phased array probe, which are both low-frequency probes. Although the curvilinear probe may visualize these views better in the authors' opinion, it does require changing probes amid the FAST examination and possibly chaotic trauma resuscitation. To obtain adequate views, the low-frequency probe should be placed just superior to the pubic symphysis with the indicator pointed cephalad. In this view, when full, the bladder will appear as a triangular anechoic (dark) structure immediately cephalad to the pubic bone, which can be identified by the shadowing created on the right side of ultrasound image (Fig. 11). To obtain the transverse view of the bladder, rotate the probe 90° counterclockwise with the marker pointing to the patient's right. You will note in Fig. 12 that the bladder now seems rectangular or even trapezoidal. Note: in the absence of possible urethral trauma, it may be necessary to instill fluid in a patient's bladder to achieve an adequate view, as imaging the pelvis with an empty bladder reduces its sensitivity. In Fig. 12, there is free fluid collecting superior to the bladder in the transverse views.

## THORACIC VIEWS

Chest radiography is commonly used in the initial evaluation of the trauma patient and can be used to detect pneumothorax and hemothorax. However, 150 mL of intrapleural fluid must be present to be detected on a chest

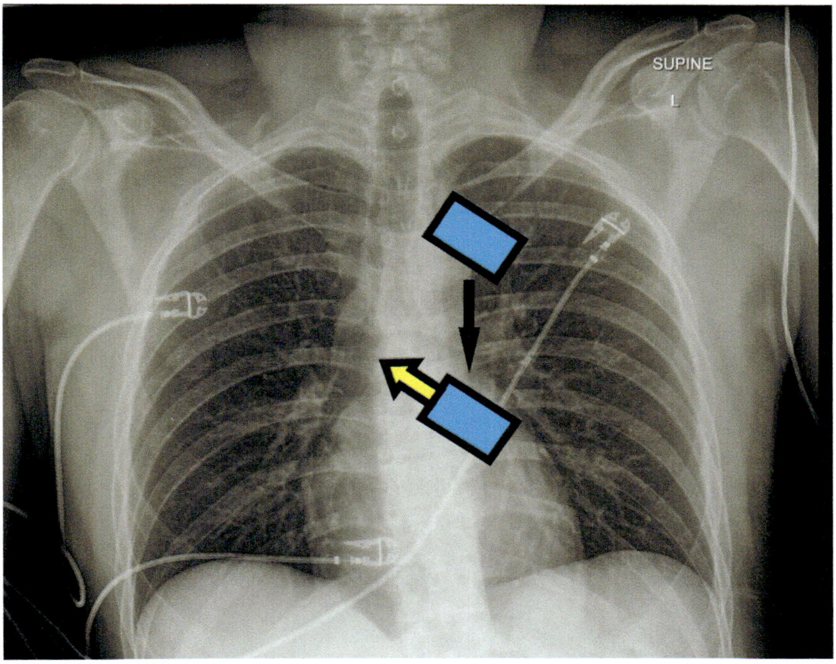


**Fig. 5.** Placement of phased array ultrasound probe (blue box) for parasternal long view as part of the FAST, with indicator pointed to the patient's right shoulder (*yellow arrow*) overlayed on a chest radiograph.

radiograph, whereas ultrasound can detect 20 mL of fluid with sensitivity of 93% [8]. Furthermore, pneumothorax can be commonly missed by supine chest radiography following trauma [11,12]. In comparison, a clinically significant pneumothorax can be detected by POCUS with a sensitivity of 95.3% and a specificity of 91.1%, and more importantly, usually much more rapidly [10].

In order to evaluate for the presence of pneumothorax, a high-frequency linear probe should be placed on the anterior chest wall near the second or third intercostal space in the midclavicular line with the marker cephalad (Fig. 13). Optimal view is when the probe is placed in between 2 ribs and shadowing is present on either edge of the ultrasound view as seen in Fig. 14 with the pleural interface in between the 2 ribs (blue arrowhead). In Fig. 15, one can see the chest wall, bright white light of the pleura (blue arrowhead), B lines (yellow arrowhead), and comet tails produced by "lung sliding," an ultrasonographic sonographic artifact of the thoracic and parenchymal pleura moving across each other. Isolated B lines can be a normal artifact, but multiple B lines can indicate increased extravascular lung water (Fig. 16). To further assess apposition of the pleura and lack of intervening air, the ultrasound should be switched to M-mode, with indicator line through the chest wall in between

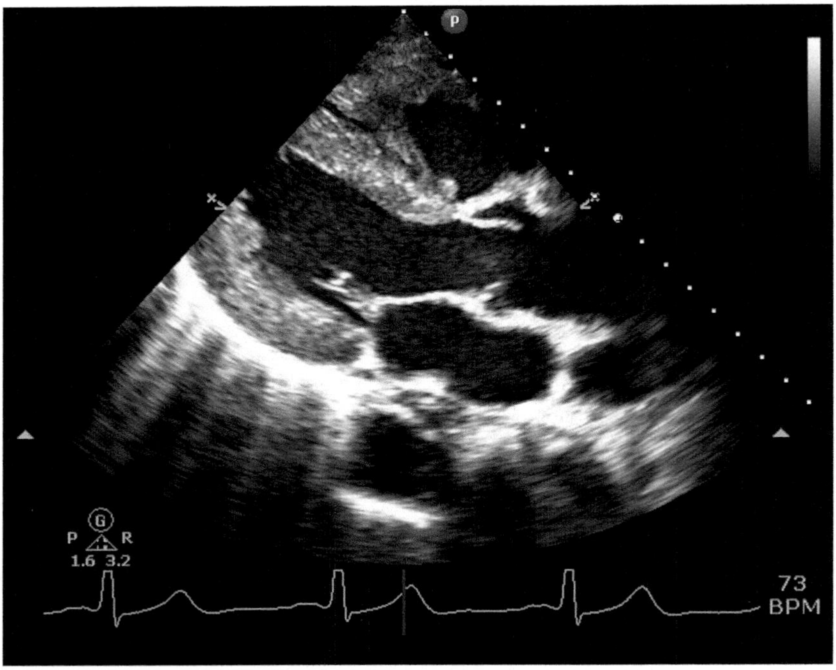


**Fig. 6.** Parasternal long view as part of the FAST to evaluate for pericardial effusion.

ribs. In this view, the lung sliding will appear as linear structures at the top of the image and then haziness below the pleura; this represents the chest wall musculature overlying the pleura line and is described as the "seashore sign." In the presence of pneumothorax, this characteristic appearance disappears, and the image is described as a "barcode sign" (Fig. 17).

## CARDIAC ULTRASOUND

Transthoracic echocardiography is a useful, easy-to-use, and immediately available tool for the surgeon for identification of cause of hypotension in both trauma and in the critically ill, as well as for hemodynamic monitoring. In addition to identification of pericardial tamponade, cardiac POCUS can assist in the evaluation of cardiac function [13,14] and fluid responsiveness [15–23] at the bedside to guide resuscitation in perioperative and critically ill patients. It can be learned easily and performed at the bedside by surgeons [16].

### Parasternal long view

A low-frequency probe (the authors' preference being the phased array probe) is positioned on the second or third intercostal space of the left parasternal border as described earlier and demonstrated in Fig. 18, moving inferiorly until cardiac structures can be identified. In the PSL window (Fig. 19), moving

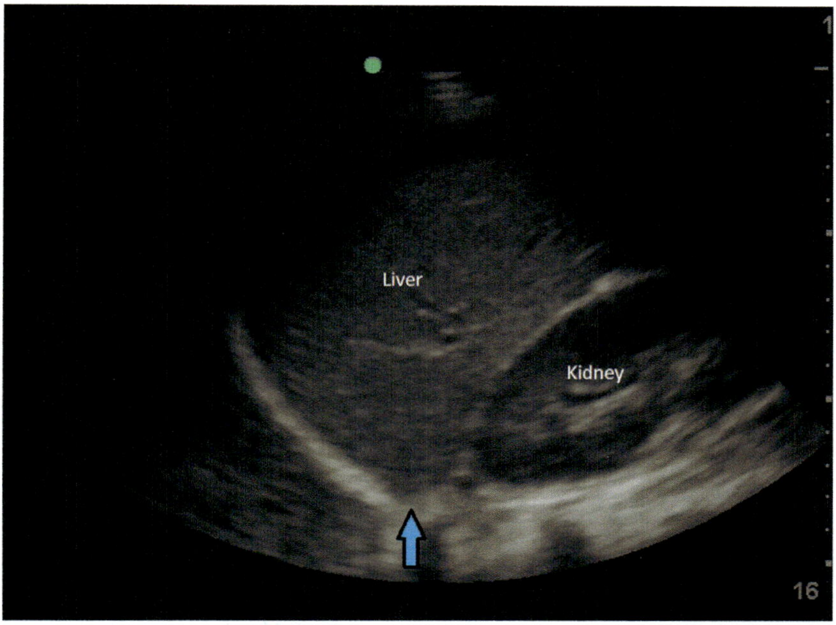


**Fig. 7.** Morison pouch: identification of the caudal tip of the liver for the FAST examination.

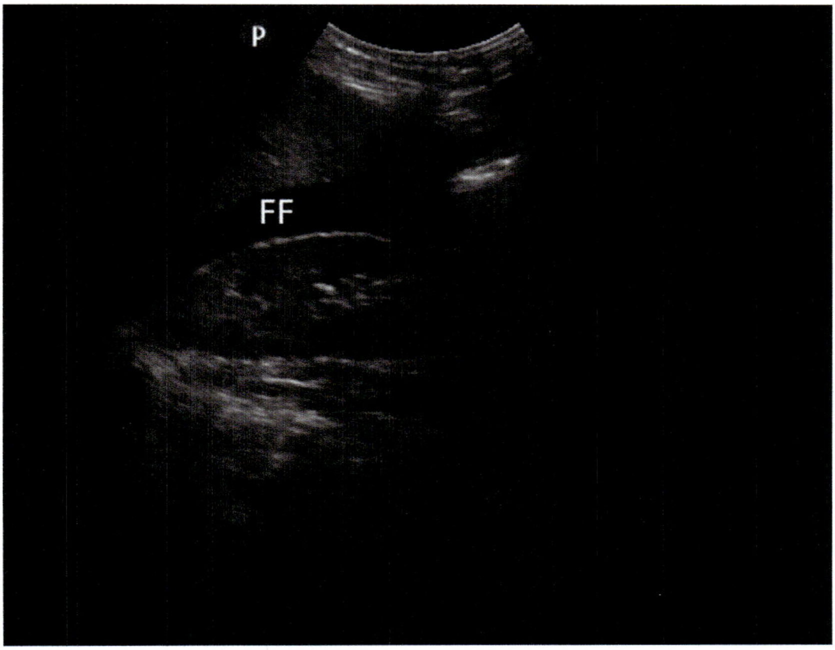


**Fig. 8.** More medial view of Morison pouch with free fluid (FF).

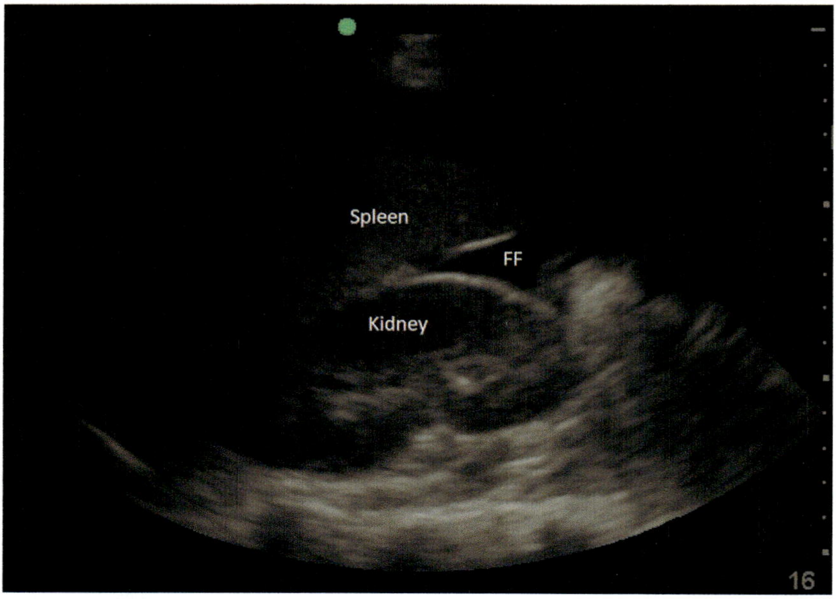


**Fig. 9.** Splenorenal recess showing free fluid (FF).

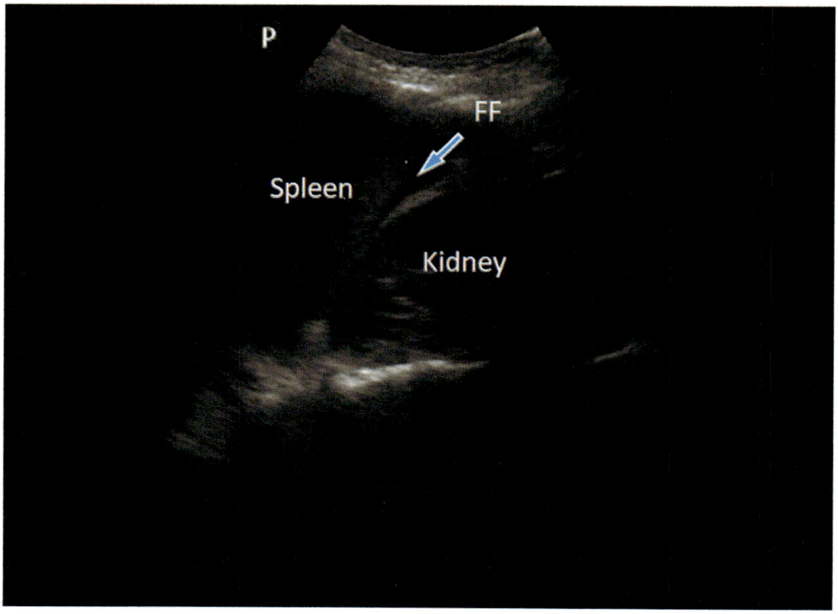


**Fig. 10.** More superior view of splenorenal recess showing free fluid (FF).

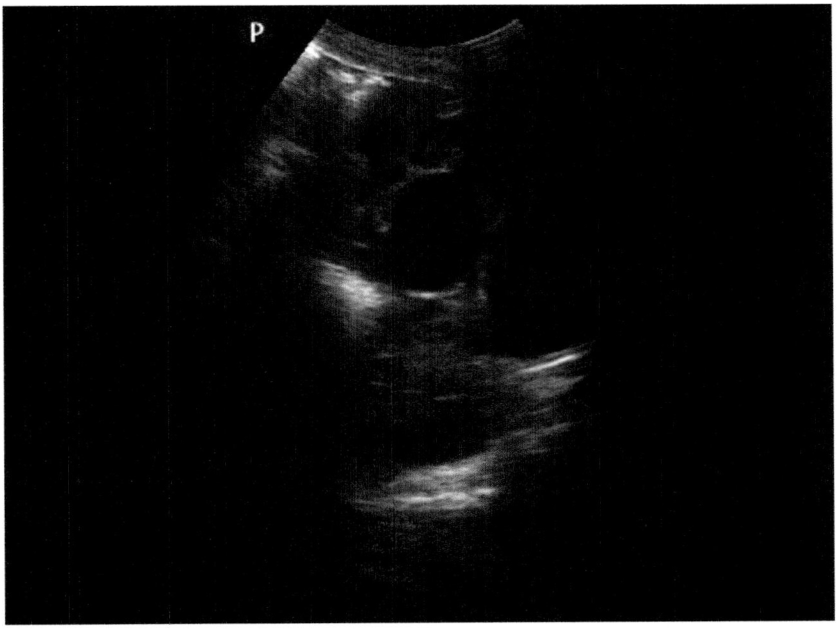


**Fig. 11.** Longitudinal view of bladder.

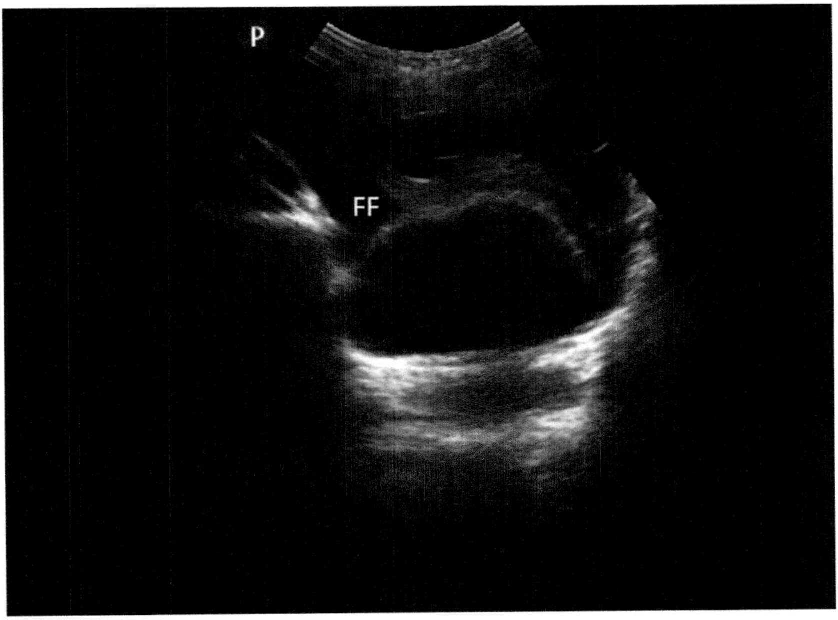


**Fig. 12.** Transverse view of bladder with free fluid (FF).

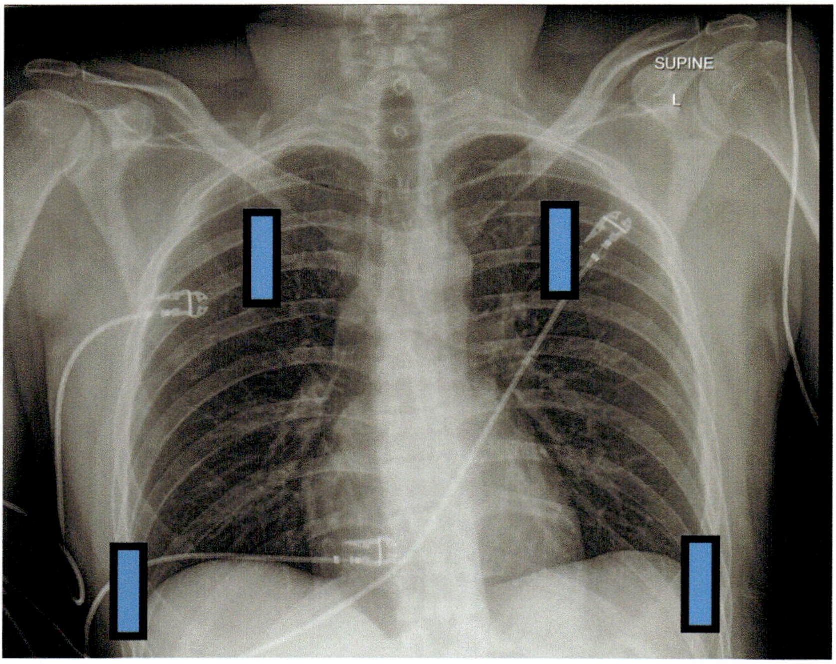


**Fig. 13.** Placement of linear array (or phased array) ultrasound probe (blue box) for "extended" thoracic imaging of the eFAST examination.

clockwise from the top to center, you can identify the RV, aorta (Ao) with the left atrium below moving through the mitral valve (MV) into the left ventricle (LV) connecting to the left ventricular outflow tract (LVOT) in the center. The descending Ao can be seen at the bottom of the image. This view allows assessment of these structures as well as the LVOT diameter (LVOTD, blue arrowheads). Along with other measurements mentioned later in the chapter, the LVOTD can be used to estimate hemodynamics including stroke volume, cardiac output, and systemic vascular resistance by cardiac ultrasound.

## Parasternal short view

In order to obtain the parasternal short view of the heart, from the placement for the parasternal long view, simply turn the probe clockwise approximately 90°, now pointing toward the left shoulder (Fig. 20) By fanning the probe from cephalad to caudad through the heart, at different levels (black lines, see Fig. 20) one can identify different structures. Immediately below the transducer is the base of the heart (Fig. 21A) showing the structures at the aortic annulus and valve. As you fan caudad toward the apex, you will identify the parasternal short mitral view (see Fig. 21B), midpapillary view (see Fig. 21C), and the apical view (see Fig. 21D). This allows reliable assessment

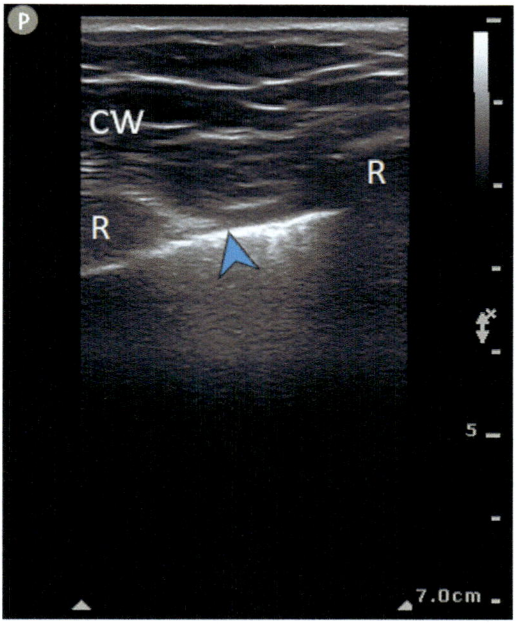


**Fig. 14.** Intercostal placement of linear probe and resulting ultrasound image showing ribs (*R*).

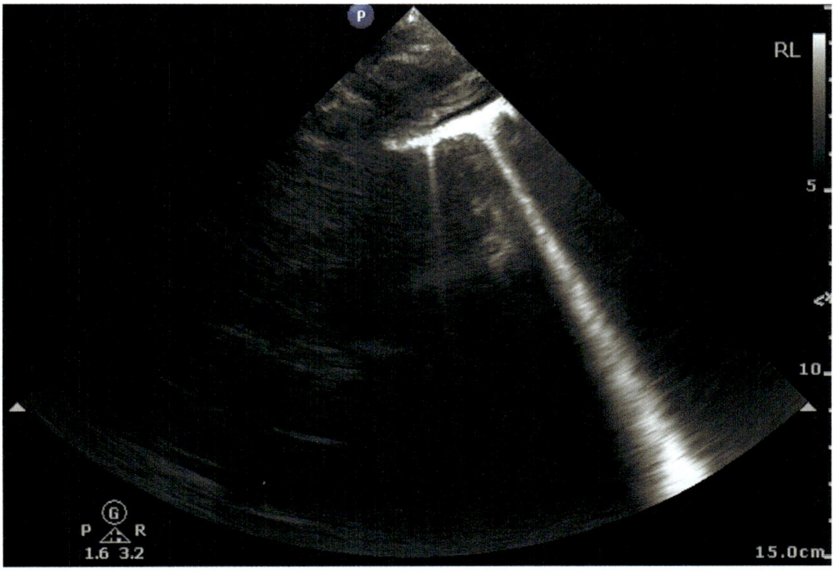


**Fig. 15.** Intercostal view of lungs with lung sliding, comet tail, and B line artifacts.

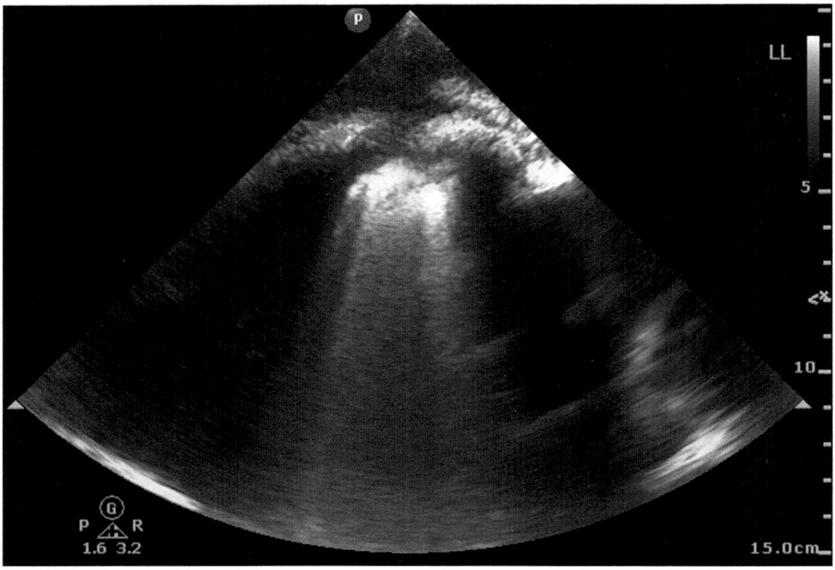


**Fig. 16.** Intercostal view of lungs with B lines, suggesting increased extravascular lung water.

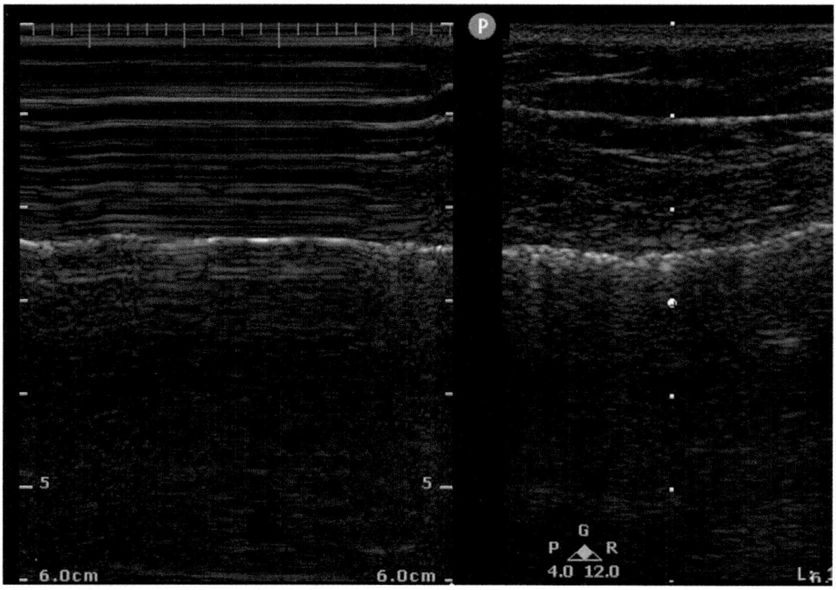


**Fig. 17.** M-mode through intercostal tissue and pleural interface showing normal appearing "seashore sign."

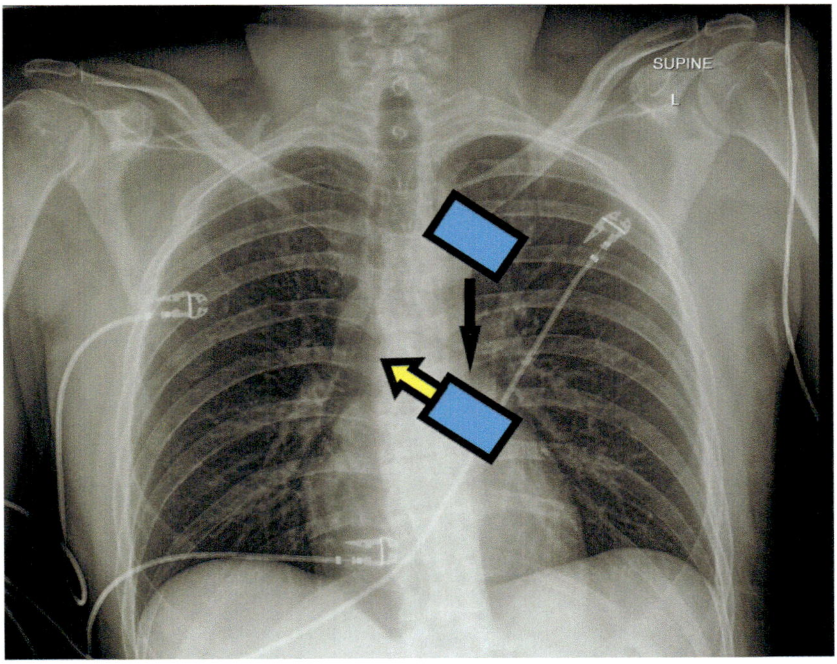


**Fig. 18.** Placement of phased array ultrasound probe (blue box) for parasternal long view, with indicator pointed to the patient's right shoulder (*yellow arrow*) overlayed on a chest radiograph.

of the left ventricular function, wall motion abnormalities, as well as the aortic and mitral valve and papillary muscles.

## Apical four-chamber and five-chamber views

Using the same phased array, or other low-frequency probe, the probe should be placed over the point of maximal impulse usually in the fifth or sixth intercostal space near the anterior axillary line. An alternate strategy is placing the probe in the midaxillary line and following the rib space anteriorly until cardiac structures can be identified (Fig. 22). The optimal apical view will have the interventricular and interatrial septa oriented vertically on the screen as seen in Fig. 23, and this allows identification of all 4 chambers of the heart, mitral and tricuspid valves, and annuli, as well as the assessment of color and Doppler flow of valvular pathology.

The apical 5-chamber view can be visualized by fanning the ultrasound slightly anterior/cephalad, revealing the LVOT as seen in Fig. 24.

By using pulse wave Doppler within the left ventricular outflow tract, the velocity time integral (VTI) can be measured by tracing the resulting waveform (Fig. 25). Using the left ventricular outflow tract diameter measured in the

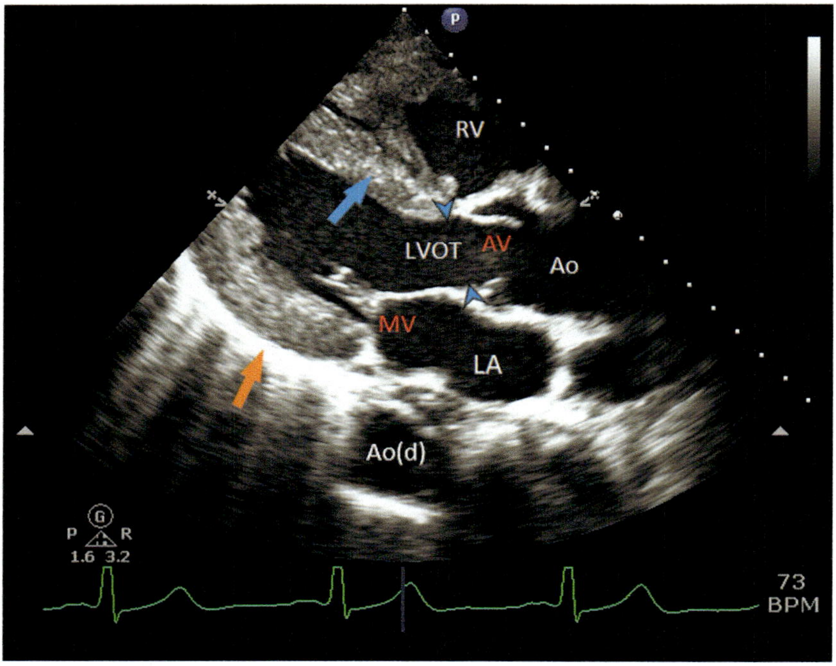


**Fig. 19.** Parasternal long view of the heart with visible cardiac structures.

parasternal long view and VTI, the stroke volume and cardiac output can be calculated easily [24].

In addition to qualitative left ventricular function assessment, right ventricular function can be assessed using continuous wave doppler through the tricuspid free wall annulus to calculate the tricuspid annular plane systolic excursion (Fig. 26). Using these simple measurements, global cardiac function can be easily measured at the bedside [25].

## Assessment of hypovolemia using cardiac ultrasound

In addition to measurement of hemodynamic indices, cardiac ultrasound can be used to evaluate the fluid status in a hypotensive or critically ill patient [13,16–18,20,22,25,26]. The most widely accepted assessment of hypovolemia and possible fluid responsiveness is evaluation of the inferior vena cava (IVC). An underfilled or flat IVC, as visualized in the subcostal view, can predict fluid responsiveness in many types of patients [21,22]. Further, variability in the IVC diameter during the respiratory cycle has been demonstrated to be effective in estimating the fluid status of ventilated patients [19,21,22,27–29]. Further calculations can be made including the IVC Distensibility Index (DI), which is calculated using measurements of IVC diameter at end inspiration and end exhalation (Fig. 27).

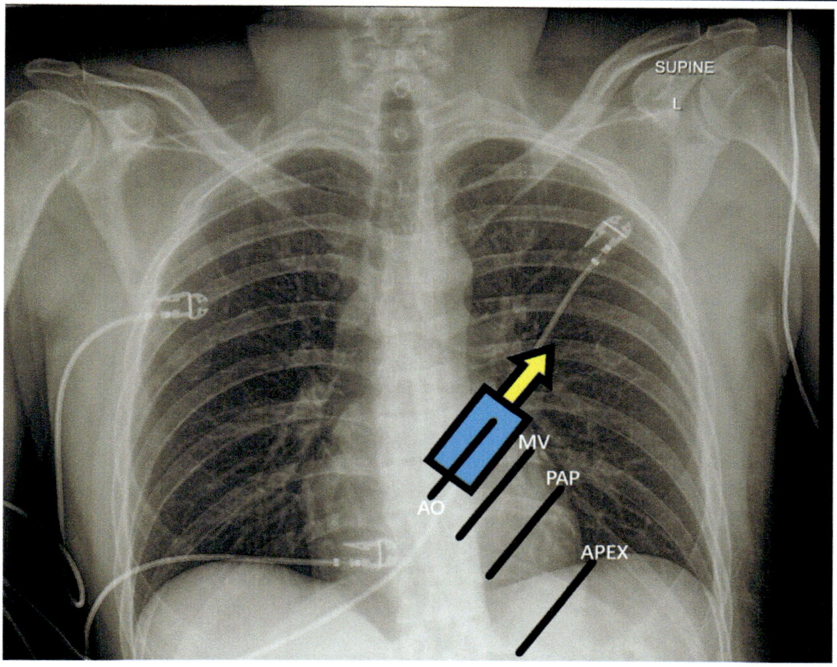


**Fig. 20.** Placement of phased array ultrasound probe (blue box) with indicator (*yellow arrow*) for parasternal short view of the heart. Black lines show levels at which probed can be fanned toward the cardiac apex to show the aortic valve (Ao), mitral valve (MV), midpapillary (PAP), and apical (apex) views.

$$DI = [(IVC^{\text{end inspiration}} - IVC^{\text{end exhalation}}) \times 100] / IVC^{\text{end exhalation}}$$

An elevated DI (>18%) predicts fluid responsiveness with a positive predictive value of 93% and a negative predictive value of 92%.

The authors' institution has published extensively on the use of cardiac ultrasound to estimate fluid responsiveness in critically ill surgical and trauma patients. Using these and other echocardiographic measurements, in addition to patient physiology, the authors have developed a protocol that is used clinically at their institution to assess fluid responsiveness [13,26].

## INTRAVASCULAR CATHETER PLACEMENT

Ultrasound has been used for the guidance of vascular access for more than 3 decades and in most cases is considered standard of care [30]. Multiple studies have shown that placement of intravascular catheters under ultrasound guidance decreases time to access, reduces the number of attempts, as well as complications when compared with blind or landmark-based procedures [31–33]. The most common intravascular lines placed by modern surgeons includes internal jugular, subclavian, and femoral central venous catheters as well as

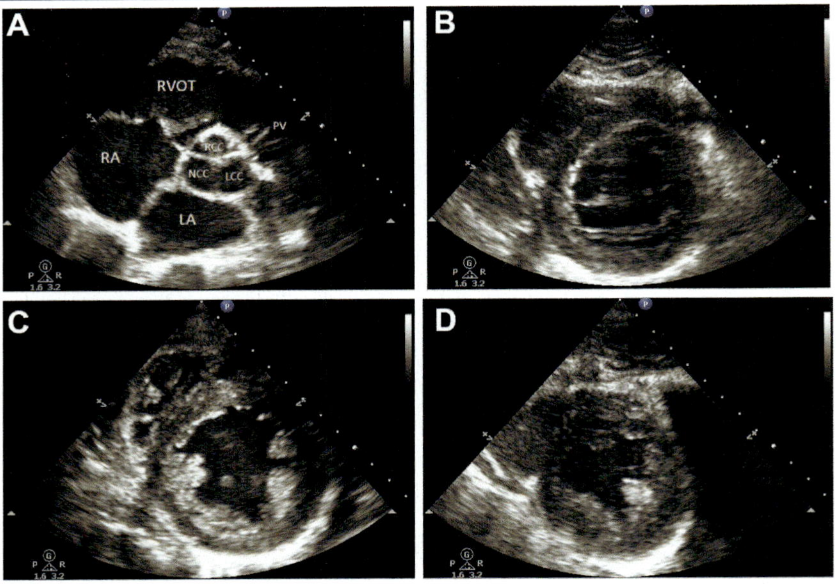


**Fig. 21.** Parasternal short axis view. (*a*) Aortic valve (Ao), (*b*) mitral valve (MV), (*c*) midpapillary (PAP), and (*d*) apical (apex) views of the heart.

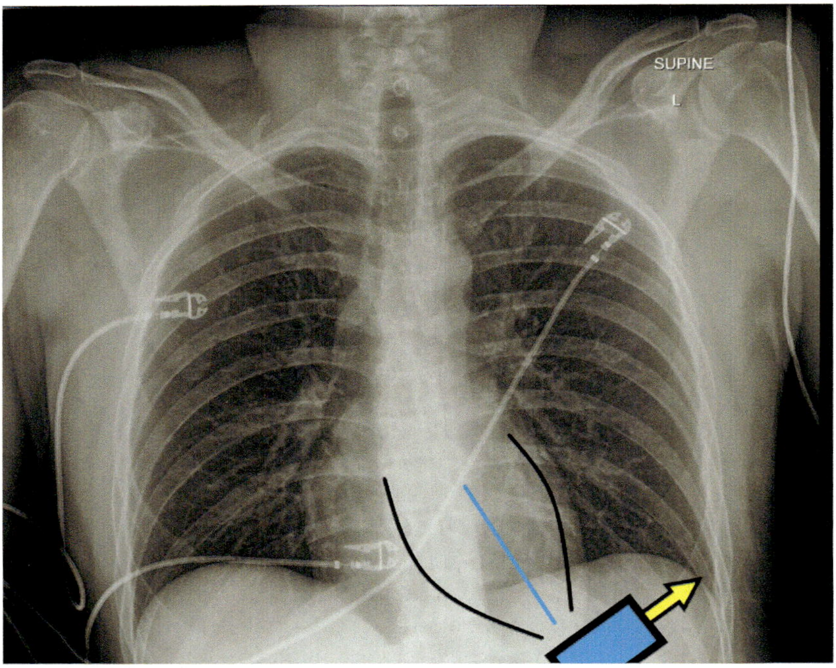


**Fig. 22.** Placement of phased array ultrasound probe (blue box) with indicator (*yellow arrow*) for apical views of the heart. The ventricular walls (*black*) and interventricular septum (*blue*) are approximated by lines.

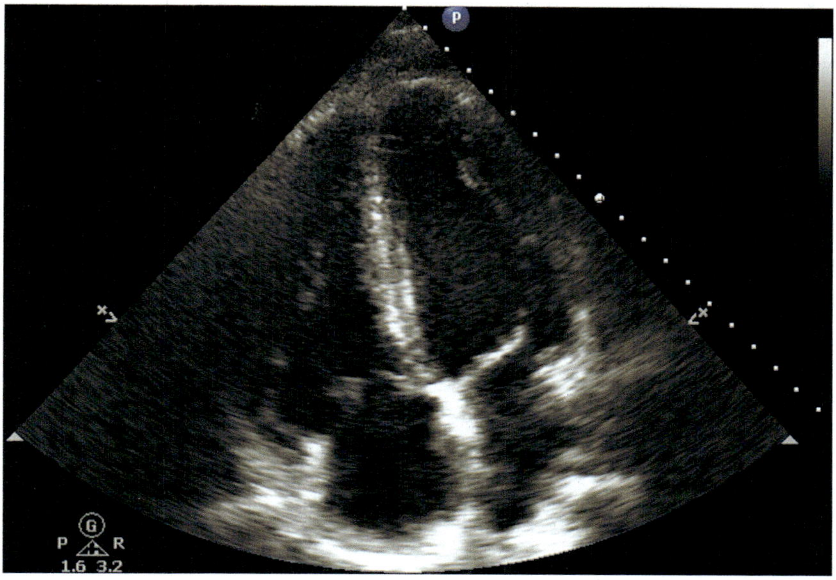


**Fig. 23.** Apical 4-chamber view of the heart.

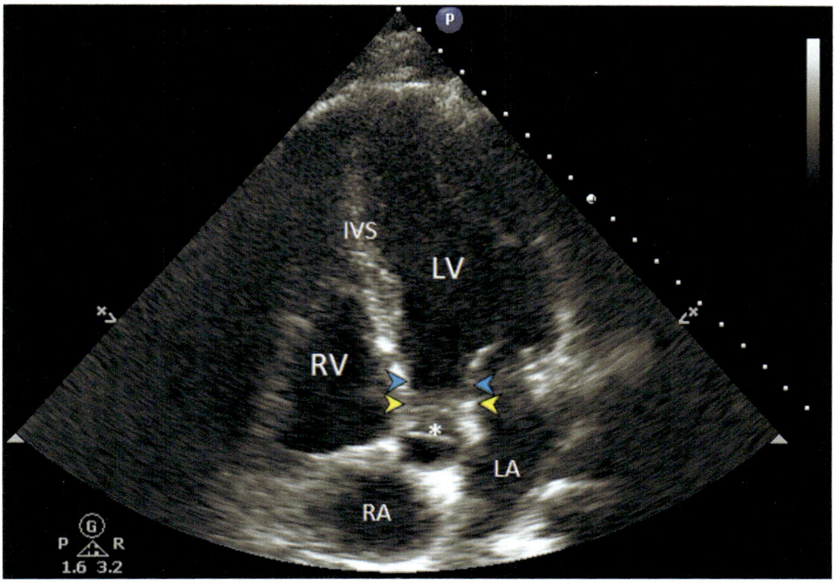


**Fig. 24.** Apical 5-chamber view of the heart showing the left ventricle (LV) and atrium (LA), right ventricle (RV) and atrium (RA), interventricular septum (IVS), level of LVOTD measurement, aortic annuls (*yellow arrowheads*), and aortic valve (*asterisk*).

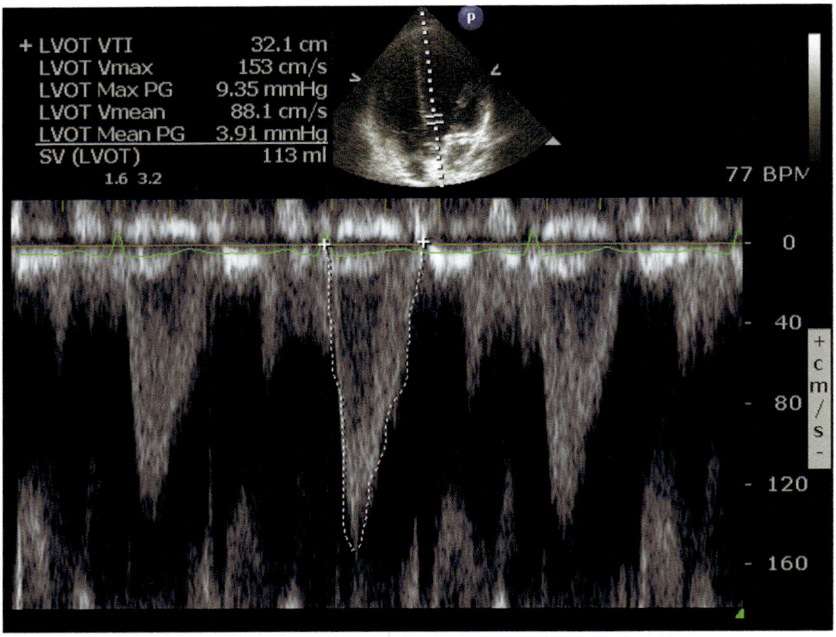


**Fig. 25.** Placement of pulsed wave doppler indicator in LVOT in apical 5-chamber view (middle top of image), tracing of LVOT PW doppler of blood traveling from ultrasound probe (bottom half) and subsequent VTI tracing (*dotted line*), with resulting LVOT VTI and stroke volume (SV) calculations.

radial and femoral arterial catheters. Good practice for insertion of intravascular catheters is similar among all these types of catheters. Although differences in cannulation of the vessels themselves is beyond the scope of this article, POCUS can be used in the localization of the correct vessel and assessment of its suitability for catheterization. Current recommendations include use of a higher frequency probe (in most cases a linear probe), the use of 2-dimensional (2D) imaging, correct placement of the ultrasound machine in direct view of the operator, and the use of recording ability when needed. The use of higher frequency probes allows for the identification of the vessels but more importantly the surrounding structures including lymphatics, bone, and nerves. Further recommendations vary based on operator experience including use of wire guides for more novice ultrasound users [30], as well as the use of Doppler functions [34,35] and in-plane technique [30,36] for only more competent users. Although Doppler functions and in-plane technique can be used, there is no strong evidence that they improve procedural outcome. Use of 3D imaging and echogenic needles has been proposed, although there is only weak evidence for their superiority over standard 2D imaging or needle types, respectively [37,38].

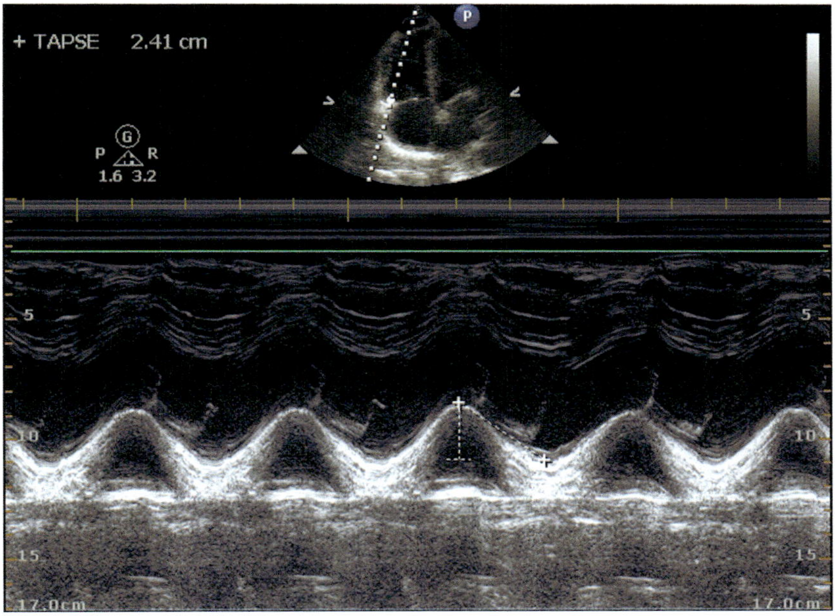


**Fig. 26.** Placement of M-mode linear indicator through the free wall portion of the tricuspid annulus (*middle top*) and subsequent TAPSE tracing (*bottom half*).

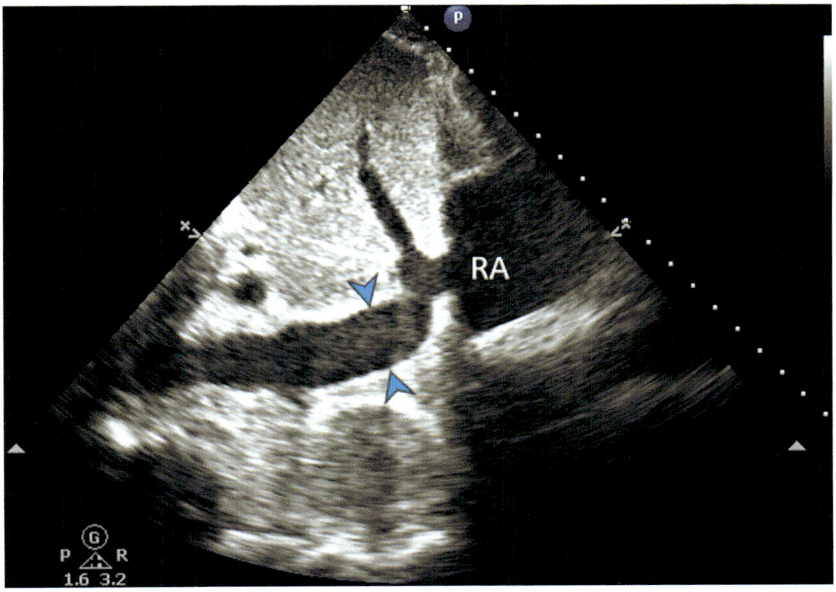


**Fig. 27.** Using curvilinear probe to show the ideal site for measurement of the IVC (*blue arrowheads*) as it empties into the right atrium (RA).

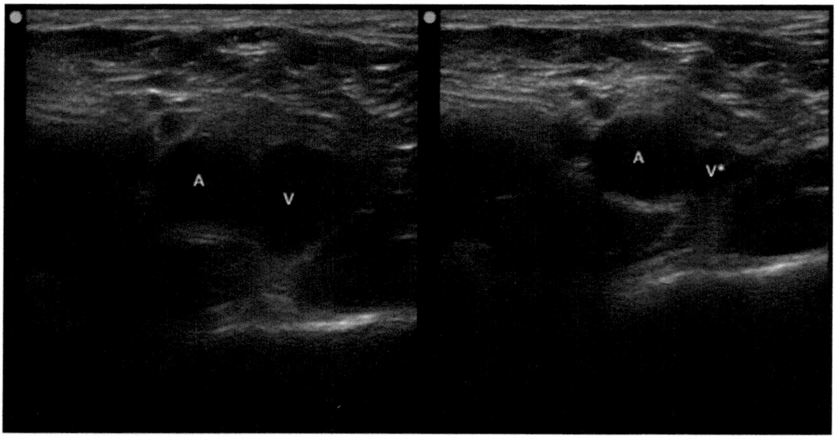


**Fig. 28.** Transverse view of the left femoral vasculature with the artery (*A*) and vein (*V*) identified. The vein can be seen in the right image after it has been compressed (V*).

In general, both venous and arterial structures will be found coursing together through the tissue, which is true for the radial, jugular, subclavian, and femoral anatomy. Note that the convention among sonographers is that the ultrasound marker will generally be placed toward the patient's right or head when selecting a proper site. Here the authors use femoral anatomy as an example. The ultrasound probe should be placed in a transverse position overlying the vessels based on anatomic principles. In this case, one can see the left femoral vasculature with the artery laterally and vein medially (Fig. 28). To further identify the difference between artery and vein (the right image of the figure) pressure has been applied to occlude the vein, whereas the artery remains open.

Most experts recommend using the Seldinger technique using serial dilation over a wire placed through the initial entry needle. It is recommended that the wire placement is confirmed by using the ultrasound in both longitudinal and transverse views to demonstrate its presence in the correct vessel. This is especially important to avoid carotid and femoral arterial dilation and with larger cannula diameters.

## SUMMARY

POCUS has evolved over the last several decades, and its use has become indispensable in the practice of surgery for the identification of intrathoracic, cardiac, and intrabdominal pathology. POCUS has become standard of practice in the evaluation of trauma, cardiac function, fluid assessment in the critically ill, and placement of intravascular catheters for a myriad of reasons. Although its use has increased, it is a tool that is only as helpful as the sonographer's ability to obtain and the interpretation of diagnostic images. As surgery advances, it is a tool that should be in the toolbox of every surgeon.

## CLINICS CARE POINTS: FAST

- The inferior poles of the kidneys and caudal tip of the liver must be visualized, as a small amount of fluid can be present.
- Serial examination may be needed in patients presenting quickly to the emergency department.
- Delayed presentation may result in mixed free fluid and clotted blood, obscuring results.
- eFAST does not rule out serious intrathoracic or intraabdominal injuries.
- eFAST can miss significant hemorrhage in the retroperitoneum.
- Ensure depth is sufficient to visualize all structures completely, especially when visualizing the pericardium, as blood collects inferiorly in a supine patient.
- Clotted blood in the pericardial space is difficult to distinguish from a pericardial fat pad, and the opposite is also true.
- Cardiac views as part of an emergent eFAST should focus on pericardial effusion "present or absent" and not on cardiac mechanics.
- Ensure all views of the FAST are evaluated by fanning through the structures, not just a single view.

## DISCLOSURE

The authors would like to thank Jesse Shriki, MD, RDCS and the Shock Trauma Ultrasonography team for selected images.

## References

[1] Kristensen JK, Buemann B, Kühl E. Ultrasonic scanning in the diagnosis of splenic haematomas. Acta Chir Scand 1971;137(7):653–7, (In eng).
[2] Asher WM, Parvin S, Virgillo RW, et al. Echographic evaluation of splenic injury after blunt trauma. Radiology 1976;118(2):411–5, (In eng).
[3] Tso P, Rodriguez A, Cooper C, et al. Sonography in blunt abdominal trauma: a preliminary progress report. J Trauma 1992;33(1):39–43 [discussion 43-4]. (In eng).
[4] Stassen NA, Lukan JK, Carrillo EH, et al. Examination of the role of abdominal computed tomography in the evaluation of victims of trauma with increased aspartate aminotransferase in the era of focused abdominal sonography for trauma. Surgery 2002;132(4):642–6 [discussion 646-7]. (In eng).
[5] Rozycki GS, Ballard RB, Feliciano DV, et al. Surgeon-performed ultrasound for the assessment of truncal injuries: lessons learned from 1540 patients. Ann Surg 1998;228(4):557–67, (In eng).
[6] Rozycki GS, Ochsner MG, Schmidt JA, et al. A prospective study of surgeon-performed ultrasound as the primary adjuvant modality for injured patient assessment. J Trauma 1995;39(3):492–8 [discussion 498-500]. (In eng).
[7] Von Kuenssberg Jehle D, Stiller G, Wagner D. Sensitivity in detecting free intraperitoneal fluid with the pelvic views of the FAST exam. Am J Emerg Med 2003;21(6):476–8, (In eng).
[8] Ma OJ, Kefer MP, Stevison KF, et al. Operative versus nonoperative management of blunt abdominal trauma: Role of ultrasound-measured intraperitoneal fluid levels. Am J Emerg Med 2001;19(4):284–6.

[9] Kirkpatrick AW, Sirois M, Laupland KB, et al. Hand-held thoracic sonography for detecting post-traumatic pneumothoraces: the Extended Focused Assessment with Sonography for Trauma (EFAST). J Trauma 2004;57(2):288–95, (In eng).
[10] Lichtenstein DA, Menu Y. A bedside ultrasound sign ruling out pneumothorax in the critically ill. Lung sliding. Chest 1995;108(5):1345–8, (In eng).
[11] Ball CG, Kirkpatrick AW, Fox DL, et al. Are occult pneumothoraces truly occult or simply missed? J Trauma 2006;60(2):294–8 [discussion 298-9]. (In eng).
[12] Ball CG, Kirkpatrick AW, Laupland KB, et al. Factors related to the failure of radiographic recognition of occult posttraumatic pneumothoraces. Am J Surg 2005;189(5):541–6 [discussion 546]. (In eng).
[13] Murthi SB, Hess JR, Hess A, et al. Focused rapid echocardiographic evaluation versus vascular cather-based assessment of cardiac output and function in critically ill trauma patients. J Trauma Acute Care Surg 2012;72(5):1158–64.
[14] Oh JK. Echocardiography as a noninvasive Swan-Ganz catheter. Circulation 2005;111(24):3192–4, (In eng).
[15] Feissel M, Michard F, Faller JP, et al. The respiratory variation in inferior vena cava diameter as a guide to fluid therapy. Intensive Care Med 2004;30(9):1834–7, (In eng).
[16] Ferrada P, Anand RJ, Whelan J, et al. Limited transthoracic echocardiogram: so easy any trauma attending can do it. J Trauma 2011;71(5):1327–31 [discussion 1331-2]. (In eng).
[17] Ferrada P, Anand RJ, Whelan J, et al. Qualitative assessment of the inferior vena cava: useful tool for the evaluation of fluid status in critically ill patients. Am Surg 2012;78(4):468–70, (In eng).
[18] Ferrada P, Murthi S, Anand RJ, et al. Transthoracic focused rapid echocardiographic examination: real-time evaluation of fluid status in critically ill trauma patients. J Trauma 2011;70(1):56–62 [discussion 62-4]. (In eng).
[19] Ferrada P, Vanguri P, Anand RJ, et al. echo: limited transthoracic echocardiogram is a useful tool to guide therapy for hypotension in the trauma bay–a pilot study. J Trauma Acute Care Surg 2013;74(1):220–3, (In eng).
[20] Ferrada P, Vanguri P, Anand RJ, et al. Flat inferior vena cava: indicator of poor prognosis in trauma and acute care surgery patients. Am Surg 2012;78(12):1396–8, (In eng).
[21] Yanagawa Y, Nishi K, Sakamoto T, et al. Early diagnosis of hypovolemic shock by sonographic measurement of inferior vena cava in trauma patients. J Trauma 2005;58(4):825–9, (In eng).
[22] Yanagawa Y, Sakamoto T, Okada Y. Hypovolemic shock evaluated by sonographic measurement of the inferior vena cava during resuscitation in trauma patients. J Trauma 2007;63(6):1245–8 [discussion 1248]. (In eng).
[23] Machare-Delgado E, Decaro M, Marik PE. Inferior vena cava variation compared to pulse contour analysis as predictors of fluid responsiveness: a prospective cohort study. J Intensive Care Med 2011;26(2):116–24, (In eng).
[24] Hunt S, Abraham W, Chin M, et al. Writing committee members. 2009 focused update incorporated into the ACC/AHA 2005 guidelines for the diagnosis and management of heart failure in adults: a report of the American college of cardiology foundation/American heart association task force on practice guidelines: developed in collaboration with the international society for heart and lung transplantation. Circulation 2009;119:e391–479.
[25] Glaser JJ, Cardarelli C, Galvagno S Jr, et al. Bridging the gap: Hybrid cardiac echo in the critically ill. J Trauma Acute Care Surg 2016;81(5 Suppl 2):S157–61, (In eng).
[26] Murthi SB, Fatima S, Menne AR, et al. Ultrasound assessment of volume responsiveness in critically ill surgical patients: two measurements are better than one. J Trauma Acute Care Surg 2017;82(3):505–11.
[27] Dipti A, Soucy Z, Surana A, et al. Role of inferior vena cava diameter in assessment of volume status: a meta-analysis. Am J Emerg Med 2012;30(8):1414–9.e1, (In eng).

[28] Barbier C, Loubières Y, Schmit C, et al. Respiratory changes in inferior vena cava diameter are helpful in predicting fluid responsiveness in ventilated septic patients. Intensive Care Med 2004;30(9):1740–6, (In eng).
[29] Stawicki SP, Braslow BM, Panebianco NL, et al. Intensivist use of hand-carried ultrasonography to measure IVC collapsibility in estimating intravascular volume status: correlations with CVP. J Am Coll Surg 2009;209(1):55–61, (In eng).
[30] Lamperti M, Bodenham AR, Pittiruti M, et al. International evidence-based recommendations on ultrasound-guided vascular access. Intensive Care Med 2012;38(7):1105–17, (In eng).
[31] McGee DC, Gould MK. Preventing complications of central venous catheterization. N Engl J Med 2003;348(12):1123–33.
[32] Randolph AG, Cook DJ, Gonzales CA, et al. Ultrasound guidance for placement of central venous catheters: a meta-analysis of the literature. Crit Care Med 1996;24(12):2053–8.
[33] Verghese ST, McGill WA, Patel RI, et al. Comparison of three techniques for internal jugular vein cannulation in infants. Pediatr Anesth 2000;10(5):505–11.
[34] Bodenham A. Editorial II: ultrasound imaging by anaesthetists: training and accreditation issues. Oxford University Press; 2006.
[35] Schummer W, Schummer C, Tuppatsch H, et al. Ultrasound-guided central venous cannulation: is there a difference between Doppler and B-mode ultrasound? J Clin Anesth 2006;18(3):167–72.
[36] Stone MB, Moon C, Sutijono D, et al. Needle tip visualization during ultrasound-guided vascular access: short-axis vs long-axis approach. The Am J Emerg Med 2010;28(3): 343–7.
[37] Maecken T, Grau T. Ultrasound imaging in vascular access. Read Online Crit Care Med Soy Cril Care Mee 2007;35(5):S178–85.
[38] Chapman G, Johnson D, Bodenham A. Visualisation of needle position using ultrasonography. Anaesthesia 2006;61(2):148–58.

Advances in Surgery 55 (2021) 299–306
ADVANCES IN SURGERY

# Breast Implant–Associated Anaplastic Large Cell Lymphoma

Melissa Camp, MD, MPH
Department of Surgery, Johns Hopkins, 600 North Wolfe Street, Blalock 609, Baltimore, MD 21287, USA

**Keywords**
• Breast implant • Breast implant–associated lymphoma
• Anaplastic large cell lymphoma • BIA-ALCL

**Key points**

- Breast implant–associated anaplastic large cell lymphoma (BIA-ALCL) is a rare type of lymphoma that is most commonly associated with textured breast implants.
- BIA-ALCL typically presents as a fluid collection surrounding a breast implant that develops at least 1 year (on average 7–9 years) after the implant was placed.
- Most cases of BIA-ALCL are diagnosed at an early stage and have an overall good prognosis if complete surgical resection can be achieved.

## INTRODUCTION

Breast implant–associated anaplastic large cell lymphoma (BIA-ALCL) was first reported in 1997 [1], and it has emerged as a distinct type of T-cell lymphoma that develops in association with breast implants. The World Health Organization initially categorized BIA-ALCL as a new class of lymphoma in 2016 [2], and the National Comprehensive Cancer Network (NCCN) established the first set of evidence-based guidelines for the evaluation and management of BIA-ALCL the same year. Awareness of BIA-ALCL has gained traction over the last several years, resulting in an increased recognition and reporting of cases. This chapter summarizes the present knowledge regarding BIA-ALCL, including discussion of the current algorithm for diagnosis and treatment as published in the NCCN Guidelines version 1.2021 (last updated October 5, 2020) [3].

*E-mail address:* mcamp@jhmi.edu

https://doi.org/10.1016/j.yasu.2021.05.019

## BACKGROUND

BIA-ALCL is a rare peripheral T-cell lymphoma that most commonly arises in association with a current or prior textured breast implant. BIA-ALCL can develop in association with breast implants that are placed for either augmentation or reconstructive purposes and can occur with both saline and silicone implants [4].

## EPIDEMIOLOGY

The actual incidence and prevalence of BIA-ALCL are challenging to ascertain due to multiple factors. Concerns exist regarding the accurate reporting of the overall prevalence of patients with implants, the level of detail recorded specifying the type of implant, the lack of robust implant and BIA-ALCL registries secondary to the voluntary nature of reporting, and the potential for underreporting due to lack of awareness of BIA-ALCL by providers and patients. Data collected over the years have estimated the risk of BIA-ALCL from 1 in a million (for all types of implants) to more recently as ranging from 1 in 3000 (for patients in Australia and New Zealand with textured implants) [5] to 1 in 30,000 (for patients in the United States with textured implants) [6].

Textured implants were initially developed with the premise that normal tissue growing into the textured surface would decrease capsular contracture, but it remains controversial as to whether the rate of capsular contracture is notably different for smooth versus textured implants. The classification system for implant surfaces ranges from grade 1 to grade 4 and is based on the surface area as well as the roughness of the surface, with 1 representing smooth implants and 4 representing the most textured surface. BIA-ALCL seems to be most associated with implants of grade 3 and grade 4 surfaces. It is postulated that the more highly textured surfaces allow for attachment of bacteria and development of a biofilm, stimulating a chronic inflammatory response and eventually leading to T-cell transformation and development of BIA-ALCL [5]. Studies have examined the bacterial biofilms of breast implant capsules in patients with BIA-ALCL as well as in patients with capsular contracture and have noted that gram-negative rods of the *Ralstonia* species are far more common in BIA-ALCL compared with *Staphylococcus* species in capsular contracture [7].

With respect to possible genetic alterations, studies have noted an association between BIA-ALCL and activation of the JAK-STAT 3 pathway leading to the overexpression of STAT-3. Compiling data from 5 studies that performed genetic sequencing of BIA-ALCL, mutations in JAK1 were identified in 3/23 patients (13%) and mutations in STAT3 were identified in 6/23 patients (26%) [7,8]. Other mutations identified in next-generation sequencing of BIA-ALCL include TP53 and DNMT3A [9].

Given the rare nature of BIA-ALCL, the US Food and Drug Administration (FDA) recommends reporting of confirmed cases to the American Society of Plastic Surgeons BIA-ALCL PROFILE (Patient Registry and Outcomes for breast Implants and anaplastic large cell Lymphoma etiology and

Epidemiology) registry [3,10], available at www.thepsf.org/PROFILE [11]. It is hoped that tracking of cases over time will allow for a more accurate assessment of the incidence and prevalence of BIA-ALCL.

## PRESENTATION

The most typical clinical presentation of BIA-ALCL is a patient with a breast implant who develops a new fluid collection surrounding the breast implant or asymmetric breast swelling, occurring at least 1 year after the implant was placed and unexplained by other causes such as infection or recent trauma to the chest [10,12]. The average length of time from implant placement to development of BIA-ALCL is 7 to 9 years [3]. Far less commonly, BIA-ALCL can present as a palpable mass, lymphadenopathy in the regional lymph node basins (axillary, supraclavicular, or internal mammary), overlying skin changes such as a rash, or capsular contracture [10,12].

## DIAGNOSIS AND WORKUP

For patients with breast implants presenting with a delayed fluid collection, asymmetric breast swelling, or less commonly a palpable mass, the initial step in diagnostic evaluation should be an ultrasound of the breast and ipsilateral axilla. Ultrasound can detect a fluid collection surrounding the implant, characterize a palpable mass (if present), and identify any lymphadenopathy. If ultrasound is inconclusive or indeterminant, then an MRI of the breast can be considered [3,10].

If a fluid collection is detected on ultrasound, aspiration of the fluid should be performed and the fluid sent for histopathologic evaluation. If there is any suspicion for potential infectious causes, a sample of fluid can also be sent for Gram stain and culture. For the most accurate diagnosis of BIA-ALCL, at least 50 cc of fluid should be aspirated and sent for evaluation by cytology, immunohistochemistry, and flow cytometry. The specific tests to request include anaplastic lymphoma kinase (ALK), CD2, CD3, CD4, CD5, CD7, CD8, CD30, and CD45 [3]. BIA-ALCL is always ALK negative and CD30 positive, and cytologic evaluation will demonstrate large anaplastic cells that express CD30. CD30 expression is nonspecific, however, and can be associated with other types of lymphoma as well as with benign inflammatory cells [7,10,12]. BIA-ALCL will have a single clone of T cells present on flow cytometry. Correlation of the appropriate clinical context in conjunction with the cytology findings of large anaplastic cells that are ALK negative and CD 30 positive is necessary for the diagnosis of BIA-ALCL [3].

Patients with breast implants presenting with a breast mass on clinical examination or detected on imaging should undergo further evaluation with core needle biopsy of the mass. Pathologic evaluation should be performed using the biomarkers listed earlier if there is clinical concern for BIA-ALCL, and other causes such as breast cancer should also be ruled out [3,12].

## TREATMENT

Following histopathologic confirmation of a diagnosis of BIA-ALCL, a multidisciplinary treatment approach involving plastic surgery, surgical oncology, and medical oncology is recommended. Further imaging evaluation with a PET-computed tomography (CT) is indicated to evaluate for the presence of any associated masses in the breast implant capsule, involvement of the chest wall, regional lymphadenopathy, and distant metastatic disease. For disease that is localized to the breast implant capsule and/or breast, the mainstay of treatment is complete surgical resection including the breast implant, total capsulectomy of the implant capsule, and resection of any masses associated with the breast implant capsule. Any suspicious regional lymph nodes should also be excised [3,10]. The implant capsule, any fluid surrounding the implant, and any lymph nodes that are excised should be evaluated pathologically for complete staging of BIA-ALCL [10]. For patients who have undergone complete surgical resection with no concern for residual disease, adjuvant therapies are not indicated. Close follow-up with clinical evaluation and examination every 3 to 6 months for 2 years, as well as consideration of annual systemic imaging with a CT scan of the chest/abdomen/pelvis or PET-CT, is recommended [3].

If BIA-ALCL involves regional lymph nodes, or if complete surgical resection is not feasible and a portion of the capsule or residual disease remains, then adjuvant therapy is indicated. Radiation therapy can be used to treat local residual disease that is not amenable to surgical resection. Adjuvant systemic therapy is recommended for patients with node-positive disease or in cases where radiation may not be possible to treat local residual disease. Systemic therapy is also indicated as first-line treatment of patients with more advanced disease for whom surgical resection is not an option. Systemic therapy regimens that are used to treat BIA-ALCL include anthracycline-based regimens such as CHOP (cyclophosphamide, doxorubicin, vincristine and prednisone) or brentuximab vedotin (a CD30 targeted therapy) in combination with CHP (cyclophosphamide, doxorubicin and prednisone) [3,10].

Although most of the cases of BIA-ALCL present with early stage disease confined to a fluid collection surrounding the implant and/or involving the implant capsule, up to about 18% of cases can present with more advanced disease such as regional lymph node involvement or distant metastatic disease [10]. As demonstrated by one study, patients with advanced BIA-ALCL were more likely to have a longer length of time from diagnosis to surgery and were less likely to have complete surgical resection compared with patients with early stage disease [13].

With respect to prognosis, there are limited data regarding the overall survival for BIA-ALCL due to the rarity of the disease and the paucity of long-term follow-up. In one study of 87 patients with BIA-ALCL, the overall survival was reported as 94% at 3 years and 91% at 5 years [12]. The ability to achieve complete surgical resection has been associated with improved overall survival and disease-free survival, as compared with incomplete surgical resection with or without adjuvant therapies [4,10]. Locally recurrent BIA-ALCL is most commonly seen in patients who undergo incomplete surgical resection or partial capsulectomy [12].

For patients with bilateral breast implants, removal of the contralateral implant and capsule may be considered, as BIA-ALCL has been identified in the contralateral breast implant in approximately 4.6% of cases [10].

## STAGING

BIA-ALCL was initially staged according to the Ann Arbor Staging System for hematological malignancies. Because of the behavior of BIA-ALCL being more in line with that of a solid tumor, the proposed staging system developed by Clemens and colleagues and included in the NCCN guidelines is based on American Joint Committee on Cancer TNM staging system [3,10]. Tables 1 and 2 depict the TNM category descriptions and associated staging.

## FOOD AND DRUG ADMINISTRATION WARNINGS ON IMPLANTS

In response to concerns regarding the association between textured implants and BIA-ALCL, the US FDA requested that Allergan recall Natrelle BIOCELL textured breast implants and tissue expanders in July 2019. The FDA's recommendation was based on the report of 481 out of 573 cases of BIA-ALCL worldwide being attributed to Allergan breast implants, resulting in a 6-fold higher risk of BIA-ALCL with Allergan textured implants compared with textured implants produced by other manufacturers. In addition, 12 of 13 deaths in patients with BIA-ALCL where the manufacturer of the implant was known had Allergan implants. The manufacturer was unknown for 20 additional deaths. Allergan complied with the FDA's request and removed the specified Natrelle BIOCELL textured breast implants and tissue expanders from the worldwide market. BIOCELL is a unique textured surface that is found only in Allergan textured implants [14].

In the United States, textured implants represent approximately 10% of all breast implants [14]. The FDA released labeling guidance for all breast implants (textured and smooth) in September 2020, with recommendations for a boxed warning stating that breast implants have been associated with BIA-ALCL, that BIA-ALCL occurs more commonly in patients with textured as opposed to smooth implants, and that deaths have occurred from BIA-ALCL. Moreover, the FDA recommends that breast implant information brochures provided to patients contain a decision checklist that indicates the risk of BIA-ALCL [15].

## MANAGEMENT OF PATIENTS WHO CURRENTLY HAVE IMPLANTS

For patients who currently have breast implants (textured or smooth) and are asymptomatic, removal of implants as a precautionary measure is not recommended. Awareness on the part of patients and providers of the existence of BIA-ALCL and its presenting symptoms, however, are key to early diagnosis and appropriate treatment [14].

**Table 1**
Proposed TNM category descriptions for breast implant–associated anaplastic large cell lymphoma [3]

| TNM | | Description |
|---|---|---|
| **T: Tumor extent** | **T1** | Confined to effusion or a layer on luminal side of capsule |
| | **T2** | Early capsule infiltration |
| | **T3** | Cell aggregates or sheets infiltrating the capsule |
| | **T4** | Lymphoma infiltrates beyond the capsule |
| **N: Lymph node** | **N0** | No lymph node involvement |
| | **N1** | One regional lymph node involved |
| | **N2** | Multiple regional lymph nodes involved |
| **M: Metastasis** | **M0** | No distant spread |
| | **M1** | Spread to other organs or distant sites |

*From* NCCN Clinical Practice Guidelines in Oncology (NCCN Guidelines). T-Cell Lymphomas, Version 1.2021-October 5, 2020. Available at www.nccn.org/professionals/physician_gls/pdf/t-cell.pdf. Accessed November 23, 2020.

## SUMMARY/CONCLUSIONS

BIA-ALCL is a rare type of lymphoma most commonly associated with textured breast implants. The precise underlying cause of BIA-ALCL is currently unknown, but it is hypothesized that the interaction between a bacterial biofilm and the textured implant surface may stimulate a chronic inflammatory response leading to transformation of T cells. Although the risk of developing BIA-ALCL is difficult to quantify, it is estimated to be 1 in 3000 to 1 in 30,000. It is hoped that ongoing registries will allow for a more accurate assessment of the risk of BIA-ALCL, as well as any potential factors that may contribute to increased risk.

In patients who present with a delayed fluid collection surrounding a breast implant, inclusion of BIA-ALCL in the differential diagnosis as well as appropriate histopathologic evaluation to confirm the diagnosis are essential. Most of the cases of BIA-ALCL are diagnosed at an early stage, and achieving complete

**Table 2**
Proposed TNM staging for breast implant–associated anaplastic large cell lymphoma [3]

| Stage designation | Description |
|---|---|
| IA | T1 N0 M0 |
| IB | T2 N0 M0 |
| IC | T3 N0 M0 |
| IIA | T4 N0 M0 |
| IIB | T1-3 N1 M0 |
| III | T4 N1-2 M0 |
| IV | T any N any M1 |

*From* NCCN Clinical Practice Guidelines in Oncology (NCCN Guidelines). T-Cell Lymphomas, Version 1.2021-October 5, 2020. Available at www.nccn.org/professionals/physician_gls/pdf/t-cell.pdf. Accessed November 23, 2020.

surgical resection (removal of the implant, total capsulectomy of the breast implant capsule, and any masses associated with the implant capsule) portends an overall good prognosis. For patients who present with more advanced BIA-ALCL, systemic therapy is recommended and radiation therapy may also be indicated.

## CLINICS CARE POINTS

- BIA-ALCL is a rare type of lymphoma that is most commonly associated with textured breast implants.
- The exact risk of developing BIA-ALCL is difficult to quantify, but it is estimated to be 1 in 3000 to 1 in 30,000.
- BIA-ALCL typically presents as a fluid collection surrounding a breast implant that develops at least 1 year (on average 7–9 years) after the implant was placed.
- On histopathologic evaluation, BIA-ALCL is composed of large anaplastic cells that are ALK negative and CD30 positive.
- Most cases of BIA-ALCL are diagnosed at an early stage and have an overall good prognosis if complete surgical resection can be achieved.
- Systemic therapy is recommended for more advanced cases of BIA-ALCL, and radiation therapy may also be indicated if residual local disease is present.

## DISCLOSURE

The author has nothing to disclose.

## References

[1] Keech JA, Creech B. Anaplastic T-cell lymphoma in proximity to a saline filled breast implant. Plast Reconstr Surg 1997;100:554–5.
[2] Swerdlow SH, Campo E, Pileri SA, et al. The 2016 revision of the World Health Organization classification of lymphoid neoplasms. Blood 2016;127(20):2375–90.
[3] NCCN Clinical Practice Guidelines in Oncology (NCCN Guidelines). T-Cell Lymphomas, Version 1.2021-October 5, 2020. Available at: www.nccn.org/professionals/physician_gls/pdf/t-cell.pdf. Accessed November 23, 2020.
[4] Leberfinger AN, Behar BJ, Williams NC, et al. Breast implant-associated anaplastic large cell lymphoma – A systematic review. JAMA Surg 2017;152(12):1161–8.
[5] Collett DJ, Rakhorst H, Lennox P, et al. Current risk estimate of breast implant-associated anaplastic large cell lymphoma in textured breast implants. Plast Reconstr Surg 2019;143(3S):30S–40S.
[6] Doren EL, Miranda RN, Selber JC. U.S. epidemiology of breast implant-associated anaplastic large cell lymphoma. Plast Reconstr Surg 2017;139(5):1042–50.
[7] Jones JL, Hanby AM, Wells C, et al. Breast implant-associated anaplastic large cell lymphoma (BIA-ALCL): an overview of presentation and pathogenesis and guidelines for pathological diagnosis and management. Histopathology 2019;75:787–96.
[8] Oishi N, Miranda R, Feldman A. Genetics of breast implant-associated anaplastic large cell lymphoma (BIA-ALCL). Aesthet Surg J 2019;39(S1):S14–20.

[9] Di Napoli A, Jain P, Duranti E, et al. Targeted next generation sequencing of breast implant-associated anaplastic large cell lymphoma reveals mutations in JAK/STAT signalling pathway genes, TP53 and DNMT3A. Br J Hematol 2018;180:735–60.
[10] Clemens MW, Brody GS, Mahabir RC, et al. How to diagnose and treat breast implant-associated anaplastic large cell lymphoma. Plast Reconstr Surg 2018;141(4):586e–99e.
[11] American Society of Plastic Surgeons BIA-ALCL PROFILE (Patient Registry and Outcomes for breast Implants and anaplastic large cell Lymphoma etiology and Epidemiology) registry. Available at: www.thepsf.org/PROFILE. Accessed November 25, 2020.
[12] Clemens MW, Jacobsen ED, Horwitz SM. 2019 NCCN Consensus Guidelines on the diagnosis and treatment of breast implant-associated anaplastic large cell lymphoma (BIA-ALCL). Aesthet Surg J 2019;39(S1):S3–13.
[13] Collins MS, Miranda RN, Medeiros LJ, et al. Characteristics and treatment of advanced breast implant-associated anaplastic large cell lymphoma. Plast Reconstr Surg 2019;143(3S):41S–50S.
[14] The FDA requests allergan voluntarily recall natrelle BIOCELL textured breast implants and tissue expanders from the market to protect patients: FDA safety communications. Available at: https://www.fda.gov/medical-devices/safety-communications/fda-requests-allergan-voluntarily-recall-natrelle-biocell-textured-breast-implants-and-tissue. Accessed November 12, 2020.
[15] Breast implants – certain labeling recommendations to improve patient communication. Available at: https://www.fda.gov/regulatory-information/search-fda-guidance-documents/breast-implants-certain-labeling-recommendations-improve-patient-communication. Accessed November 12, 2020.